SECOND EDITION

THE COMPETITIVE EDGE

Advanced Marketing for Dietetics Professionals

SECOND EDITION

THE COMPETITIVE EDGE

Advanced Marketing for Dietetics Professionals

Kathy King Helm, RD, Editor

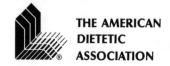

THE AMERICAN
DIETETIC
ASSOCIATION

Acquisitions Editor: Betsy Hornick
Copy Editor: Cynthia Fostle
Designer: Maureen Ulicny
Managing Editor: Diane Culhane
Production Manager: Carolyn Rand

Library of Congress Cataloging-in-Publication Data

The competitive edge: advanced marketing for dietetics professionals/
  Kathy King Helm, editor – 2nd ed.
    p. cm.
  Includes bibliographical references and index.
  ISBN 0-88091-138-7
    1. Dietetics – Marketing.   2. Dietetics – Practice.   I. Helm, Kathy King.
  RM218.5.C66 1995   94-34425
  613.2'068'8 – dc20   CIP

Foreword

A Leader Without a Vision of the Future Is but a Manager of Today's Affairs.
Jeffrey Heilbrunn

We can no longer depend on the ways we have traditionally practiced our profession. Rather, we must develop the knowledge and skills necessary to anticipate how changing practice environments will affect our customers, our organizations, our businesses, and our lives. Further, we must learn to identify opportunities and challenges posed by micro and macro trends and to build strategies that will take us into exciting new practice areas in the future.

While Mr. Heilbrunn was directing his remarks to corporate leaders, his advice is equally important to those of us affected by changes in the health-care delivery system, food environments, and health and disease prevention areas. Today's world rewards those who are customer-driven and accessible, who provide real value as defined by the customer, who understand that new collaborative networks and partnerships are necessary survival strategies in a competitive marketplace, and who can document the cost-effectiveness of their services. To navigate effectively through changes in the food, nutrition, and health environments will require looking to the future, approaching change with a marketing mindset, adapting proactive entrepreneurial solutions, and developing a culture that encourages the acceptance of risks.

The Competitive Edge, Second Edition, will prepare you to manage the impacts of all those rapidly changing environments. Its purpose, as the authors emphasize, is to help dietetics professionals better prepare for the future. To this end, a variety of marketing experts from our profession – private practice, business and industry, acute- and long-term-care organizations, wellness programs, and commercial food companies – have shared their expertise, experiences, and insights and provided stimulating case studies you can use as models for building your own practice environment.

This book is so full of thoughtful ideas, case studies, and practical "how-to" strategies that you will refer to it for guidance for many years to come. The case studies and practical applications of marketing theory will stimulate your thinking as you change your existing practice roles or create new opportunities.

Kathy King Helm had the challenging task of organizing the papers of our contributing authors within a meaningful framework. The material has been organized into five sections: internal and external trends affecting the profession; the business of marketing; marketing strategies within primary market segments; the development of marketing plans; and practical "how-to's." The overall theme is that knowledge, techniques, and technologies exist to develop and implement effective marketing strategies in virtually every area of dietetics practice. Members can achieve their objectives of entering and surviving in a dynamic marketplace.

The major message to be carried away from reading *The Competitive Edge* is that opportunities for dietetics professionals are limited only by their creativity. This book can help you outline appropriate and visionary marketing strategies. I am pleased that The American Dietetic Association has made it available to you as it provides a cornerstone to your future. The future is yours – the time to capture it is now!

Sara C. Parks, MBA, RD
President
The American Dietetic Association, 1993 – 1994

ABOUT THE EDITOR

Kathy King Helm, RD, of Lake Dallas, Texas, has been in private practice since 1972, specializing in preventive nutrition, weight loss, and advanced business and counseling seminars for dietitians. Her entrepreneurial activities include marketing new food products for corporations, writing numerous books and articles, hosting her own radio talk show, consulting for the Denver Broncos Football Team, and speaking nationally and internationally.

DEDICATION

For my husband, Carter, and daughters, Savannah and Cherokee, who give me quality of life when I finish working. Also, to all my family for supporting me enthusiastically and for embracing entrepreneurism as a way of thinking so that new ideas and ventures keep our lives interesting.

ACKNOWLEDGMENTS

Acknowledgments go to all the dietitians and diet technicians from around the world who shared so freely in the development of this book. Through their efforts and sharing of information, this book will offer new, exciting marketing strategies for practicing in the food and nutrition and health-care arenas. Take these ideas and assess them, embellish them, apply them to your own markets, nurture them, and then come back and show us how to do it better!

Special thanks are due to the following reviewers for their contributions:

Deborah Canter, PhD, RD, Associate Professor and Director, Coordinated Program in Dietetics, Kansas State University, Manhattan, Kansas;

Susan Calvert Finn, PhD, RD, Director, Nutrition Services, Ross Laboratories, Columbus, Ohio;

Marsha Hudnall, MS, RD, Nutrition Communication Specialist, Ludlow, Vermont;

Gill Robertson, MS, RD, Nutrition Consultant, Sun Prairie, Wisconsin;

Kristine M. Westover, MS, RD, Nutrition Consultant, The Westover Group, Idaho Falls, Idaho

Contents

Contents

Introduction

By Looking at the Trends

Affecting Our Markets,

We Can Anticipate

the Future Better.

Introduction

Chapter 1

Change: The Dynamic State of the 1990s

Kathy King Helm, RD, Private Practitioner, Lake Dallas, Texas

The fact that the 1990s are the last ten years of this millennium may mean, if history repeats itself, a decade to remember! Looking back through history, the last ten years of each century have been a time of unusual or unique occurrences, creations, and awakenings, according to small business adviser and speaker Jean Yancey. Universities were first started in Paris in the 990s; exploration was big in the 1490s; Galileo and others made revolutionary scientific discoveries in the 1590s; and there was a surge toward big business and recognition of the problems it created for people in the 1890s.

In fact, we don't have to wait for historians to tell us this is a memorable time that will change our lives forever. Communism is dissolving around the world; the cold war as we knew it is over; adversarial factions in countries like South Africa, Israel, and Ireland are starting to negotiate, while wars rage in once quiet countries; population migration is at an all-time high; and capitalism and global trade are growing.

In America we are experiencing the end of the effects of the Industrial Revolution, when people moved from farms to cities to work for large corporations, especially manufacturing ones. As Tom Peters, author and business analyst, stated in his syndicated column in the *Dallas Business Journal:* "We are coping with the biggest economic change in two centuries. Amazingly, the churn caused by the Industrial Revolution has just ended. We needed 150 years to work through the last big upheaval – even though most of the core technologies were put in place during the first 25 years or so." (1) He goes on to state that it may only take 25 years to get the new technological advancements in place, but it may take society 100 more years to adapt to the shakeout.

The technological revolution that is presently taking place is eliminating jobs and job security (software has been and will continue to replace workers with jobs requiring routine tasks). It is setting up communication channels that make a home-based business run by a dietitian in Omaha as accessible to world markets as a multinational company. New technologies and research make keeping up with the current body of nutrition knowledge a full-time challenge.

And if that isn't enough, the total health-care industry – our profession's largest employer – is in a state of flux unparalleled in history. Changes in the delivery and payment of health care are being debated in Congress and at every hospital and medical office in the United States. Hospital visits are getting shorter, locations for care are changing to outpatient services and the home, and prevention and managed-care programs like HMOs and PPOs are growing. The food industry, our other big employer, is exploding with interest in nutrition, labeling, and how to meet the needs of its changing customer base.

So what do the experts suggest we can do to survive while all of this is going on? The consensus is that we should remain flexible, develop a tolerance for ambiguity, and become more independent and entrepreneurial. In fact, the December 29, 1993, issue of *Kiplinger's Washington Letter* reports: "Business schools are finally discovering entrepreneurship . . . how to create a new product, start a business, nurture it, see it grow. Students are demanding it. Applications for

MBA programs are down because fewer good jobs exist in large industries. Many MBA programs are adapting to this change in the marketplace by making their programs teach practical business skills and instinctive approaches, like when to take risks, listening to customers, and making business deals. The result will be graduates with broader skills, more real know-how." (2)

People who anticipate trends, react quickly to changes in the marketplace, offer excellence in their products and services, and expect to remain responsible for their own careers will still prosper in today's markets. As you will read throughout this book, the dietetic profession has a wealth of dynamic, creative individuals who fit that description. Their interest and proficiency in marketing helped them reach their customers better, which in turn opened new doors and generated more revenue and self-satisfaction.

MARKETING: THE BOTTOM LINE IN BUSINESS

Fifteen years ago marketing was seen as the functions businesspeople performed to promote and sell their products and services. We discussed logos, color palettes, brochures, ad layouts, dressing for success, the features of the service or product, and how to give a sales pitch.

Today, we see marketing as an integral part of the entire business process. Marketing involves everything it takes to make the customer want your product or service more than any other. In other words, when we instruct the secretary how to answer the phone, or ask the custodian to clean client restrooms better, or change the weight-loss group to a room on the first floor because it's easier to find, or keep the cafeteria open 30 minutes later for our customers' convenience, we are paying attention to details that make our products or services more attractive to our target market.

We are trying to please our customers. Why? Because it makes good sense. It increases demand, which usually increases our income and power (internally with our boss and administrator, or externally as we gain competitive advantages), and improves our image. It also makes good sense because satisfied customers will return to buy again, and they will send their friends. In counseling, satisfied clients may feel we are trying harder and in turn may try harder themselves.

THE CHALLENGE

In reaction to many of the previously mentioned trends and changes, the way we market has to change. According to Rapp and Collins, authors of *The Great Marketing Turnaround,* the 1990s will be the decade when individualized marketing changes the way businesses, big and small, reach their customers. (3) They define *individualized marketing* as "any integrated program of sales communications directly from the advertiser to selected members of the public, whether by letters, brochures, audiocassettes, videocassettes, telephone messages, computer disks, advertiser-sponsored events, or any other means of direct contact."

There are many profound reasons why mass advertising doesn't work as well as it used to, such as too many products, clutter and overkill in advertising, too many discount stores, less brand loyalty, and weaker national TV networks. But closer to home, another reason is the changing demographics and lifestyles of consumers, which affects us all.

Demographics show that more women around the world are working away from home or in home-based businesses and have little free time to watch TV and advertisements. There is a dramatic increase in homes run by single parents and people living alone. This creates the next great problem – lack of personal time, which has contributed to the interest in buying through catalogues, direct mail, home shopping networks, and one-stop-shopping stores. As Rapp and Collins state, "Advertisers must almost literally run down the street to catch up with and button-hole the hurrying customers." On top of this, the marketplace now includes more minorities, teenagers, and golden agers, and they don't want the same things as the former average consumer. So now the "one size fits all" mass message and many utilitarian products aren't as attractive to customers as they used to be.

Since lifestyle influences what people eat, these demographic changes greatly affect the dietetics profession. Instead of wives and mothers buying the groceries and making family nutrition decisions, it may be the teenagers or husbands. The average consumer eats half of all meals away from home and a high portion of already prepared food at home. Fewer meals are made from scratch, and therefore fewer young people know how to cook. Consumers want fast, healthy food that tastes good. When we say healthy, we also mean lower in fat and calories, since a growing percentage of the population has weight problems. Also, a growing percentage of the population is going hungry every day, and making adequate food available to them is also our concern.

We are answering these changes with changes of our own. A growing number of dietitians and dietetic technicians work with the manufacturers and producers of food. We own, consult for, and work as chefs at restaurants, spas, and corporation food services. We bring nutrition education to students in school systems and to consumers in grocery stores. We are creating "social marketing" campaigns like 5-A-Day and Project LEAN to educate consumers. We invent or help market new, healthier foods. We conduct weight-loss classes, and manage food pantries and hunger programs. This book will present you with role models who display the skills needed to successfully pursue these new markets.

A CLOSER LOOK AT TWO MAJOR TRENDS

Throughout, this book will discuss trends that particularly affect a topic. Two trends bear further investigation at this time: global markets and dietetics around the world, and the growth in entrepreneurship. These topics will be discussed in the next two chapters.

References

1. Peters T. In search of excellence. *Dallas Business Journal.* September 17, 1993.

2. *The Kiplinger Washington Letter.* December 29, 1993, p. 1.

3. Rapp S, Collins T. *The Great Marketing Turnaround.* Englewood Cliffs, NJ: Prentice Hall; 1990.

Lauren Swann, MS, RD, President, Concept Nutrition, Inc., Bensalem, Pennsylvania

Like many dietitians, I began my career in a hospital. Yet even as a Coordinated Undergraduate Program (CUP) student, I wanted to creatively apply nutrition in a nontraditional role to effectively influence food choices and dietary habits. I saw food advertising and product labeling as powerful means to achieve this, and my inclination was reinforced during my brief clinical dietetics career. As I attempted to counsel people with diabetes and hypertension at hospital bedside, I discovered that calorie-controlled meal plans and low-sodium modifications never held nearly as much appeal as appetizing food commercials and glossy print ads.

After earning a master of science in nutrition communications in 1981, which included an internship in the public relations department of an advertising agency, I freelanced for a few months, then landed a job in the Consumer Affairs Department of Kraft, Inc. As a Communications Specialist, I developed and promoted informational materials, programs, and educational kits. Around the mid-1980s, when Kellogg's anti-cancer claim on their All-Bran cereal package sparked the already controversial debate over nutrient and health claims on food labels, I applied for a position in the Regulatory Compliance Department at Kraft. My communications background was an asset to a department conventionally filled with food scientists and chemists, and I was promoted to Labeling Compliance Specialist.

This laid the groundwork for my future consulting business. For the next five years at Kraft, I developed labeling information and managed product-disclosure issues for a wide variety of retail and food-service brands. I was an integral part of the marketing team, and my function was indispensable to them. They simply could not get a product to market without label copy that complied with food regulations. During those years, while working with product developers, brand managers, package designers, and food law attorneys, I tracked the progress of food-labeling reform as it picked up steam.

On a personal note, I felt a growing desire to relocate back home to the Philadelphia area. I originally wanted a nice, safe, presumably secure job near my family. That's when I discovered the potential business opportunities. The Philadelphia area, also known as the Delaware Valley, encompasses southeastern Pennsylvania, southern New Jersey, and northern Delaware, and has hundreds of food companies because of its agricultural abundance. When I initially contacted some of the companies about jobs, I learned that the vast majority weren't large enough to employ a nutritionist full time, but could benefit greatly from my expertise on a consulting basis. As labeling reform heated up and came to tangible fruition with the NLEA introduction to Congress, I recognized that there was a lucrative market of small to midsize regional food manufacturers who previously had little need for a labeling specialist, but now could utilize my services.

I saw the NLEA as a window of opportunity to establish myself as a food-marketing nutrition consultant. Nutrition labeling on every food package would result in an indispensable role for nutrition expertise in the food-marketing system. The new food label would indisputably influence marketplace positioning, prompting companies to evaluate product composition, nutrient profiles, and promotional qualities for modifications necessary to remain competitive and profitable. The NLEA was a chance to establish a consulting relationship with clients, particularly in a suppressed economy. Nutrition public relations programs and marketing campaigns are expendable when budgets are cut, but food labeling must be managed to legally sell a product.

With the helpful guidance of an excellent career counselor, I left my job at Kraft at the end of April 1990, moved to the Philadelphia suburb of Bensalem, and spent the first six months establishing Concept Nutrition, my new consulting business. I incorporated upon the advice of an attorney; designed a logo, letterhead, and business cards; and developed a brochure. I also attended several small business and consulting seminars, wrote an informal business plan, and compiled a database that included company names, major products, key personnel, and addresses and phone numbers of potential clients within a manageable geographic area.

The NLEA was signed into legislation by President George Bush in November 1990, around the same time I was ready to implement my first major marketing effort. I started with a direct mail campaign, sending a letter to every company in my database, requesting an opportunity to meet with them and discuss their needs and plans for complying with new labeling laws. I spent days making follow-up phone calls, which resulted in several initial meetings and a few requests for proposals and fee quotes, but no actual contracts. Enactment of the NLEA merely meant that FDA had to publish a proposal for new labeling rules by November 1991. Most companies, particularly the smaller ones, saw little reason to take action before then.

To publicize my new business, I sent press releases that described my consulting specialties to trade and professional publications. I also attended nearly every food-labeling and nutrition-marketing conference I could and found this to be an excellent networking tool. Good networking leads to referrals — the most powerful and effective means of marketing consulting services.

Promotional Materials for Concept Nutrition.

(Copyright Concept Nutrition, Inc. Reprinted with permission.)

Within ten months of starting out (about four months after NLEA enactment), I was asked to speak at a conference entitled "Marketing and Positioning Healthy Foods." International Business Conferences contacted me after reading an article in *Food Technology* that featured my new consulting business. The article was picked up from a press release I had sent. My marketing efforts had begun to take root!

I continued to pursue prospects from my database and discovered that the first meeting with a potential client was really a time to probe and learn as much about the company operation as possible. The direct mail efforts I initially intended as a marketing campaign actually served more value as a research tool to learn about company structure, operational procedures, internal responsibilities, and product management. As I reviewed the findings from each meeting, I recognized some common areas where small to medium-size companies could benefit from consulting. I developed a systematic procedure that I offered as a consulting service to enable manufacturers to preliminarily prepare for the new labeling regulations internally, minimizing a last-minute scramble, and ensuring that product and ingredient records accurately supported labeling declarations.

In November 1991, the FDA published its proposal for labeling reform, and I implemented another direct mail campaign. This time I marketed with more savvy. I had kept my database current with results from the first effort and news clippings about local companies from consumer and industry publications. For this mailing, I sent the literature to prospects who expressed interest from my first contact or had been cited by FDA for labeling violations, and I invited them to visit my exhibit at a local Institute of Food Technologists Supplier Night. Using my recent public-speaking engagement as news, I sent another round of press releases to local publications and radio stations, and successfully generated more article placements and media interviews.

While attending a conference that same month, a colleague who had seen my picture and business publicized in *Food Technology* referred me to a packaging consulting group for subcontracting on a food-labeling project. I landed the contract for development of a nutrition-labeling seminar for the Institute of Packaging Professionals (IoPP), and continued to market my business by attending and speaking at food-labeling conferences, writing product-labeling and nutrition-marketing articles for industry publications, and following up on qualified leads from a slow but growing trickle of referrals (see sample business flyer).

I made numerous contacts while developing the IoPP conference and was a keynote speaker at the seminar, which turned out to be the first public forum held after the new labeling format proposal published in the *Federal Register*. That was in July 1992, two years after I had incorporated Concept Nutrition, Inc., and less than four months before the final rulings for the new label were to be published in the *Federal Register*.

In retrospect, I recognize that my timing had been nearly impeccable. I had quit my job to start a consulting business when the NLEA was introduced into Congress. By the time the NLEA was passed into legislation in November 1990, I had laid the foundation for my business and developed a prospective client list. I launched my initial marketing effort right after that, and it inadvertently turned out to be an extremely valuable research tool for developing specific client services and strategies for future marketing plans. Subsequent efforts through direct mail, press releases, and public speaking kept Concept Nutrition, Inc., in front of prospective clients, particularly when the proposal published in November 1991 prompted more companies to "stay tuned."

I continued to update and add to my prospective client database by attending trade shows and checking annual industry directories. I also focused on networking with prospects by joining food trade and professional organizations, frequenting their functions, and volunteering for committee work.

By the end of 1992, I had built a small but solid following of clients and had reached the vast majority of prospects in my geographic area with publicity about my business. I had planned a new marketing campaign to implement when the final rulings were published in January 1993, but suddenly it seemed that the "floodgates had opened!" On January 6, the new labeling regulations became available, and I immediately got calls from prospects — people who had seen me speak at conferences, saved an article I had written, collected my business card at a professional function, received my literature via direct mail, clipped an advertisement for my services, or been referred by a colleague.

By July 1993, the third anniversary of the incorporation of Concept Nutrition, Inc., my business had grown from a struggling start-up to an established consultancy with a solid client list. Its growth and prosperity directly correlated with the three-year progression of the NLEA from congressional introduction to final rulings. Opportunities abound for dietitians to expand professionally. We need only make the most of viable opportunities, many of which result from developments in the food system and newly created needs for innovative nutrition services.

Chapter 2

The Growth of Entrepreneurship

Anne Rejent-Scholtz, RD, Consultant, Chef, St. Louis, Missouri

If there is one coefficient of entrepreneurial success, it is energy. You may have all the ambition in the world, gobs of capital, a gambling man's soul, and business degrees covering an entire wall, but if you are not a human dynamo, forget it.
Joseph R. Mancusco (1)

Entrepreneurship and intrapreneurship (creating new ventures as an employee) have come to full bloom in dietetics in the last decade. Dietetics professionals are finding their way, as they try to stay one step ahead of ever-changing nutrition and health-care job markets. This is not an easy task! However, academic instruction, practical and job-related experience, plus a bundle of energy and vision have allowed some dietitians to seek careers outside the realm of traditional tasks with greater ease.

WHY WOULD DIETITIANS WANT TO BE ENTREPRENEURS?

With the job market fluctuating and job stability and security questionable at best, why would dietetics professionals leave their salaried positions with benefit packages for an unsure undertaking without benefits? Most are drawn by what entrepreneurship offers: more independence, more opportunities, and potentially more profits. Others choose it after being laid off from their clinical or management positions. Many want to work in new settings with well people who love to work out and eat beautiful foods. Some see self-employment as the natural step for them to take as highly trained and experienced practitioners who have outgrown their present jobs and seek new challenges. For whatever reason, dietitians are reexamining their career choices and finding new ways to market themselves.

Dietetic students seem drawn to the excitement of entrepreneurship. In surveys in 1990 (2) and 1994 (unpublished), 58 percent and 60 percent, respectively, of dietetic students said they wanted to pursue nontraditional careers in dietetics one day.

CHARACTERISTICS OF ENTREPRENEURS

What makes a successful entrepreneur? According to James McHugh, an associate professor of business at St. Louis Community College Forest Park and co-author of *Understanding Business,* (3) certain personality traits are needed to assume the risks, create a vision, take the initiative, and motivate others to follow your lead. These traits are more difficult to learn or acquire than are managerial or leadership skills.

Hundreds of studies and books have tried to identify the attributes that make successful entrepreneurs. Some of the most consistently mentioned traits are:

- *Self-directed.* Since you will be responsible for your business's success or failure, you should be self-disciplined and self-driven.
- *Self-nurturing.* You must be able to replenish your enthusiasm for your ideas.

- *Action-oriented.* Great ideas are not enough to make your business successful. You must have the drive to realize, actualize, and build your ideas into a successful business plan.

- *Highly energetic.* Because it is your business, you must have the emotional, mental, and physical ability to work long hours.

- *Tolerant of uncertainty.* Successful entrepreneurs must take calculated risks. Remember, entrepreneurship is not for persons bent on security.

Entrepreneurs of today resemble only slightly the entrepreneurs of the past. Look for entrepreneurs of the future to be:

- *More educated.* Entrepreneurs of the future will most likely have postgraduate degrees.

- *More experienced.* New entrepreneurs will have a vast array of experiences to draw from.

- *More mature.* Future entrepreneurs will be older because they will start their new careers later in life.

- *More organized.* More planning, organization, and control will be used, in contrast to past tendencies to make decisions by reflex or instinct. (3)

DIETITIANS AS ENTREPRENEURS AND INTRAPRENEURS

Women in general have found the path of the entrepreneur to be highly attractive as they try to juggle the demands of both work and home. According to the Small Business Administration, women start their own businesses at twice the rate of men. The flexible schedule and home office allow greater leeway for meeting personal or home obligations without interfering with productivity.

The financial rewards vary. Some entrepreneurs earn far more income than they could in a traditional job (although while starting their businesses, they may have earned far less). Others test the market with consultant positions while continuing to work full or part time. Still others barely break even and return to work for others.

The disadvantages of entrepreneurship most often cited are long hours and lack of benefit packages. There is no disputing that becoming an entrepreneur requires that you work longer and take more financial responsibility for your own needs.

Today, there are new options and new markets. There is also a new attitude among employers – they want business-minded, dedicated, and creative people to use their talents to develop new ventures, attract more customers, and generate more revenue. Many persons with entrepreneurial skills work as intrapreneurs in hospitals, creating out-patient clinics; in food services, adding delis and catering services; and in corporations, launching new food products. For years we called them aggressive managers, now they are called intrapreneurs.

MARKETING THE ENTREPRENEUR

Because the lines of communication in nontraditional job markets are less formal and unstructured, you must learn new ways to market yourself. Networking, speaking, publishing, volunteering on committees, and becoming involved in organizations that include peers or potential employers are the best ways to become known and find jobs. Some consultants report that 70 to 80 percent of their new work comes from networking.

How do prospective employers or consulting clients find you? Usually, it is your role as an entrepreneur to make yourself known through the methods mentioned above. Your personality may be your biggest asset when making new contacts and nurturing present and past clients. Since most new jobs are likely to arise from personal interaction and word of mouth, mutual friends and new or old acquaintances can do much to further your promotion.

FUTURE JOBS WILL REQUIRE MORE BUSINESS SKILLS

Dietetics professionals will benefit from having a more global understanding of the business world. Employers no longer feel obligated to provide career paths, offer job security, or hold the hands of nonproductive employees. More jobs are expected to change from full-time to consultant (without benefits) and to on-call or part-time. To upgrade our career ladders to include more management opportunities, and more marketable skills, we need a working knowledge of what it takes to start and run a successful business. More specifically, we need skills in writing a business plan, marketing our services and products, reading and preparing financial statements, writing proposals, and understanding contracts and letters of agreement (most of which will be covered in this book). Any prior business experience is beneficial and can help the dietetic entrepreneur parlay her dietetic skills into new markets.

WHAT DOES THE ENTREPRENEURIAL RD OR DTR DO?

The dietetic professional should have one or more areas of expertise. If you have diverse knowledge and abilities, you should still be known as an expert in some field. Consider what you like to do or what skills seem to come easiest for you – for example, writing or public speaking, negotiating or selling, counseling, food demonstrations, communications, wellness programs, research and food analysis, clinical specialties, or culinary arts cooking.

Many entrepreneurs find their niche and a successful career as well by combining two areas of expertise. For example, some dietitians succeed in wellness or sports nutrition by combining nutrition with physical fitness. Others combine dietetics with journalism to become freelance nutrition or health writers. Still others combine nutrition with culinary skills to become recipe developers, cookbook authors, or consultants to the food industry. The sky is the limit.

Satisfied entrepreneurs find work they enjoy. They have come to realize that if they enjoy it, they will be good at it. If they are good at it, people will pay them well to do it. But the motivation must come from within. Then they truly have a career of choice and vision.

References

1. Mancuso J. The right stuff: Do you have what it takes to start your own business? *The Wall Street Journal's Managing Your Career*. Spring 1991:15-19.

2. Helm KK. Finding nontraditional jobs in dietetics. *J Am Diet Assoc*. 1991; 91(4):419-420.

3. Nickels WG, McHugh JM, McHugh SM. *Understanding Business*. 3rd ed. Burr Ridge, IL: Richard D. Irwin, Inc.; 1993.

Cyndi Weis, RD, Co-owner of FIT COMPANY of Rochester, Inc.,
Rochester, New York

My partner and I founded FIT COMPANY of Rochester, Inc., starting in 1986 in an effort to tap into the expanding corporate fitness market. Prior to starting FIT COMPANY, we both worked several years as fitness instructors in health clubs. (Neither of us had formal education in nutrition or exercise physiology, but by taking advantage of the few nationally recognized exercise-certification programs, we acquired credible fitness training.)

Initially, we formed our business to provide on-site exercise programs to corporations. Our mission statement evolved over the past eight years through trial and error in various ventures, and through improved understanding of the needs of our market. Companies utilized our exercise classes while contracting nutrition programs from providers such as Weight Watchers, Nutra/System, and others. We realized early on that there was a definite need to combine fitness with nutrition services in the corporate arena. By combining both exercise and nutrition in a single program under one provider, FIT COMPANY could offer the depth and continuity necessary for long-term change in eating and exercise habits.

Given our small size, it was impractical for FIT COMPANY to hire the necessary nutritional expertise required to design a credible program, so I enrolled in a coordinated dietetic program at a local university. After I graduated and passed the registration exam, FIT COMPANY began adding such services as lunch-time lectures, eight-week weight-management programs combining exercise and good nutrition, and consulting to corporate food-service operations. The response to these new services has been phenomenal! In fact, we have plans to hire additional dietitians to enable us to expand this segment of our business.

FIT COMPANY has made the transition from a corporate fitness business to a full-service corporate wellness business. Not only do our combined services better equip participants to progress toward their individual fitness goals, but the combined concept is also quite exciting to market to our corporate clients. Because of the poor success rate of most weight-loss regimes, the consumer is becoming more aware of the necessity of combining a well-planned, moderate exercise program with a change in eating behaviors.

If FIT COMPANY's success with a total approach to employee wellness is any indication of the opportunities awaiting those who can successfully blend a nutrition and exercise background, then dietetics professionals should be scrambling to acquire the necessary skills and training. A solid fitness background gained by certification from such organizations as the Institute of Aerobic Research and the American College of Sports Medicine would provide a foundation. Speaking and presentation skills are obviously a plus. These skills, coupled with a knowledge of how to get your foot in the door, will enable you to tap into the corporate market.

Linda Schuessler, MS, RD, LD, Director of Nutrition and Public Relations,
CIMA, Dallas, Texas

By capitalizing on the increased emphasis on marketing in health care, dietetics professionals may find new career possibilities. In today's health industry, combining nutrition and marketing provides unique employment opportunities not available with either specialty alone. The climate for taking this concept into the physician's office may become increasingly favorable. Only a very large medical practice can afford a full-time nutrition counselor; however, a moderate-size practice may consider hiring a dietitian with versatile skills.

Such was the situation at Cardiology & Internal Medicine Associates in Dallas, where I was hired to perform a variety of duties. The five-physician group originally approached me to do some nutrition counseling and classes, and to write a newsletter — all on contract. After some negotiation, however, the physicians were convinced by their senior partner that the practice could indeed benefit from the services of another full-time employee, if that person could wear several hats, including that of marketing manager. Both the nutrition counseling and the marketing efforts would produce the revenue needed to cover the increased expense.

Today, as managed care continues to grow, 40 to 50 percent of the patients I instruct come from the 36 PPO accounts and one HMO account our practice serves. I also instruct patients with private insurance, Medicare, and no insurance coverage. We find that the managed-care accounts cover my fees more often than do private insurance companies.

A closer look at how this position evolved reveals that several factors were working.

1. *Dietitians bring to the table a number of transferable skills that have been honed in dietetic practice.* We have numerous opportunities to gain experience in marketing. As I looked toward the proposed position in the doctors' office, I reflected on how my career in dietetics had prepared me.

As a consultant in private practice, I had several years of marketing experience. I had built informal networks, visited physicians to discuss my services, made presentations to industry and community, and promoted myself through brochures and phone calls.

In my practice in an internist's office years earlier, I had proposed writing a health newsletter, with the physician paying for publication and distribution. It was sent to my patients outside his practice as well as to his patients. This ultimately resulted in a contract to edit the newsletter, *Healthstyle,* which I did for ten years. This newsletter, as it turned out, was the tool that later opened the door for a marketing position.

During part of the time the newsletter was in process, I also was fortunate to work closely with the marketing vice president of a large Dallas weight-management program. It was there that I was first exposed to focus groups, marketing surveys, media events, and the importance of analyzing the competition.

During that time, I also began developing computer skills that would increase my attractiveness as an employee. Such skills are important to the marketing function. Desktop publishing can be valuable for producing brochures and other marketing materials, and a database program allows efficient tracking of marketing efforts. For example, in our cardiology practice, I can use a database to gauge the frequency of referrals from physicians and to maintain a mailing list for promotional materials. Most multiphysician practices have a patient database that can be accessed for targeted mailings.

2. *The initial job offer was made because I am a nutrition professional.* Never forget your roots or that dietetics is your primary profession. It is the ticket that will get you in the door. Physicians are increasingly aware that as nutrition professionals, dietitians can help market a medical practice merely by offering nutrition counseling and/or classes. Nutrition education is perceived as a value-added service that can raise the status of the practice in the eyes of the patient.

3. *The basic job description was expandable.* The position expanded to full-time because the physicians believed I had further skills that would be valuable to their medical practice. In addition to experience in developing a nutrition program from the ground up, I brought the added dimension of marketing ability. With my writing and design background, I would be able to develop promotional materials, such as a practice brochure, educational pamphlets, and a newsletter to referring physicians. Developing relationships with hospital administrators, managed-care contractors, and referring clinics and physicians would also be part of my job.

Along with nutrition and marketing, a third dimension of the job would be to assist the administrator of the medical practice in such areas as personnel and patient relations. I could also help the practice develop systems to streamline its operations. These administrative skills were a natural extension of my management experience with the Women, Infants, and Children's (WIC) Program and in hospitals.

4. *The power of networking cannot be underestimated.* Through the years, I used every opportunity to hand out my *Healthstyle* newsletters and to tell people about my occupation. The physician who was responsible for my nutrition/marketing job offer had seen the newsletter and had heard me speak enthusiastically about my work. It pays to be vocal about what you do well.

Dietitians who have an interest in marketing have a unique opportunity to fill a growing need in the moderate to large medical office. Physicians are scrambling to position themselves in the rapidly changing arena of managed care. As never before, they must face the need to market their services, create a niche, and fine-tune their operations for optimum patient satisfaction. The dietitian who can offer both traditional and innovative nutrition services along with expertise in health-care marketing is more likely to be perceived as an asset to a medical practice.

Chapter 3

Global Markets Ahead

Bernadette Feist-Fite, PhD, RD, President, Feist Associates, Santa Fe, New Mexico, and Alexandria, Virginia

The shifting of nations, alignments, and borderless markets demonstrates that competitive market issues are heating up. These include

1. Rapid technological growth (size and rate comparable to those experienced during the Industrial Revolution of the 1800s)

2. Changes in population (citizens of the third world immigrating to more affluent countries, world population increasing at an alarming rate, and more people living longer)

3. The influence of global markets on economics (new alliances with neighboring countries opening boundaries and cutting tariffs, and companies expanding from mature local markets with slow growth into new overseas markets with growing interest in consumer goods and services)

RAPID TECHNOLOGICAL GROWTH

Rapid technological growth has cross-pollinated markets and accelerated changes. Hot areas include biotechnology, information systems, and global networks. The new technology adds to an industrialized nation's competitive edge. However, the ability of an industrialized nation to maintain a competitive edge depends on the quality of its workforce and its ability to generate new ideas. Another factor is the nation's ability to educate and train its domestic workforce, thus allowing its industries to keep pace with global competitors.

Changes and challenges from global markets will be one of the most burning economic issues the United States faces for at least the next fifteen years. This affects most U.S. industries, markets, and professions. Examples affecting dietetics are the explosions of communication technology and biotechnology, such as biochemical nutritional analysis of the human body. Traditional jobs that have not been upgraded to keep pace with the new technology may be eliminated. Repetitious tasks may be replaced by computer software or taken over by lesser-trained employees. Middle-management positions may be handled remotely by one manager who oversees several sites through telecommunications and more group decision-making. It is very conceivable that foreign corporations will one day become major employers in the U.S. health-care market.

CHANGES IN POPULATIONS

Another crucial factor facing the world today is changes in the global population. At this time, the world is facing the largest population shift in history as millions of people, usually from developing countries or countries torn apart by violence and war, move to safer, more prosperous countries. This mass migration brings in new labor forces, who may or may not be appropriately educated and trained. This can be positive in countries like Japan, West Germany, and the United States, where residents are unwilling to perform low-paying, manual labor. In the short term, however, such shifts can have a destabilizing effect, especially if new immigrants settle in large numbers in a few areas, where they may exhaust local resources for schools, health care, and social support. Dietetics professionals who speak the languages of these new immigrants will often find work in government programs, patient education, product development, and marketing programs.

The changes and challenges introduced by more affluent migrating and traveling populations affect domestic and international markets, affording the profession of dietetics tremendous opportunities. The marketing of products and services can be targeted to domestic and international needs. Foods of other countries become popular here, and our products find new markets in other countries when people return home.

Chronic diseases in our aging population and infectious diseases like AIDS impose an excessive drain on world health-care resources. They affect health standards and the stability and growth of dietetic jobs. At the same time the market needs more health-care providers, including dietitians and dietetic technicians, it is faced with the need to "right size" and critically evaluate every expense and each employee's position and contribution to the final outcome. Experts have predicted a shift in dietetics to more out-patient, managed, and home health care. Dietitians who work in prevention and wellness may contract with corporate buying groups and insurance agencies to work with their client accounts to help reduce health risk.

THE INFLUENCE OF GLOBAL MARKETS ON ECONOMICS

As global competition increases, there will be new challenges to the U.S. way of doing business. In response, the United States must educate and train its people to meet the challenges this competition affords.

Undoubtedly, markets throughout the world are influenced by this competition. Some would like to solve market challenges through collaborative efforts, like those of the European Union and the nations of the Pacific Rim. One way in which the United States is collaborating and meeting this challenge is through the North American Free Trade Agreement (NAFTA). This agreement can be viewed either positively or negatively.

On the positive side is the reduction or elimination of trade barriers, such as tarrifs and subsidies, that discourage the sale of goods between Canada, Mexico, and the United States. With the reduction of these barriers, the resulting internal competition and cooperation would ensure that more goods could reach larger markets at lower costs.

On the negative side, people in all three countries are concerned that currently successful companies will not be able to compete with lower-cost foreign-made goods and that jobs will be lost or markets totally taken over by better products that previously had limited distribution. The question from either viewpoint is whether the U.S. domestic market can keep up with global changes.

DIETETICS AND THE GLOBAL MARKETS

Dietetics as a profession will be influenced by both the global markets and changes in domestic markets. When taken as a challenge, the issue of change can help dietetics professionals learn to be more entrepreneurial in the new environment. New jobs will become available as our management and food companies expand into foreign markets. Language skills, strong management skills, and experience are seen as crucial to upward mobility.

It is important to understand global marketing methods. These include: (1) maintaining a domestic market while exploring internationally; (2) knowing about international issues, such as cultural differences, finances, economic stability, costs of mailing, and protecting intellectual property; and (3) how to gain access to domestic and international networks to market services and products.

To maintain a competitive edge requires both personal and business growth. Valuable resources that can help you explore importing and exporting are available from the Department of Commerce in Washington, D.C., and your state economic development office or state international trade representative.

DIETETICS PROFESSIONALS AROUND THE WORLD

The first step in developing liaisons and relationships with other nations is to learn more about them. The following short sketches will provide insight into the dietetic professions and markets in a sampling of the countries and regions that belong to the International Committee of Dietetic Associations (ICDA): Australia, Canada, England, Europe, Israel, Japan, the Philippines, and South Africa.

The ICDA holds a four-day international symposium every four years in one of its member countries. Dietetics professionals are invited to submit ideas for presentations and poster sessions. Attendees may rent booth and bookmart space to display their products and services. The opportunities to network, share strategies, sell to global markets, and learn about other cultures make the International Congress of Dietetics (ICD) unique. Look for meeting announcements in the *Journal of The American Dietetic Association* and at ADA's Annual Meeting and Exhibition.

A PROFILE OF DIETITIAN-NUTRITIONISTS IN AUSTRALIA

Sally Evans, BHSc, MDAA, Former Director of Food and Nutrition Services, Princess Alexandra Hospital, Brisbane, Australia

Dietitian nutritionists traditionally work in metropolitan and provincial centers along the east and southwestern coasts of Australia. The Federal Department of Human Services and Health is currently developing a Rural Workforce Strategy to help rural centers recruit more health professionals, including dietitians.

The Dietitians Association of Australia (DAA) has a total membership of 1,551, with 94.4 percent female members, 5.6 percent male, and 68.5 percent under 35 years of age. The majority of dietitians work in hospitals and nursing homes (54.4 percent), followed by private practice (16.4 percent), community health (11.5 percent), education (6.5 percent), government (3.3 percent), industry (3 percent), and other (5 percent).

THE EMPLOYMENT MARKET

Australia maintains its socialized health system (Medicare) by assessing all income earners 1.5 percent of their gross income as a Medicare levy. This levy supports Primary, Secondary, and Tertiary Health Services. Less than 33 percent of the Australian population has private health coverage. Private practice dietetic consultations are reimbursed by the Private Health Funds, but not by Medicare.

There are two major trends in the dietetics workforce:

1. The percentage of dietitians employed in hospitals is decreasing — a drop of 10 percent in the last ten years.

2. Increasing numbers of dietitians are going into education, food and food-service industries, health promotion, private practice, and sports and fitness. Dietitians are increasingly functioning as marketing and public relations consultants, journalists, food-service managers, and food-production and retailing-industry consultants.

Few dietitians are unemployed in Australia; thus, there is potential to increase the number of dietetic graduates each year.

EDUCATION

Dietetic programs vary from a four-year undergraduate program at Newcastle University to an eighteen-month graduate diploma at Queensland University of Technology to a two-year master's program at Deakin University. DAA recently developed its competency standards for graduate dietitians.

An increasing number of dietitians are completing other kinds of graduate degrees, such as Master of Business Administration, Master of Health Administration, and Master of Public Health. Similarly, an increasing number of dietitians are completing PhD degrees.

References

Dietitians Association of Australia. *Annual Report* 1993.

Scott J, Binns C. A profile of dietetics in Australia: part 1 — demography and educational characteristics. *J Food and Nutrition.* 1988; 45:3, 77-79.

Scott J, Binns C. A profile of dietetics in Australia: part 2 — employment characteristics. *Aust J Nutrition Dietetics.* 1988; 46:1, 14-17.

About the Author

Sally Evans is a New Zealander who graduated from Otago University in 1980 and became a registered dietitian in 1981. Sally has worked as a clinical dietitian in New Zealand, Australia, and the United Kingdom. Sally recently resigned from the position of Director of Food and Nutrition Services from the 1,100-bed Princess Alexandra Hospital in Brisbane, Australia, to take a position as Contract Manager with a commercial catering company (Gardner Merchant) in Hong Kong.

THE CANADIAN PERSPECTIVE

Anne Carlson, BSHEc, RD, The Salvation Army Grace Hospital, Calgary, Canada

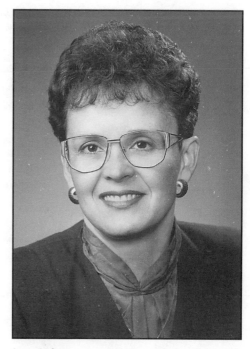

Anne Carlson

The job market and marketing opportunities for registered dietitians are changing in Canada. Currently, approximately 5,100 dietitians are members of the Canadian Dietetic Association. Thirty-four percent work as clinical dietitians, 15 percent in administrative/food service, 10 percent in public health, 4 percent in education, about 6 percent in private practice, 19 percent in fields other than dietetics, and the rest are retired or not working. (1)

Registration of professionals is in the jurisdiction of provincial governments. Each of the ten provinces has a body that registers dietitians. Membership in the Canadian association is voluntary and does not provide registration. Regulations for registration can vary from province to province. As of January 1994, dietitians practicing in Ontario must be members of the College of Dietitians, which means a dietitian must write an exam to become registered (to be implemented in 1995). A quality-assurance program will be implemented within the year, and members will need to meet new standards to maintain registration. Also, Ontario province is the first to discontinue paying stipends to all health-care interns; therefore, economic factors may determine who can obtain practical training in that province. Other provinces are expected to follow similar cost-cutting measures shortly.

Health care in Canada is paid for primarily by the provincial governments, federal government, and supplementary group plans. At present, the contribution by the federal government is decreasing, and this trend is expected to continue. Health reform means regionalizing health care in many provinces. Alberta is using case mix systems (similar to diagnosis related groups in the United States), and other provinces are developing other means of resource allocation.

Methods of coordinating acute care, long-term care, public health, social services and other programs, and communication across these sectors within the dietetic profession become of paramount importance as the system moves to regional planning. This shift in resource allocation has the potential to significantly alter the base upon which institutional dietetics is founded. Health-care costs are paid by governments, and no reimbursements can be made over and above government payments, except for some cosmetic services, some dental services, and upgrading of specific services. The group plans, such as Blue Cross, cover additional services and higher levels of service that are not part of insured services, for instance, private hospital rooms and ambulance costs. Group plans are usually available at the worksite or can be purchased by the individual at higher rates. Social Services provides some additional health-care coverage for the poor, such as prescription drugs.

CANADIAN DIETETICS IS CHANGING

Dietetics is indeed changing in Canada. The hospital length of stay is shortening to the point where it is difficult to provide adequate nutrition consultation for inpatients. These patients go home needing care that will be provided by community services, agencies such as home care, public health departments, or private practice dietitians. Thus, jobs will shift from hospitals to the community.

There is a shift away from treating illness to providing health promotion and prevention strategies, such as wellness. Hospital-based prevention programs also are growing in numbers. Subsequently, there is ongoing need for highly specialized practitioners for acute care patients, as well as generalists who will work in the community sector. There is increasing demand for registered dietitians in private practice to consult with individuals and industry. Registered dietitians are developing important relationships with industry, including food manufacturers, food service companies, pharmaceutical companies, and industries specializing in marketing, research, and development.

Dietitians are using innovative ideas to market more to the public, other health-care professionals, and industry. Dietitians are developing videos, nutrition displays, restaurant guides, packaged weight-control programs, franchises, television and radio programs, and advertisements. They are writing trendy cookbooks, newsletters, and nutrition books in the style of the popular press. They are writing for magazines and professional newsletters, and developing brochures for clients. They are giving grocery shopping tours and doing more public speaking. Dietitians are becoming more visible in their communities by initiating activities or participating in local activities.

PUBLIC POLICY

Currently, many dietitians at both the provincial and the federal levels have become more politically involved to influence national health policy for the benefit of all Canadians. This arena will require dietitians to enhance their skills in marketing, lobbying, negotiating, communicating, and interpreting information. The recent upsurge in research in dietetics demonstrates that the Canadian Dietetic Association, and its members, are beginning to respond to the importance and implications of scientific and technological change. The newly formed Canadian Foundation for Dietetic Research should serve to enhance the research base for the professional.

THE FUTURE

Future growth for dietitians appears to lie in private practice, community health, and joint ventures with industry, government, and local businesses. Dietitians will need to design products and services that are appropriate for their target markets and then market effectively to create demand. It is important for dietitians to prove that their services are making a difference and are cost effective. The focus is on health outcomes and total quality management (TQM). It is critical for dietitians to work together to proactively deal with the current changes.

Reference

1. Canadian Dietetic Association. *Roadmap for Success for the 90s and Beyond.* Toronto, ON: Canadian Dietetic Association; 1992.

About the Author

Anne Carlson, BSHEc, RD, is currently employed as a Health Consultant Registered Dietitian at Women's Health Resources, Grace Hospital Women's Health Centre. Anne also has an active private practice. She has been a speaker or consultant in university, corporate, community, and hospital settings. Anne's other interests include her family, curling, hiking, raising purebred Hereford cattle, and running. She recently completed the Honolulu Marathon.

Anne earned her B.S. from the University of Saskatchewan, and completed her internship at University Hospital in Saskatoon. She is a member of the Canadian Dietetic Association, Alberta Registered Dietitians Association, Calgary Sports Nutrition Specialist Group, Cardiac Dietitians Special Interest Group, and American Dietetic Association.

ENGLAND

Paula Hunt, Bsc, SRD, Health Education Authority, Oxford, England

There are approximately 3,000 State Registered Dietitians (SRDs) in the United Kingdom (U.K.), of whom the vast majority are women and members of the British Dietetic Association (BDA). Of the BDA members who are practicing, the most recent data show that almost two-thirds (60 percent) work in a hospital-based role for the National Health Service (NHS), doing clinical, therapeutic dietetics with minimal food service. Twelve percent do community-based NHS work, with 2 percent in private practice, 2 percent in non-NHS teaching, 2 percent in industry, 1 percent in research, 1 percent freelance, 1 percent in government departments, and the remainder not working or working outside dietetics.

The British National Health Service is funded by the federal government, and everyone is entitled to good quality health care through this system. A small proportion of people opt to buy additional private health care through insurance companies.

CHANGES IN DIETETICS

Dietetics in the U.K. is becoming increasingly diverse and more highly specialized. There is growth in community-based NHS work, with an emphasis on health promotion. Much of this work is being done by general practitioners (family physicians) and the multidisciplinary primary health-care team. There is also an increase in opportunities for dietitians to work outside the traditional NHS role, in industry, or in a freelance/consultancy capacity. Dietetics is becoming more business-oriented and client-centered, with an increased emphasis on needs assessment and evaluation of work.

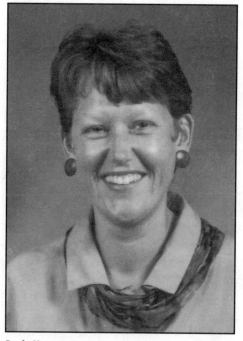

Paula Hunt

INCREASED MARKETING

The BDA recently employed a part-time public relations officer to market the role of the State Registered Dietitian, particularly via the print and electronic media. This position was funded directly through a significant increase in members' dues, which illustrates dietitians' clear recognition of the need for marketing their professional role.

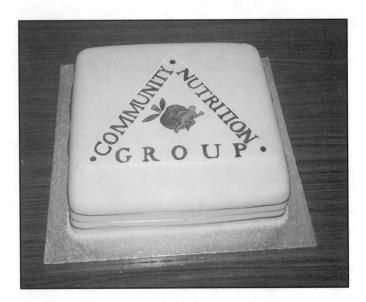

The Community Nutrition Group, a practice group of the BDA, recently launched a new logo representing a positive, progressive image. The group launched the logo by designing T-shirts, new letterhead, and new brochures that promote the varied roles of dietitians working in the community. To publicize their new logo at their spring conference, the group invited news photographers to take photos of members with a large iced cake displaying the logo.

Dietitians work closely with their local media, especially radio and television, to ensure that the public has increased exposure to SRDs. NHS Dietetic Service Managers are lobbying to secure funding for more dietitians, particularly in the community and primary-care setting, as studies increasingly show that health professionals require, and welcome, further training and ongoing support from SRDs. This interest from health professionals is being harnessed as a marketing opportunity for dietitians.

THE FUTURE

The future is likely to bring growth in the total number of dietitians, especially those working in health promotion and public health nutrition, industry, freelance consultancy, and private practice.

The government's 1992 Health of the Nation strategy presents nutrition targets for the year 2005, including a reduction in both total fat and saturated fat and a reduction in the prevalence of obesity. The Nutrition Task Force, which is creating a framework and driving implementation toward meeting these targets, holds the role of SRDs in very high regard and sees dietitians as the key professional group for nutrition education in the U.K.

About the Author

Paula Hunt, BSc, SRD, works for the Health Education Authority in Oxford, England, is a member of the Council of the British Dietetic Association, and is an active member of the Community Nutrition Group of the BDA.

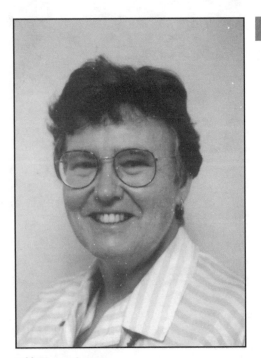

Hilde M. van Oosten

EUROPE

Hilde M. van Oosten, Honorary Secretary, European Federation of the Associations of Dietitians, The Hague, Netherlands

European dietitians, like their American counterparts, are beginning to branch out and work in more nontraditional fields. Ideally, dietitians should be able to work throughout the European Community (E.C.) in the spirit of the E.C.

Dietitians, while cooperating in diet therapy with physicians and hospital staff, do not limit their sphere of activity to that field. More and more they are acting as advisers for large-scale feeding of healthy people and take part in the nutrition education of the public. For this purpose, dietitians must receive special training recognized by national diplomas. They respect professional rules concerning their sphere of duties.

Dietitians in Europe work in many different areas: in administrative, clinical, and scientific research fields; in hospitals, pediatrics, psychiatry, and community health centers; and in catering. Most dietitians work in clinical areas that have recently become highly specialized — for example, renal nutrition and oncology nutrition. In some countries, dietitians are working in food-service positions. In other countries, the idea of food service is still new. The food industry has begun to hire dietitians and to recognize the value of their work. There are some private practice dietitians, and their number is increasing. However, most dietitians in Europe are employed in government health-care positions.

THE EUROPEAN FEDERATION OF THE ASSOCIATIONS OF DIETITIANS

The European Federation of the Associations of Dietitians (EFAD) represents about 22,000 dietitians in Europe. It was established on February 21, 1979. The aims of the federation are to encourage a better nutritional situation for the populations of the member countries of the Council of Europe; to develop dietetics on a scientific and professional level in the common interest of the member associations; to promote the development of the dietetic profession; to improve the teaching of dietetics and to standardize the criteria for qualification in the dietetic profession; and to pursue these objectives with the help of international organizations, and especially with the Council of Europe. The Federation does not pursue any political, religious, racial, or financial ends.

MEMBERSHIP

Full membership is open to one association from each country that is a member of the Council of Europe. As of March 1994, the members of the Federation are national associations of dietitians representing Austria, Belgium, Denmark, Finland, France, Germany, Greece, Iceland, Ireland, Italy, Luxembourg, the Netherlands, Norway, Portugal, Spain, Sweden, Switzerland, Turkey, and the United Kingdom. Affiliated membership, which would be open to other associations, has not been implemented yet. EFAD has two honorary members who have distinguished themselves in the service of the federation.

ORGANIZATION AND STRUCTURE

The General Meeting is made up of representatives of each of the member associations. The Federation is directed and represented by an Executive Committee, made up of five members elected by the General Meeting of EFAD: the Honorary President, who is elected in a personal capacity, and four member associations. The General Meeting elects members as representatives to the Council of Europe and to the World Health Organization Regional Office for Europe.

ACTIVITIES

The EFAD has assessed and made reports on educational requirements and training programs for dietitians in its member states; members' organizational structure, membership, goals, and activities; ethics of the dietetics profession; and dietitians' career avenues now and in the future.

To improve the transition into an integrated Europe, a European Forum for dietitians will be established for the exchange of experiences and professional knowledge to improve and maintain the high standards of the dietetic profession. European dietitians will communicate through a network. The Forum should cover all levels of dietitians' work: scientific and applied, clinical and administrative, dietetics and nutrition. At seminars and workshops, the participants will discuss specific topics and present their work. The Forum will promote the profession, increase awareness of training programs, and encourage new fields of employment. It will also strengthen contact with the Council of Europe, the European Community, and the World Health Organization Regional Office for Europe.

About the Author

Hilde van Oosten studied home economics and dietetics in the Netherlands and received her degrees in 1968. As an on-the-job Trainee, she experienced the diverse work of registered dietitians in a large hospital in Dayton, Ohio, from 1969 to 1970, and worked in a retirement home as an assistant foodservice director till 1976. She returned to the Netherlands and is employed by the Netherlands Bureau for Food and Nutrition Education. She is an active member of the Dutch Association of Dietitians. She served as secretary of the board (1982-1986) and delegate at the General Meeting of European Federation of the Associations of Dietitians (EFAD). Since 1988, she has served as Honorary Secretary of EFAD.

Yaakov Levinson, MS, Nutritionist, Director, The Israel Nutrition Institute, Jerusalem, Israel

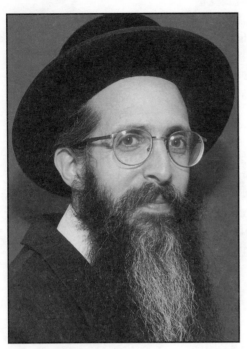

Yaakov Levinson

The Jewish people lived in Israel until about 2,000 years ago. Since the destruction of the temple in Jerusalem at that time and the beginning of the Diaspora exile, we have been hosted by and been living in almost every nation in the world. Because of this background, we witness today, with the return of the Jewish people to the Land of Israel, a society that combines the lifestyles and eating habits of virtually all parts of the world. Our citizens have come from all continents and have recently included massive immigrations from Russia and Ethiopia. It is in relation to this historical and international backdrop that Israeli dietitians face both an immense challenge and an exclusive opportunity for innovation and interesting professional development.

The full potential for nutrition and dietetics in Israel is only just beginning to be recognized. We share the usual health problems, seen in the United States and other developed countries, such as cardiac disease, obesity, diabetes, and cancer, which indicate that nutrition is a critical component in total health care. We have a developing market economy, with our citizens striving enthusiastically to achieve Western-style living, including all of its positive and negative implications. The potential market for nutrition services is therefore vast but largely untapped.

We have just one school of dietetics in conjunction with the Faculty of Agriculture in Rechovot that offers a bachelor's degree in nutrition. Advanced degrees, when sought, are generally earned in other related fields. Our Ministry of Health has a Department of Nutrition. We also have the Israel Dietetic Association (IDA), which focuses mainly on sponsoring educational opportunities and employment development. The IDA has approximately 600 members, and the membership is predominantly female, except for five males.

To date, most dietitians (56 percent) work in hospitals, 40 percent are employed by Kupat Cholim in one of the various health funds, and a very few work in supervisory capacities in the health ministry. An occasional dietitian works for a business, generally one of the pharmaceutical companies. A handful of private practitioners are forging their way through unplotted territory.

There is, however, a growing consciousness about nutrition in Israel that is quite exciting. Nutrition labeling on food products has gained popularity and is becoming mandatory. Health consciousness, in general, has been increasing, and people are seeking more natural alternatives to health care.

In short, the field of nutrition in Israel is wide open for dynamic, well-trained, nutrition professionals willing to take ground-breaking responsibility for raising public and professional awareness and for developing their own new markets.

About the Author

Yaakov Levinson received a BA in biology from Hamilton College in Clinton, New York, and an MS in clinical nutrition from Case Western Reserve University, Cleveland, Ohio. He was a registered dietitian and worked as a clinical nutritionist at Memorial Hospital, Albany, New York. In Israel, in 1978 to 1983, he was the Instructor in Nutrition at Zefat School of Nursing and Internship Supervisor at Zefat Hospital. He has worked at the Hadassah University Hospital and Neve Simcha Geriatric Hospital in Jerusalem.

In 1989, Yaakov founded the Israel Nutrition Institute in Jerusalem, where he educates the public on nutrition via publications, lectures, classes, media, personal patient consultations, and research.

Professor Mitsuo Arai, Journal Committee of Food and Nutrition Topics, *Japan Dietetic Association*

S ince history is so important in Japan, it is fitting that Japan's dietetic organization be described from the beginning. The National Institute of Nutrition and the Saiki School of Nutrition, established to oversee research in nutrition and to train nutritionists, respectively, were founded by a Yale University-trained physician, Dr. Tadasu Saiki, in 1926. Graduates of the school were given the title *Eiyoshi,* or Nutrition Professional.

In 1945, the Dietitian Law was enacted. Graduates of the Saiki School of Nutrition organized the Japan Dietetic Association. The President was the Commissioner of the Bureau of Health within the Ministry of Health and Welfare.

In 1952, the Nutrition Improvement Law was enacted, setting standards for nutrition services at health centers, a national nutrition survey, nutrition services for mass feeding, and the labeling of food for special dietary uses.

The 1993 classification of nutrition professionals called *Eiyoshi* had 26,291 members. These people must complete a two-year program in a junior college or vocational school. After two years of practical experience, an *Eiyoshi* may take the state examination to become a more highly qualified *Kanri-eiyoshi.* A person can also become a *Kanri-eiyoshi* by graduating from a four-year university program in dietetics and passing the state examination.

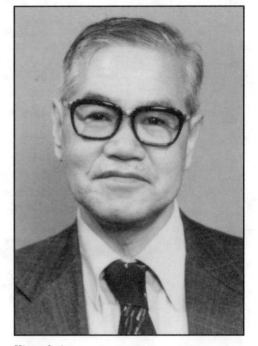

Mitsuo Arai

THE JAPAN DIETETICS SOCIETY

The annual meetings of the Dietetics Society are operated by the Japan Dietetic Association (JDA). At the Thirty-Ninth Annual Meeting, held in Kyoto in 1992, 2,500 members were in attendance and 350 original papers were presented.

The primary activity of the JDA is the continuing education for its members. This year's focus is on the training of clinical dietitians.

The classification of members by job title in 1993 was

School food service	5,455
Educator, university or vocational	1,496
Correctional institution	29
Government health agency	2,397
Research	189
Industrial food service	2,419
Hospital	1,507
Welfare	5,690
Defense forces	243
Private practice, homemaker, etc.	6,641
Total (95% female and 5% male)	41,402

MEDICAL COST PROBLEMS

All Japanese citizens are covered by the Social Health Insurance System, which is managed by the government and funded by employers, employees, and the government. The allowance for hospital meals has been fixed at 1,950 yen (about $18.75) per patient per day to cover food costs, labor, heat, water, and maintenance. Due to rising national medical costs, the government plans to require direct payment of food costs by the patient. Our Hospital Dietitian Group has declared its opposition to this plan.

THE MOVEMENT OF THE MINISTRY OF LABOR

The Total Health Promotion Movement has developed to protect the health of workers. One health problem that is causing growing concern is *Karoshi,* or sudden death resulting from job stress.

The Ministry of Labor has prepared short courses to help industrial physicians, nurses, sports trainers, psychological counselors, and dietitians protect the health of workers.

LOCAL GOVERNMENT DIETITIANS

About 1,100 dietitians are newly employed in the public health services of city, town, village, and other local governments.

About the Author

Mitsuo Arai is the former Liaison Director of the Japan Dietetic Association, former Vice President of the Tokyo Dietetic Association, current President of Registered Industrial Dietitians, and Director of *Japan Nutrition News,* a biweekly newsletter. He has written two books, *Food Acceptance Study in Mass Feeding,* and *How To Be a Dietitian,* and has translated into *Japanese Food Service in Institutions,* by West, Wood, and Harger.

THE PHILIPPINES

Betty Dykes, MEd, RD, LD, Professor and Chairperson, Dietetics and Nutritional Management Department, Sinclair Community College, Dayton, Ohio

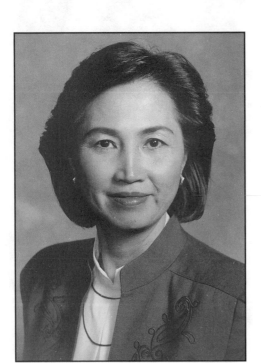

Betty Dykes

The Philippines is made up of 7,107 islands covering a land area of 115,739 square miles. The main island groups are Luzon, Visayas, and Mindanao. The population of 65 million is made up of Indo-Malay, Chinese, and Spanish descendants. Although there is a national language (Tagalog), the existence of many regional dialects impedes communication. English, the medium of instruction in schools throughout this tropical country, is the usual means of communication.

The Philippines was a colony of Spain for over three centuries. In 1895, it was ceded to the United States as the result of the Spanish American War, and on July 4, 1945, it obtained its independence. During its 50-year presence, the United States developed a democratic form of government and established schools patterned after its own.

DIETETIC EDUCATION

Dietetic education in the Philippines can be traced to 1939, when a U.S.-trained dietitian introduced a baccalaureate degree in home economics with a major in foods and nutrition at the University of the Philippines. Because of World War II, however, the first class did not graduate until 1948. Graduates were recommended for, and received, dietetic internships in the United States.

Upon their return to the Philippines, these ADA-qualified dietitians were recruited to develop an internship program at the Philippine General Hospital, an affiliate of the University of the Philippines. This was in 1952, and the following year saw the first internship class of eight.

Dietetics is one of the most popular academic programs in the Philippines. Invariably, most of those who complete their coursework in the Philippines obtain dietetic internships in the United States. Over the years, many schools have followed the lead of the state university and now offer baccalaureate programs in home economics with a major in foods and nutrition.

To ensure that hospitals employ qualified dietitians, legislation was passed in 1960 to license all practicing dietitians through examination. (Prior to this, nurses supervised dietary departments.) A 1977 law provided for the integration of practical training into the undergraduate programs and established the title *nutritionist/dietitian* for graduates who successfully meet the requirements.

DIETETIC PRACTICE

Nutritionists/dietitians typically are employed in hospitals and other health-care institutions. However, others prefer to work in community or public health agencies. Other employment opportunities exist in schools (the first school mass feeding was at the University of the Philippines), industry (Proctor and Gamble Company in the Philippines had the first in-plant cafeteria), and restaurants and clubs (the early ones were the Aristocrat Restaurant and U.S. Employees Seafront Dining Room).

In the past, very few dietitians ventured into entrepreneurship or more nontraditional areas, but that is starting to change. Several dietitians have started home-based consulting practices. Some work for shipping lines as on-board food-service managers. Others work for weight-loss centers to help the more affluent public lose weight and control diabetes or heart disease.

At present, approximately 50 percent of employed dietitians work in community or public health settings, 30 percent in hospitals, and 20 percent in teaching and research.

PROFESSIONAL DIETETIC ORGANIZATIONS

The Nutritionists/Dietitians Association of the Philippines (NDAP) provides its membership with continuing education, newsletters, and social events. It works very closely with the Board of Nutrition of the Professional Regulations Commission (PRC).

RECIPROCITY

The training of Filipino dietitians is comparable to the coordinated dietetic programs in the United States. To practice, dietitians must successfully pass the two-day examination administered by the Philippine Professional Regulation Commission, a governmental agency. Continuing education is required, and licensure is mandatory to practice.

September 29, 1993, marked the culmination of negotiations between the Commission on Dietetic Registration and the Philippine Professional Regulation Commission. The agreement permits Filipino licensed nutritionists/dietitians to write for the dietetic registration examination without having to return to school or complete the supervised dietetic practice (internships or AP4). Likewise, any U.S.-trained registered dietitian who wishes to take the dietetic licensing examination in the Philippines may do so. In both cases, complete verification statements from the respective agencies must be obtained.

Bibliography

Corpus A., ed. *Nutrition and Dietetics in the Philippines*. Quezon City, Philippines: Nutritionists/Dietitians Association of the Philippines (NDAP); 1985.

Karnov S. *In Our Image*. New York, NY: Ballantine; 1989.

Tourist Research and Planning. *Philippines*. 2nd ed. Manila: Lorenzo Martinengo; 1982.

Meetings with Esther Feliciano, NDAP President, October 1993.

About the Author

Betty Dykes, MEd, RD, LD, is a Filipino-American dietitian. She is Professor and Chairperson of the Dietetics and Nutritional Management Department of Sinclair Community College in Dayton, Ohio. Betty is a very active member of The American Dietetic Association.

Jane Badham, Dietitian, Director and Marketing Specialist for
The Association for Dietetics in Southern Africa, Randburg, South Africa

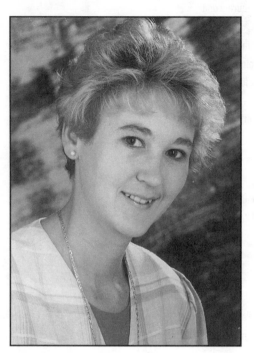

Jane Badham

Relatively speaking, dietetics in South Africa is still in its infancy — the first local degree course having started in 1945. Until 1986, dietitians shared an association with home economists. In 1987, they formed The Association for Dietetics in Southern Africa (ADSA).

Since then, the Association and the profession have grown and become highly visible among the public, industry, the media, the medical profession, and the allied health professions. Dietetics as a career has also expanded, with nine universities offering the bachelor of science degree as well as postgraduate courses.

There are some 700 dietitians registered with the South African Medical and Dental Council, and approximately 550 of these are members of ADSA. The majority are women, but the interest among men is increasing. There is still a need for Black and Indian dietitians, but here too a steady growth has been seen.

South Africa has not only a diversity of population groups, but also a mix of first and third world that makes dietetics an interesting, broad, and challenging field. There are roughly twenty dietitians for every one million people. The statistics show that about 40 percent of the white population suffers or dies from diseases of overnutrition, such as ischemic heart disease. At the other end of the scale, it is estimated that one-third of Black children under five years old are underweight and stunted for their age, and two-thirds of their deaths are related to undernutrition.

With this in mind, the sky can be the limit when it comes to where dietitians can and should be working, from policy making to teaching basic nutrition to clinical work in hospitals that can match those found anywhere in the world.

Private practice, clinical work, community work, education and research, and food-service management are the main areas of work, but dietitions are also involved in industry, marketing, and journalism. In the past, the public sector, such as public hospitals, public health departments, the defense force, and corrective services, employed the majority of dietitians. However, with a growing awareness of the value and versatility of dietitians, more private-sector companies, such as those in the food and mining industries, private hospitals, gyms, research organizations, and media services are employing dietitians on either a full-time or a consultancy basis.

Traditionally, South Africa has had both government-sponsored health care (usually for the less wealthy) and private health care. In recent years, the private health-care and medical insurance industries have grown dramatically. However, the government must still provide substantially subsidized health services (at both the preventive and therapeutic levels) for the majority of the population. Because South Africa is undergoing dramatic political and social changes, it is inevitable that its health-care services will also change — how is still a matter of debate and question.

In a changing society, dietetics too must change. There has been and still is a shift toward community dietetics. There will always be a need for dietitians to be involved in specialized, clinical work, but increasingly, the need is at the community and preventive levels. Intervention at an early stage is vital if we are to achieve ASDA's mission of optimal nutrition for all South Africans. Community dietetics itself can have a number of broad meanings and applications. Community nutrition can range from teaching vegetable gardening and the making of simple oral rehydration mixtures to largely illiterate populations in rural areas to providing the media with accurate and scientific facts on topics such as food irradiation and preservatives.

MARKETING CHALLENGES

Dietitians are constantly challenged to market themselves in innovative ways that emphasize the vital roles they can play. Marketing has had to reach the medical profession, which saw the dietitian as a glorified cook, the person in the kitchen preparing the patients' food; the public, who saw the dietitian as a luxury for only the overweight and the wealthy; and the media, which saw the dietitian as a recipe consultant or a conservative person with some knowledge about food. The Association has worked hard and continues to work at changing these perceptions. Campaigns have included

- The creation of a national office and a post for a public relations dietitian,
- A series of advertisements in the lay press,
- The development of topical fact sheets, position papers, and booklets that are widely circulated,
- A newsletter that is sent not only to members, but also to the media, industry, and members of the Nutrition Society,
- A badge that dietitians can wear to identify their profession,
- A biennial congress for everyone interested in nutrition and dietetics,
- Running of a food intolerance databank,
- An attractive nutrition calendar,
- A comprehensive list of privately practicing dietitians that doctors, gyms, and pharmacists can use for referrals,
- Developing relations with key people in the media and making dietitians available to assist with articles and programs,
- Representation on important forums, committees, and other bodies,
- Visibility in the form of having booths or giving lectures at medical congresses and career exhibitions,
- Involvement with other health-related associations and organizations.

Dietitians in South Africa are actively involved in marketing themselves and their profession, and in so doing are affecting the community as a whole. Dietetics in South Africa is a dynamic, different, and dedicated profession that is growing and adapting to meet the needs and challenges of the community.

About the Author

Jane Badham has a three-year bachelor of science in dietetics and a postgraduate diploma in hospital dietetics. In 1989, Jane planned and set up the Catering and Dietetics Departments of a new 200-bed private hospital. In 1991, Jane joined The Association for Dietetics in Southern Africa (ADSA) to run their national office and handle the public relations and marketing.

In 1993, Jane set up her own consultancy business. In addition to the ADSA, Jane's clients include an international pharmaceutical company involved with diabetes and overweight patient management. She developed an educational weight-control program aimed at addressing the cause for weight problems, rather than just dealing with the symptoms. Jane often appears on radio and television, is frequently quoted in the media, and regularly gives lectures to a variety of groups on a wide range of nutrition topics. Jane believes strongly in a total lifestyle approach to the management of nutrition problems.

The Business of Marketing

The Business of Marketing

To Be Successful in

Answering the Needs

of Target Markets

and Achieve Your

Business Goals,

Good Marketing Requires

Research, Creativity,

Planning, Managing,

and Evaluation.

Chapter 4

Marketing: The Challenge

Kathy King Helm, RD, LD, Private Practitioner, Lake Dallas, Texas

Marketing is not an exact science. There are no guarantees that you will attract more customers than you can handle by having the right slogan, or the most expensive brochure, or the best product in the marketplace. Timing, customer whims, competitors, and competitive positioning of your product or service make marketing more a game of strategy. These variables and others can make or break a new product or service in the marketplace. Miller Lite (Miller Brewing Co., Milwaukee, Wisconsin) was actually the third or fourth lower-calorie beer tested in the market, but it was the first one not called "diet" beer. Consumers were ready to hear that beer could have fewer calories and still taste essentially the same, so timing for the product was on target.

CUTTING THE RISK

There are no magic formulas, but you can improve your chances for success by doing your homework, learning as much as you can about the target market and your product, and then investing the effort and resources necessary to make it go. The process is dynamic. You make the best decisions you can as you begin, but you adapt and adjust along the way to keep on track to your goals. Put your plans in writing. Creating a written marketing plan will force you to anticipate needs and problems, plan your strategies, and evaluate the competition, as well as to forecast your financial income and expenses. (See Chapter 20 for details on how to write a business and marketing plan.)

OVERVIEW OF THE PROCESS

Assume you work for a hospital and want to start a weight-loss program for the public and hospital employees. How would you go about it? The following will give an overview of the systematic creation of the program and its marketing.

Enlist Organizational Support

Write a proposal explaining the project and what you hope to accomplish with it (see Chapter 34). You are seeking preliminary support to see if there is any interest in the idea. At this time, you should offer to develop the business and marketing plans for the venture. Management will use the plans to evaluate the idea and allocate funds for the start-up, or they will request more clarification. They may also turn the project down, but your organized presentation and plans will surely leave a lasting good impression.

For this example, remember that weight-loss groups are best started in the fall and after the new year, when the weather improves. Therefore, start five to six months ahead to allow sufficient time for planning, approval, and marketing.

Write Your Mission Statement

Your mission statement sets your course. It helps you decide what your goals should be so you can keep your allocation of resources focused. For this example,

---

Using Numbers to Sell Your Ideas

Kennon Moffitt, MS, RD, LD, Director: Nutrition and Food Services, St. Paul Medical Center, Dallas, Texas

In today's health-care market, and that of the future, *change* is the key operative word. Additional operative words for all dietitians, irrespective of their area of practice, are *profit and loss statement, return on investment (ROI), financial projections, capitation,* . . . The list goes on. All of the key words have one thing in common: they deal with a financial outcome and, therefore, the viability of the organization in which you work.

Business managers don't just want to hear how well customers will like longer hours in the cafeteria, the new outpatient nutrition clinic, or the convenience of having a sports nutritionist on staff. They mainly want to know how much that new service will cost as compared to how much new revenue it will generate. The difference is the ROI. Even with the cutbacks at hospitals today, dietitians justify new positions using the business principle of return on investment (ROI).

Continued page 27

your mission statement could be "To provide high-quality nutrition-education programs to the people of Centerville and employees of Memorial through the Clinical Nutrition Office staff at Memorial Hospital."

Identify Your Major Product and Target Market

Describe your product (your proposal may already offer the appropriate wording). Now answer: Who will buy it? Describe who your target market is. Consider age, gender, income, educational level, profession, and the newest parameters experts use, which are lifestyle and buying habits. The more you know about your target market, the more you can custom fit your program and marketing to its needs. Also, you will want to market the benefits of your program from the clients' point of view, so you must know your customers' perspective.

Describe your target market's feelings and history with weight-loss programs and obesity in general. Are obesity, eating disorders, fitness programs, wellness, and disease prevention major or minor concerns to your market? Who cooks the food at home? How often do they eat out? Who does the grocery shopping?

Consider what other items or services you might sell to members of the weight-loss group, such as a grocery store tour, a gourmet low-fat cooking series, cookbooks, a fitness component, and so on. Experts agree that it is usually easier to sell something to a satisfied customer than it is to find another customer. Some of these items might also be included in the program as value-added extras to beat the competition.

Conduct Market Research

This step will help you find out if your idea for a weight-loss class is a good one. Primary market research is the research you conduct yourself through private conversations, telephone interviews, and surveys. Today, mailed surveys must compete with mounds of junk mail and other demands on recipients' limited time. If you decide to mail a survey, call beforehand to identify to whom it should go. Don't address it to "Hilldale Clinic"; instead, put "Dr. Mary Alexander, Hilldale Clinic." Also, consider adding a cover letter from a respected physician colleague or some other incentive for recipients to read it and respond. Allow a week for a local survey and then start calling people to remind them how important they are to your results. If they won't take the time to fill out a survey, ask permission to quickly ask them a few questions over the phone.

Secondary market research consists of statistics and information collected by someone else, such as the Chamber of Commerce, business organizations, and trade and university groups. To be assured that you have thoroughly researched your concept, use both primary and secondary research.

Evaluate the Trends Look at market trends both locally and nationally to see what is happening in weight loss and to your target market (for example, women 35 to 50 years old). You may feel this step isn't too important, but you are wrong. Did you know that commercial weight-loss programs are experiencing a backlash to the diet mania of the 1980s? Even professional programs are trying to assess where the market will go and what will sell in the future. Is it happening in your area? Are your potential customers looking for a "new" diet, or do they prefer a healthy lifestyle change that doesn't mention diet, or are they using over-the-counter meal replacements on their own? It's crucial to know for your marketing.

General Situational Analysis What are the general characteristics of the

Continued from page 26

For example, a dietitian in Washington State wanted to create a new managed-care half-time staff position. To do so, she used statistics to show that the hospital had to absorb an average of \$7,500 for every Medicare patient who returned to the hospital after being discharged. She then researched why the patients had to return and showed that nutrition intervention at the patient's home (for postsurgical malnutrition, diabetes management, chemo-induced diarrhea, and so on) could have kept at least three, and maybe four, patients each month from returning to the hospital, for a gross savings of \$22,500 to \$30,000 per month. If the half-time dietitian is paid \$1,400 per month in salary and benefits, the hospital's ROI for that position is a savings of \$21,100 to \$28,600. Expressed as a percentage, such a figure will give an idea of the financial marketability of a request for proposal. In this example, the ROI for this dietitian's keeping three patients healthier at home is 1507 percent. No wonder the hospital approved the position!

The same reasoning can be used to assess a new cafeteria line, a new outpatient clinic office, a new line of picante sauce, or whatever. Each organization has a general rule on ROI expectations that can be obtained from the Chief Financial Officer.

market where you want to start your weight-loss class? Do most of the women in your area work? What is the economic climate? What does your target market spend its money on? Is adolescent obesity an even bigger problem in your area, with fewer competing programs? Talk discretely to potential customers and trusted referral agents. Ask open-ended questions.

Conduct a SWOT Analysis A SWOT analysis is a realistic, honest examination of your internal *strengths* and *weaknesses,* and your external *opportunities* and *threats.* In other words, what do you or your department do well that could make this project successful? What weaknesses will you delegate, subcontract, or work around? What opportunities and threats are in your environment or marketplace? An opportunity might be the opening of a hospital-based fitness center or a new insurance carrier that recognizes the value of avoiding obesity in the prevention of disease. Threats could be posed by another local hospital that is planning to begin or expand its weight-loss program, or a local psychologist who is approaching the same medical community for weight-loss referrals.

Competitive Analysis Go deeper in your analysis. Identify your competition, its locations, its products or services, and any advantages or disadvantages it may have. The purpose is to find niches or weaknesses in the competition that will enable you to position your program as different or better.

When entering the marketplace, it's important to determine if you are the leader or the follower. A leader usually owns the largest share of the market, has the greatest name recognition with its target market, and sets the standards of service. A follower looks for and tries to capitalize on the leader's weaknesses. For example, if the leader is a large commercial weight-loss chain that requires customers to buy only its food, your program could say, "Are you tired of cooking a separate meal for yourself when you want to lose weight? Learn how to lose weight by eating foods the whole family will love!" (See Chapter 5 for more information on how to evaluate your competition.)

Plot Your Product on the Product Life Cycle Curve Through your evaluation, you will be able to determine which stage the market is in and what kind of market your product is entering. The curve of the product life cycle is shown in Figure 4.1.

Figure 4-1. Product Life Cycle

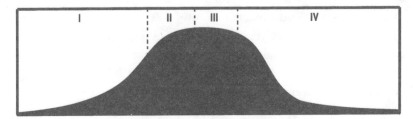

Graph by Marty Waugh, M.B.A.

In stage one, infancy, the idea is new and the competition is often lighter and not well established. Not many people are making a living selling the product or service. The idea does not have mass appeal, and little money is required to become established at this point. True entrepreneurs love this stage. They thrive on the untapped potential of the emerging trend.

Stage two, growth, begins when the idea becomes more popular and demand grows for the best services, products, and leaders from stage one. Profits rise, and the new idea starts to attract the attention of other possible providers (your competitors). Competitors copy or improve on the best ideas and add lots of marketing dollars. As the market matures, it becomes expensive to enter with a new product or service. Ineffective and marginal services, products, staff, and marketing strategies are let go. The venture is honed to a lean, well-functioning revenue-generating business.

Saturation becomes a problem in stage three, maturity, as too many competitors vie for a piece of the market. Sales are at the highest level since the product or service was introduced, but growth declines. As James Rose, MS, RD, stated in his Cooper Lecture in 1987, "During stage three the business becomes fairly routine, so many entrepreneurs lose interest. A person with good management skills is needed at this stage to keep the product or service consistent in quality and efficiently produced." Marketing is especially competitive at this stage, with each competitor trying to attract the same shrinking target markets. There also may be fewer buyers because everyone who wanted the product or service has already purchased it.

Finally, stage four, decline, arrives. The trend and its attractiveness to its present target market decline. Sales drop, and the market is no longer competitive. There are three options at this stage. The first is to continue selling the product or service as long as it is profitable. The second is to reformulate and introduce a "new and improved" item. The third, while pursuing either option one or option two, is to invest a percentage of resources into a new, cutting-edge concept in stage one or early stage two. Most businesses offer several products or services, each fitting into a different stage of the life cycle.

Most people would call the weight-loss market mature (stage three), with some segments, like extreme fad diet programs, in stage four. In a month or a year, however, a new "magic" answer might revive the industry and take it back to stage two.

Develop Your Strategic Assumptions Strategic assumptions are statements about what you expect the market to do. For example, based on your research, your strategic assumptions may be: (1) the local market hit a slump in attendance at weight-loss programs in 1993 and is now recovering to near levels reported in 1987, and (2) indications show that the industry has fewer competitors, but the target market is feeling negative about dieting and skeptical of expensive, quick weight-loss programs. By deciding what the strategic assumptions are for your business area, you can better anticipate what will sell and how to sell it. You should review your assumptions yearly to see if they must be altered or if new ones must be added.

Set Your Goals and Objectives

Define what you want to achieve, given the mission statement you wrote. Make goals and objectives as succinct and measurable as possible. Write specific objectives that will help you reach your goals, including profit and marketing. (See Chapter 20 for more details.)

Determine Major Strategies

Now is the time to determine the specifics of your marketing strategies, or marketing mix, also known as the 4 P's of marketing: product, price, place, and promotion.

Product You know the program you want to sell, but take a few minutes to describe its positioning in the marketplace: What is its market niche? What benefits will the consumer get? How is the program unique? What unique aspects really appeal to the target audience? When you market a service, never forget that you are part of the total package. This means your personal presentation, communication, interpersonal interaction, and appearance are important to the success of the program. There are many chapters and case studies in this book that deal with this topic.

Price What are your pricing strategies? (See Chapter 21.)

Place You need to give thought to how you distribute your product or service. This includes the location where customers buy your product or attend your group classes. This variable could be particularly important if the room is poorly lighted, drafty, or difficult to find. If parking is expensive or inconvenient, it can affect your program's success. The key is to make your products and services as convenient for consumers as possible.

Promotion Specifically explain what you plan to do to promote your weight-loss program. Think of as many ways as you can to spread the name and story of your program: send press releases requesting interviews to local newspapers and radio stations; buy space for ongoing ads in local newspapers; write a brochure and cover letter to send in a direct mail campaign; choose free giveaways with the program name or logo, such as mugs, T-shirts, sweat bands, gym bags, and pens, to offer attendees. To encourage sign-ups in the hospital, consider paycheck stuffers, articles in employee newsletters, brochures in nursing stations and employee lounges, and signs on bulletin boards. To make the system work smoothly, ensure that the phone number used in promotional materials is staffed every day during normal business hours by someone who knows how to answer the phone professionally and take care of customers and their needs. (See Chapter 12 for more ideas on promotion.)

In their book, *The Great Marketing Turnaround*, Rapp and Collins state, "Individualized marketing recognizes, appreciates, and responds to the special needs and interests of individual consumers." They see sellers using more database names and buying preference information to generate direct mail promotions. They see the most successful companies as ones that continually carry on dialogues with their target market. In other words, success is built on continuous market research and relationship-building activities.

Many changes are taking place in mass marketing: the once creative universal advertisement that was repeated to the saturation point is being replaced by asking customers about their needs and wants. An analogy closer to home for dietitians is how clinical counseling has changed from giving information according to the diagnosis to finding out what the patient wants and needs.

In our weight-loss example, you could glean names of prospective group members from earlier cooking or wellness classes, inpatient lists, diabetes education classes, and prenatal classes. A stack of response cards for people to indicate their desire for more information on weight loss or a free booklet on the subject could be left in lobbies and waiting areas, given to local physicians, and distributed at clinics without competing programs.

In a mature marketplace, where competitors look a lot alike, it can be difficult to stand out or stand above the crowd. Years ago marketers used U.S.P. – unique selling proposition – such as a dental association's stamp of approval on a toothpaste tube, to distinguish themselves, but today, such tactics are no longer unique. So what can you offer that gives you a competitive advantage?

Tapping the Marketing Capabilities of ADA

Marty Yadrick, MBA, MS, RD,
Training Consultant, Computrition,
Chatsworth, California

A multitude of opportunities exist within The American Dietetic Association that can help you market your product or service, or help you gain exposure:

• Submit your program proposal to ADA's Meetings Department in November of each year for the next year's Annual Meeting and Exhibition. You can merely suggest other people as speakers, or suggest yourself as a speaker or moderator.

• Each spring, submit your application to ADA for an original presentation (ten minutes) or poster session at the AME.

• Rent booth space at AME in the member Product Marketplace.

• Rent exhibit space for three days as an exhibitor at AME.

• Sign up for ADA's Nationwide Nutrition Network to obtain referrals.

• Rent booth space that Dietetic Practice Groups like SCAN (Sports, Cardiovascular and Wellness Nutritionists), CN (Consulting Nutritionists), and DBC (Dietitians in Business and Communications) offer their members, or take an ad in their product catalogs.

Continued page 35

In the 1990s, an E.V.P. – extra-value proposition – can be the best way to gain a unique advantage, according to Rapp and Collins. Simply put, an E.V.P. is a supplementary service accompanying a product or service that is so attractive to consumers, they develop a favorable mindset about the product and remain loyal. In our example, an E.V.P. could be child-care services for attendees during meetings or a month's free membership at the hospital fitness center.

You can easily recognize the E.V.P.'s used today in the food industry: 800 number consumer phone lines, product recipe booklets, free employee education videos with major equipment purchases, and so on.

When considering promotion, the term *integration* is very timely. It means that you think holistically about whatever is necessary to identify, contact, activate, and cultivate individual customers and increase market sales and share. Today, Rapp and Collins believe the most successful marketers will choose integration. Decisions will be made according to which means of promotion reaches the consumers best. All marketing functions will use a common client database so that one hand knows what the other is doing concerning messages and contacts with the clients.

Integration also means presenting a unified image and consistent voice when providing messages to your customers, according to Elaine Cibotti, MBA. Another key is being a good listener, which builds relationships. A good listener actively seeks input from the audience. Such incoming information gathered through surveys and focus groups is key to understanding integration. Databases provide a useful means to store and retrieve this feedback. By examining this data, you can assess how you are doing and whether customers are satisfied.

Develop Action Plans and Assign Responsibilities

In this step, you break down the actions in this chapter into specific activities and arrange them on a timetable showing dates, resources required, budget allocation, deadlines, and so on. Assign responsibilities if someone other than yourself, such as a graphic artist, printer, or publicist, is contributing to the project. Don't assume anything. Stay on top of the project because whatever happens will reflect on you.

Establish a Financial Reporting System and Measure Results

These topics are handled very completely in Chapter 20.

Now you are ready to return for final approval of your plan and go forward with a lot more wisdom and confidence . . . and much less risk.

Bibilography

Cibotti E. Integrated marketing. 1993. Unpublished.
Crull T. Integrated marketing? It's synergy. *Advertising Age*, March 3, 1993.
Rapp S, Collins T. *The Great Marketing Turnaround*. Englewood Cliffs, NJ: Prentice Hall; 1990.

Continued from page 34

• Submit publication ideas to DPGs for patient education and professional growth materials in your specialty area.
• Get involved, become known, and submit your name for committees and speaking opportunities.
• Talk to DPG newsletter editors and offer to write an article for an issue.
• Incorporate the ADA member logo on your letterhead and business card. Some DPGs offer this too.
• Frame the ADA membership or DPG certificates and hang them on your office wall.
• If you have an idea for a book, study kit, or other publication, consider submitting a proposal to ADA's publication department.
• Submit an application for a research grant from ADA Foundation, if you have interest and expertise in the designated topics.
• Submit articles and research to the *Journal of The American Dietetic Association* for possible publication.
• Submit your application for ADA Ambassador or your state-sponsored Media Representative when the opportunity arises.
• Volunteer to your incoming state and national officers for their committees and work groups.

As you can see, the list is impressive. The resources and opportunities are there. Take advantage of these important and useful benefits of ADA membership.

Mary Donkersloot, RD, Owner, Personal Nutrition Management,
Beverly Hills, California

I n 1983 I left Pritikin programs to start a private practice. I decided to offer lower-fat dietary-restructuring programs to individuals and families in their homes.

RESPONDING TO A MARKET NEED

One of the first things I noticed was that people needed healthy recipes that tasted good and were simple to prepare. Since I chose dietetics as a career because I loved to cook and eat good food, I was delighted to respond to my clients' needs. I developed a recipe collection called "Fast Food at Home." Clients could add their own recipes to mine and begin a collection. It went right along with my philosophy of building new eating habits. Little did I know that this idea would lead to much bigger things. In fact, it would be the base for my other projects over the next ten years.

My former secretary at the Pritikin program suggested that I talk to her friend, who was a marketing executive for a high-tech firm that made computer-storage containers. Her $45 hourly fee was the best money I've ever spent. She met with me in her home on one Sunday afternoon a month. She advised that I put the recipes in a red box — for the same reason that Tide comes in a red box — to ATTRACT ATTENTION. I consulted with a graphic designer and came up with a box and label that carried my logo and the title "Fast Food at Home." The recipe boxes cost $5000 to produce, so I went to the bank and took out a loan against my car.

My adviser suggested I hold a "Fast Food at Home" tasting reception at my home and make it a media event. Together we wrote several press releases, which we sent to all the local newspapers and radio and TV stations to invite them to send reporters to the reception. The response was terrific. One TV station even gave out my telephone number so people could order the recipe boxes. I was inundated with calls, not only for the recipe box, but also for my nutrition counseling services.

The local interest in my recipe collection convinced me that I should launch a national marketing campaign. I sent recipe boxes and press releases to all the appropriate national magazines. The product was reviewed by *Shape*, *Glamour* and *American Health*. I received orders for the boxes from all over the country. So far I have sold over 10,000 boxes.

ONE SUCCESS BUILDS ON ANOTHER

The success of the recipe collection and my track record in working with the media, led me to a publishing agreement with Simon and Schuster for my book, *Fast Food Diet: Quick and Healthy Eating at Home and on the Go*. It had the same basic information as my recipes and taught people how to prepare quick, healthy foods at home. Due to my former sales, the publisher gave me a much larger advance than they normally give first-time authors. I decided to go with a publisher and take my advance and small royalty instead of self-publishing because I wanted to gain access to their national distribution channels.

The book was marketed through Simon and Schuster's publicity department. It was released in hard cover in 1991, then as a paperback from Fireside, their trade paper division, a year later. Their press releases on my book were picked up by countless publications. A review in *USA Today* caught the attention of Taco Bell, who asked that I assist them in developing a line of new, healthier menu items. I have since consulted with numerous other food companies who learned about me through my book.

The lessons are many. First, develop a good product (food always interests people), and then let people know about it. The outcome of that little box far exceeded my expectations. And it all happened as a result of marketing.

How to Evaluate Your Competition

Chapter 5

*Mindy Hermann, MBA, RD, President, The Hermann Group, Inc.,
Mount Kisco, New York*

A dietitian had a successful consulting practice at the city headquarters of a major corporation. Suddenly, budget cutbacks forced him out of a steady position. What should he do – open an office near his home in a densely populated suburban area, or set up shop in a high-rent, upscale business district one hour from home? Renting office space in the suburbs is less expensive; rents in the business district are very high. Several dietitians have private practices near his home; only one dietitian serves the business district. After evaluating his competition in each location, the dietitian decided to sublease office space in the business district. His practice is booming.

The dietitian immediately improved his chances for business success by taking the pulse of the competitive environment. He determined that the suburban market, while attractive, would be too difficult to break into because it was so saturated with well-established dietetic consultants. On the other hand, the business district offered far more opportunity, even though start-up costs were higher. By jumping into a wide-open market, the dietitian not only avoided the competition, but also achieved a competitive advantage over other professionals who might decide to compete with him at a later point in time.

COMPETITION – WHY WORRY?

Good marketing practices require constant assessment of the competition. It is essential to know who you are up against in the competitive market, how their businesses are similar to or different from yours, and which unique consumer needs you fill that your competition does not. In every nutrition market – food service, counseling, consulting, writing, educating – successful dietitians and companies have developed distinct advantages over their competitors by meeting specific customer needs. Those who do not fill a unique need or maintain their competitive edge are at high risk for failure. The dynamic nature of the marketplace also requires constant surveillance of the competition to enable you to change and adapt your practice based on what your competitors do.

FINDING THE COMPETITION

Competition includes not only those businesses that are exactly like yours, but also those that are similar in one or more of three areas: products or services, customer base (target market), and geography. The grid in Figure 5-1 illustrates the ways in which a dietitian who specializes in high school food service could define her competition. The better you have defined your own business, target markets, products, and services, the easier you will find it to define and identify your competition.

Keep in mind that your competition extends beyond other dietetics professionals. Physicians, chiropractors, non-RD nutritionists, food-service-management companies, practitioners of alternative therapies, and even health food stores may be competing with you for the same clinical clients. All eating establishments within a certain radius may compete with your corporate cafeteria for employees or with your campus dorm dining room for students.

Figure 5-1. Competition Grid

MAJOR PLAYERS	PRODUCT OR SERVICE	CUSTOMER BASE	GEOGRAPHY
Close competitors	Sack lunches 7-11 fast food Vending snacks McDonald's	Students at Central High	Stores and fast food within 1 mile radius
Broad competitors	All restaurants, fast food, vending, home cooking	All teenagers	In the same county

The next step is to get as much information as possible about competitors who appear to fit the product or service, target market, and geographic profiles of your business. For a general but incomplete list of potential competitors, start with the *Yellow Pages*. However, the limitations of the *Yellow Pages* are that they give little or no specific information and can be time-consuming to use. Instead, for a clinical business, speak to as many local health professionals as possible – physicians, nurses, physical and occupational therapists, and pharmacists – to get a feel for who the major players are and how saturated the market is.

Market research can help identify unmet customer needs, such as nutrition services that competing practitioners currently do not offer or catered foods that clients like but no one offers. Consider developing a brief market research questionnaire to distribute to members of your target market or referral sources.

One of the best ways to get information on the competition is to network, network, network. Talk to friends, neighbors, and local merchants to learn about private practitioners in your area – who they are, how well-known they are, and what they do. Talk to colleagues in dietetic practice groups. Telephone contacts and potential clients in public relations, advertising, food-service management, nursing-home management, home care, or other fields related to your area of business. Each call should generate the name of at least one additional person to call.

Bonnie Taub-Dix, RD, a nutrition consultant with private practices in New York City and Long Island, New York, attributes the success of her Long Island office to networking. After each new client appointment, she sent letters to both the referring physician and the primary physician, whom she did not know. Her mailing to the primary physician included a nutrition report on the client, along with a letter of introduction, a résumé, and a business card. Every letter was followed up with a phone call. Taub-Dix used this type of networking to introduce herself to potential sources of new clients and to keep her name prominent in the physicians' minds for future referrals.

Identify at least one dietetics professional who has firm roots in the professional community, is not a direct competitor, and can be trusted. Ask in confidence about the scope of business, professional reputation, and image of each potential competitor. This dietitian confidant should be asked to keep your business plans private to prevent competitors from knowing your ideas.

Dietetic practice groups are another good source of information on competitors. Look at newsletters and directories for names of both contact persons and potential competitors. Contact one or more prominent practice group members for additional information on who is doing what type of business. Information on competitors can be documented in a log book or on a computer. Include information on type of business, target market, approximate size (big, medium, small), strengths and weaknesses (for example, well-connected in food industry [strength] or not available for evening counseling [weakness]). Finally, add an assessment of perceived threat, that is, how much your competitor's business overlaps yours. You can then use this information to define and modify your own business.

FITTING INTO THE COMPETITIVE ENVIRONMENT – POSITIONING

Armed with a comprehensive profile of your competitors, you can now structure and market your business, or position your products and services competitively, to fill unmet consumer needs better than anyone else.

First, decide how broad to make your product or service line. A nutrition consultant, for example, could offer a full line of counseling services if no other competitors serve the same geographic market. Consultants in highly competitive markets should look for specific market segments whose needs are not being met, for example, pregnant women or overweight teens.

Seeking out windows of opportunity where you will encounter little or no competition improves your chance of success. Leni Reed, founder of Supermarket Savvy, spotted a window of opportunity in supermarket tours. Although other dietitians had been conducting supermarket tours for years, none had developed a formal program. Reed turned Supermarket Savvy into a marketable product that included instruction kits for dietitians, slide sets, and a newsletter. Julie Hagan, a nutrition consultant in Mount Kisco, New York, became an expert in counseling children because few, if any, services were available for children with nutrition-related medical problems.

Use information on your competitors' price structures to set up or fine-tune your own pricing. In a saturated market with an abundance of competition, lowering price may seem the only way to build your business, but use it as your choice of last resort! To grow strong in the marketplace, you and your products or services must have some inherent competitive advantages other than price! If you are the only player in the market, you have the luxury of charging higher prices, as long as clients will pay. Higher prices often, but not always, connote higher quality. Conversely, some markets respond only to lower prices.

Linda Jones, a consulting dietitian in Sandy Hook, Connecticut, worked for one of two local fitness centers. Whereas the other fitness center attracted a wealthy, older crowd, the center employing Jones was frequented by young singles. Jones set lower prices and package deals for multiple visits to appeal to her unique market. However, to be profitable, it is important that Jones keep her overhead low and offer more products or services that appeal to her market so that a higher volume of sales makes up for lower profit on each sale.

Evaluate how you are most likely to succeed and remain profitable: getting into the market first, making your product or service different from the competition (differentiation), or focusing on a market segment that others are unlikely to go after. The first in the market (the leader) has the most time to iron out bugs and build a loyal customer base. Theoretically, the longer you have been in the market, the more you have learned from your experience; the more you know about your business and market, the better able you are to compete.

Product or service differentiation works well if you have satisfied a previously unfulfilled need or desire in your target market. For example, you develop a comprehensive nutrition therapy protocol for weight-loss clients that calls for collaboration and individual patient consults with experts in exercise and psychology along with your services.

The final course of action is to focus on a specific market segment that competitors are unlikely to go into, for example, a particular immigrant population not fluent in the English language. Dietetic professionals fluent in less widely spoken languages may encounter little if any competition.

KEEPING AHEAD OF THE COMPETITION

Business environments constantly change. Outside factors, such as DRGs, the proliferation of HMOs, health-care reform, and peaks and valleys in the economy, have catalyzed change in the food and nutrition business. Competitors have dropped out, new products and services have entered the market, businesses have folded, and other businesses have merged. The goal of any business is to remain competitive in spite of shifting forces in the marketplace. Businesses usually fall into one of four competitive categories: market leader, challenger, follower, or niche marketer.

If you are the biggest in the market, you are the market leader. When the target market needs a particular product, they think of the leader first. This can make the leader very powerful in setting the standards by which products and services are measured. But on the downside, lack of competition may make leaders lazy and complacent. Market leaders continually must fight off competitors and keep costs under control. It is expensive to be the market leader because keeping competitors away usually means cutting price, increasing advertising, or adding promotions. Market leaders are forced by competitive pressures to introduce new products and services, improve existing products and services, set appropriate prices, and strengthen weaknesses.

The number two spot in the market is held by the challenger, or runner-up. Challengers often try to go head-to-head and overtake the market leader, even though it is expensive and difficult to do. One strategy is to offer the same services or products as the market leader does, but at a lower price, with a different flair, or with a different distribution channel. For example, the market leader in nutrient analyses may offer 15-nutrient computerized diet analyses for $30 per diet; the challenger charges $25 for the same analysis and offers a 24-hour turnaround time.

Followers are providers of products and services who are not positioned to become market leaders. As a follower, your strategy is different. A follower tries to capitalize on the leader's weaknesses or satisfy needs in the target market that the leader overlooks, albeit not for long, if the strategy is successful. Many followers are comfortable with the size and scope of their businesses; for example, a freelance magazine writer with small children at home who decides to accept only one article assignment a month, or a private practitioner who limits counseling to two days a week. The follower's main challenge is to keep business at a steady level.

Niche businesses are so specialized that they are not in conflict with the market leader. The owners of such businesses are faced with the challenge of finding a niche that is profitable, has growth potential, and is not in direct competition with the market leader. For example, you consult to food services that are ready to convert from full-service cafeterias to salad and sandwich preparation only.

LEARNING FROM OTHERS' MISTAKES

The competition can be a valuable source of information on which factors lead to business success. Carefully evaluate your competition – what they are doing right, what they did wrong, what made them succeed. Use that information to modify and build your own business. Remember that a one-time look at the competition is never enough; follow your competitors throughout the life cycle of your business.

Bibliography

Kotler P. *Marketing Management.* 3rd ed. Englewood Cliffs, NJ: Prentice Hall; 1976.

Corey ER. *Marketing Strategy: An Overview.* Boston, MA: Harvard Business School Case Services; 1978.

Chapter 6

Internal Marketing:
Identifying Moments of Truth with Clients

Connie Mobley, MS, RD, Department of Community Dentistry, University of Texas Health Science, San Antonio, Texas

I nternal marketing is the act of practicing good communication enhanced by effective marketing strategies *within* our present organization to our patients, clients, peers, employees, and managers. It could range from things as simple as greetings in the hallways, respectful attention at meetings, and acknowledgment of others' accomplishments to more organized and deliberate internal newsletters, presentations at staff meetings, awards banquets, direct mail promotions, and telemarketing.

To be successful in business, dietitians and dietetic technicians in all settings need to be as concerned about marketing to and supporting the people who already come as clients, contribute to the overall function of the organization, and act as referral agents as they are about reaching new prospects.

The following is an example of how an outpatient dietitian (J.T.) could change a consultative style to better meet the needs of a private client and, in doing so, improve her effectiveness and image in the marketplace:

The previous session with Mr. Smith was peppered with praise for the many ways J.T. had suggested that he adjust to his low-fat diet. Like a dutiful student, he had been attentive to instructions. The food diary he had brought with him was extensive, and his probing, though hesitant, questions gave J.T. ample opportunity to explain how his diet could change a lipid profile associated with heart disease. J.T. felt that his fears about being unable to follow his special meal plan were unfounded. Why had he not returned for his follow-up visit? He seemed very interested when J.T. talked about the supermarket tour, but he had not even bothered to call to cancel the scheduled appointment.

It had been difficult for J.T. to convince the hospital administrator to allow the establishment of an outpatient clinic with fees for services. J.T. had spent months marketing this new program to the medical community, and the referrals had increased slowly the first few months. However, now things seemed at a standstill. Patients weren't keeping their appointments. New referrals weren't coming in. The monthly newsletter was still being mailed out. What was the problem?

MISTAKEN BELIEFS

For many years, health educators, including dietitians, have held the belief that if clients are provided knowledge, they will adopt appropriate lifestyle behaviors. However, with the advent of Health Objectives for the Year 2000 and the benchmarks to monitor the achievement of those objectives clearly identified, we realize that it is change in health status rather than knowledge gained that will be the focus of successful measures.

Knowledge empowers, but individuals control change. Dietitians do not change a person's diet. Each person changes his or her own diet. What we do is collaborate with clients to create realities in which change can occur. J.T. had been constructing her own reality. She'd forgotten that marketing is an activity embedded in how we interact with peers, clients, employees, other health professionals, and the public at large. It is a dynamic process that continues over time. Such internal marketing is what dietitians do to make services unique. We not only provide knowledge, but act as resources to foster the choices people make based on the knowledge provided.

Conceptually, dietitians have considered compliance with directives as the ultimate achievement. If clients are compliant, they have acted out what was prescribed. What does *compliance* mean? It means to yield to others. Is that the objective? No, what we truly want is *adherence,* which means a moral or mental attachment to an act or quality.

We want clients to make changes not because they must yield to them, but because they value those changes. Values do not change because one declares change. Values are a reflection of beliefs and attitudes coupled with knowledge. Those attitudes and beliefs grow out of the interactions that occur relative to change. It is at this juncture that dietitians play an important role. They create an atmosphere that accommodates what could be labeled internal marketing. How does one practice internal marketing that acknowledges these concepts and promotes change?

COMMUNICATION VIA FACT

Internal marketing is the result of communication via FACT. The act of communicating is central to marketing. The elements of FACT, illustrated in Figure 6-1, make communication effective. Each moment with a client is an opportunity to communicate with FACT.

Figure 6.1. FACT

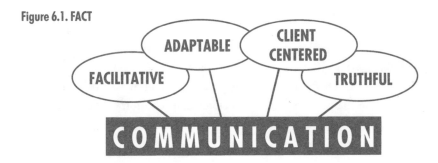

Facilitative

The major role of a good communicator is to facilitate a continuing dialogue. It is not the ability to talk to people, but *with* people. In fact, a good communicator is always a good listener. Frequently, dietitians are anxious to share nutrition knowledge. We rush in with all the pearls of wisdom that can be crammed into a time frame. We make notes to prompt our memory and gather written, audio, and visual material to reinforce what we say.

In today's world, being the source of knowledge is not always a dietitian's asset. Technology has made knowledge accessible to everyone. Yet, being a facilitator who identifies appropriate sources of knowledge and matches needs with knowledge is an asset. A facilitator is one who makes things easier. To do that, dietitians must let the client describe the problem and then identify resources that address the problem. Often we forget to ask clients what they want to talk about or know. By asking, we create the opportunity to identify those moments of truth.

Maybe J.T. focused on personal goals rather than on what Mr. Smith wanted to know. What he really wanted to know was how to get variety into his meal plan rather than why the plan would lower his lipid levels. He wanted nutrition counseling that was feasible for him.

Internal marketing requires a facilitative approach that incorporates feasible messages designed to meet individual needs. Remember the feasibility must be defined by the client, not by the dietitian.

Adaptable

Have you ever heard the saying "The customer is always right"? To some extent, clients who seek the services of dietitians may be described this way. They are right about what they can do and what they want to know. Dietitians, like other health educators, tend to use the medical model of diagnosis and prescription. As authorities on diet and nutrition, we often take control of the situation. Furthermore, we tend to want to outline directives for dietary behavior that are precise, detailed, and, oftentimes, standardized.

Dietary modification does not occur because dietitians prescribe it. Stages of change described in theoretical models often represent spans of time that far exceed the one or two visits a client may share with a dietitian. Thus, good communication to promote a satisfied customer requires that dietitians be accepting of cultures, opinions, concerns, and issues. Knowing where the client is in the change process is critical. This means approaching each interaction with an open mind, recognizing that the plan may not be followed, being adaptable, and being a good learner. After all, it is the good learner who makes the best teacher and counselor.

J.T. did not accept Mr. Smith's fear of being able to follow his meal pattern. She wanted to be able to schedule the supermarket tour at his next visit. It was important to dispel his fears rather than explore them. It is the dietitian's ability to accept what the client brings to a given situation, and to adapt to the need of both the situation and the client, that enhances both communication and marketing strategies. Being sensitive to the client's perspectives precipitates those moments of truth, those internal marketing opportunities.

Client-Centered

What are dietitians marketing? The answer to this question is diet and nutrition knowledge, interpretations of food technology, and skills and techniques for making positive lifestyle choices. But even beyond these specifics, we are ultimately empowering the client with useful tools for achieving positive individual or community dietary habits that are in concert with healthy lifestyles. Being client-centered means stepping outside the clinical realm of nutrition as a means to good health. It means broadening that realm to encompass the client's world, which is not clinical. Each client's world is full of real-life experiences, demands, and desires that may appear to have nothing to do with nutrition.

Let us take a moment and revisit the definition of a client. It may be the patient who comes to the dietitian for dietary counseling. It may be the physician and nurse who are colleagues at the hospital. It may be the community volunteers who share responsibility for the annual health fair. In each case, internal marketing requires us to cultivate a relationship that focuses on the client, the client's identified needs, and the client's identified desires.

For example, one of the most successful community nutrition-awareness campaigns in Austin, Texas, was chaired by a dietitian who focused on networking with business community leaders (clients). Chefs, restaurateurs, work-site directors, grocery-chain executives, school administrators, produce purveyors, nurses, physicians, and dietitians planned and executed a city-wide program that featured a healthy menu designed to decrease risk of developing cancer. Over a one-year period, this dietitian focused on facilitating each individual contributor's agenda, maintaining a constant dialogue with everyone involved, and scheduling social events in conjunction with meetings to enhance participation. Relationships were developed and sustained by periodically sending personal notes or making phone calls to each participant to acknowledge that person's contributions. Five years after the completion of the project, members of this group continue to come together in other forums to promote nutrition. Collaborative opportunities for not only this dietitian, but others as well, have grown out of this project. The dietitian viewed the community leaders as clients.

The same principles are effective at the individual level. Attention to individual client needs and desires can be one of the most effective tools in promoting communication that can lead to change. Clients generally are interested in two specific things: they want foods to taste good and to be affordable. Nutrition messages that focus on taste and cost can be more effective than those focused on restrictions. Furthermore, everyone needs to be respected and acknowledged as a unique person. In this society, finding someone who will take the time to smile, offer a courteous comment, take an interest in jobs and family, and remember special days, such as birthdays, is extremely important. Dietitians who are client-centered take the time to share those special moments, those moments of truth, and sustain client relationships over time. The best referral comes from a satisfied client.

Truthful

Over the years, nutrition knowledge has vastly expanded. A few basic concepts have become overwhelming volumes of information. The consumer has been bombarded with conflicting messages about food choices, supplements, and diet-disease connections. The resulting confusion has evolved into a challenge for the dietitian. Others portray themselves as nutrition experts and offer simple, untruthful advice that appeases the client. Sometimes that advice is cloaked in scientific jargon that adds to listeners' frustration and confusion. Being truthful results in realistic expectations for the client and the dietitian. It is one of the most powerful rapport builders in existence and is the basis for the dietitian's credibility. When dietitians are able to transmit knowledge in a respectful, truthful manner, they are practicing effective internal marketing strategies. Clients appreciate nonjudgmental, truthful advice that is prefaced by a discussion of the client's unique situation.

SUMMARY

In summary, internal marketing positions you, your products, and your services in a positive light with those closest to you. Often their support and goodwill are a result of your high-quality services and products and successful internal marketing.

The services dietitians market are intangible. They are not visible to the naked eye, and they cannot be taken off the shelf and observed. Because services can constantly change, be reinterpreted, or be controlled by the user, they must be constantly marketed. Internal marketing is the act of practicing good communication enhanced by facilitative, adaptable, client-centered, truthful (FACT) marketing strategies. It is essential to our success, and to J.T.'s success with Mr. Smith and all future clients.

How to Market a Professional Service

Denice Ferko-Adams, RD, President, Denice Ferko-Adams and Associates, Coopersburg, Pennsylvania

You provide a service so wonderful that the right clients will reap many benefits, . . . but how will potential clients know? Any businessperson will tell you that marketing a professional service is different from marketing a product. Examples of services are providing nutrition counseling, consulting to a nursing home or wellness program, being a management consultant to a food service, and acting as a labeling consultant to a food manufacturer.

A service is intangible – it cannot be held, looked at, or tested for quality in advance of purchase or use, as a product can be. Your challenge is to make the service seem interesting, high quality, and worth every cent to consumers before they buy it. Surrogates, or substitutes, that represent your service, such as brochures, proposal binders, business cards, advertising, business image, and your personality, image, and reputation, take on far more importance.

Providers of professional services often become so caught up in providing their services that they fail to market effectively. Everyday, we see nutrition programming with technically correct information and costly audiovisuals that does not attract enough customers to cover the rent. Often the reason is inadequate or inappropriate marketing – not reaching the target market with the right message often enough for the consumer to get the message.

One overall marketing goal for service providers is to build an image and presence in the minds of their target market. Providers of nutrition services want their target customers to think of them first whenever they want anything related to nutrition. Another marketing goal is to create a distinction between your services and your competitors' and to convince customers that your professional performance is superior.

In this chapter, we will explore three primary areas of service marketing: (1) identifying a marketing niche, (2) using market signals or messages to build your presence, and (3) developing a market network.

IDENTIFYING YOUR NICHE

How can you make sure customers know what you have to offer? One technique is to identify and understand your market niche – the narrow segment of the total market that shares similar needs and desires. You must know what customers expect from you. Who are you really selling to? Is it physicians or their patients? Is it the food-service director or the personnel director? Is it the weekend athlete or the elite competitor? Every service has a niche – a market segment that needs or could use that service more than any other.

It is important to recognize that you cannot be everything to everyone. Determine what services you perform better than your competitors. You may have expertise or particularly enjoy working with certain nutrition problems or with a certain age group, gender, economic group, literacy level, and so on. How are your services unique and different? When you create a service, it is often a mixture of what you like to do and what your market research tells you someone will buy. The process is dynamic. Trial and error may influence what you offer more than all your initial market research.

What type of relationship do you have with your customers? When you buy a product, such as a pair of shoes, you rarely develop a formal relationship with the sales clerk. However, when customers desire nutrition counseling, they want to know and trust you. Your customers are present for the delivery of the service, and they help determine the outcome of the counseling session. For your own evaluation, write a description of the typical customer you presently attract to your business. Then write what customers typically say they like or dislike about your services. You can find this feedback in notes, letters, follow-up evaluations, or interviews. Analyzing such information helps you to understand your niche. Once you clearly identify your service niche, you are ready to detect and use market signals to create a strong basis for effectively marketing your services.

MARKET SIGNALS

The term *marketing signal* first appeared in an article by A.M. Spence in 1974. (1) He described it to mean the observable attributes (like surrogates, mentioned earlier) that help customers draw conclusions about something they cannot see or have incomplete knowledge of. In other words, setting a high fee for your service is a signal to customers that your service is higher quality – and they will expect it to be so. A more expensive brochure or advertising campaign signals that you are successful, presumably because you offer good services.

Signals are used by competitors to let each other know their intentions or capabilities. If you are an industry leader and you make strong statements in the media against a newly developed liquid protein diet being marketed through physicians' offices, you signal competitors where you stand.

Unfortunately, consumers' use of signals to make decisions can sometimes be exploited by sellers. For example, customers usually want to buy soft bread because they believe softness signals freshness. Sellers may respond by adding chemicals to bread to keep it soft longer instead of working harder to ensure that fresh bread is always available. (2)

The use of signaling has increased over the past decade. The reasons are many: product complexity and service content are increasing; the service sector is expanding; media clutter is increasing; shopping time is growing scarce; and technology is rapidly changing. Therefore, the necessity of transmitting attractive signals is growing. In general, the more complex and intangible a product is, the more crucial it becomes to pay attention to the signals that are sent. (3)

USING SIGNALS TO MARKET SERVICES

Marketing a service usually requires a combination of many different approaches. This section focuses on using signals to market a service. Herbig and Milewicz describe four marketing characteristics: intangibility, perishability, inseparability, and heterogeneity. (2) This is a brief review of those signals, with applications and personal examples of marketing the services of a registered dietitian.

Intangibility

You cannot pick up or hold professional services. It is difficult to examine a service without first experiencing it while simultaneously consuming it. This intangible quality makes it important for sellers to signal the tangible aspects of their services. If you have your own office for nutrition counseling, decorate it to appeal to the type of customers you desire. A dietitian who works with obese adults needs large, not-too-soft seating, while the office of a pediatric dietitian needs small chairs and colorful diversions. The way you dress, speak, and present your comments at a meeting to discuss a wellness program with a Fortune 200 company sends many signals about your competency and level of success. Another tangible signal is the quality of your teaching materials, which essentially serve as calling cards for your other services. Identify the many tangible components of your business and signal your customers clearly. In other words, take time to develop the image you want to portray.

Perishability

Perishability means that you cannot stockpile or sample services in advance. This means that matching seasonal demand (or lack of demand) with your capacity is difficult. You cannot store your excess services the way you would store an inventory of self-published books in your basement or extra cookies in your freezer. How do you handle the periods when your phone rings constantly and other times when it is silent for weeks? When business is booming, it can be great, up to the point where staff gets tired and quality of services decline. This can push customers away.

You will never recover the time and money lost when a client does not show up for a counseling session. However, you can do something to prevent these pitfalls – during off-seasons, by creating more demand, and during peak seasons, by signalling customers that your business is sensitive to their needs. You can create pricing strategies for low times, such as bring a spouse or friend for free; develop an appointment and reminder system; and broaden your service capabilities to include new items. During peak times, such as the New Year's resolution months or pre-summer swimsuit season, hire part-time dietitians to handle increased demand. Upgrade reservation systems to improve scheduling and responsiveness to consumer calls. Make clients feel as if they are your number one business interest!

Inseparability

Simultaneous production and consumption is called inseparability. Do you both deliver your service and market it? Such inseparability makes it difficult for your business to grow because to provide service, you must always be present. Possible solutions are to teach group sessions, to focus on large-group corporate programs, or to hire dietetic technicians to perform some of the assessment functions of a counseling session. Professional services are people-oriented, and inseparability creates the problem of consumers' only wanting you as the provider. However, another alternative is to hire reputable, well-trained, conscientious dietitians to assume some of your responsibilities. Slowly assimilate them into your practice: announce their arrival and specific areas of expertise, and introduce them to your clients. Help your clients accept them as capable of providing services similar to yours.

Inseparability from your clients can also cause problems. Much of your success as a counselor or consultant depends upon the cooperation and commitment of your clients. Unsuccessful clients can reflect on your services, even when you did all you could.

You can signal your commitment to your clients in many different ways, such as a ready smile, a friendly handshake, and positive body language. You can signal "humanness" by cracking jokes or chatting about families and hobbies prior to the consultation. Pictures on your walls or desk and special artwork or antique furniture show your interests. You can hang awards or diplomas on your walls to signal "business." (2)

Heterogeneity

Lack of consistency, or heterogeneity, means you don't give each client the same quality of service. Standardizing business procedures is very important, whether you are working with consumers, physicians, or companies, because individuals will interact and compare notes on your services.

Service providers need standardized quality-control procedures. Follow-up will set your business apart from the competition. For example, after you finish coordinating and implementing a cafeteria program, remember to use response cards, interviews, and surveys to evaluate customer satisfaction. Provide a written report to let your corporate client know the level of customer satisfaction achieved through your program. For individual counseling, have a third party call to check on customer satisfaction or use a short survey on a return-postage-paid postcard. Such attention to detail signals that you care about your clients' satisfaction. Even customers who suggest improvements are more likely to retry your services because of your evaluation efforts.

CHARACTERISTICS OF PROFESSIONAL SERVICES

Certain characteristics help distinguish professional services from all other entities: specialized knowledge, licensing requirements, and technical competency. In addition, services are usually provided by small businesses. These characteristics also give signals to customers.

Specialized Knowledge

Specialized knowledge sets dietitians apart from other health providers and the lay public. It can also be a limiting factor in that consumers do not know the full scope of our professional abilities and may think of us only as working on hospital floors or in dorm cafeterias. A dietitian's specialized knowledge of diabetes management or weight control can both attract new clients and turn people away, depending upon whether they want such services.

Possessing similar work experience to what the consumer is looking for is a highly desirable quality. If you must have surgery for a sports injury, you are likely to choose an experienced surgeon who is skilled in your type of injury. Similarly, your clients want to know your success record, and they will ask around. You can help yourself by building a credible reputation in the local community, the media, business networks, and your health professional circle for delivering reliable and effective services.

The need to have experience to obtain clients is not only a problem for new practitioners, but also for professionals who try to change their areas of expertise. In the ranks of professional service providers, being a newcomer is not always favorable.

Credentials/Licensing Requirements

Being a registered dietitian signals consumers that you have met a certain level of professional standards. Place framed certificates and licenses in your customer waiting area. If you also have state licensure or other professional achievements, such as a master of science in exercise physiology, then your perceived credibility and level of proficiency will increase. If you work cooperatively with other licensed counselors and health professionals, be sure to promote this to your customers. To further boost your image, everyone involved with your business must exude professionalism. Customers form opinions as a result of everything they encounter in the process of receiving your service. This includes how the telephone is answered, how the person is greeted upon arrival, and even how they are invoiced. Be professional!

Technical Competency

Why are your services better than those of less-educated competitors? If consumers do not understand the technical aspects of the nutrition services you provide, then they probably do not feel they need you. An inability to understand the technical aspects forces buyers to focus on the more qualitative components of your services. To counteract this, you must educate clients at multiple levels about your services. Effectively communicate the specific characteristics and advantages that give you a competitive edge!

Small Business Entities

Most professional service businesses are considered small entities. The size of a business can send signals to customers. Large companies may signal that they are more stable, successful, and prestigious. However, smaller size signals personalized service and better rapport.

Most clients like to meet and assess the person from whom they will receive professional services. For that reason, it is very hard for someone else to market your services for you. Some of the most successful dietitians are ones who learned to market themselves early in their careers. Professionals who improve their selling skills and actively market themselves usually surpass their competition. In fact, evaluating how competitors signal consumers can help you plan your marketing strategy more effectively.

BUILDING A MARKETING NETWORK

One difficult aspect of marketing a service is adapting to continuous changes in population and trends. As a business leader, you need to develop a network that not only promotes your services, but also keeps you informed of changing needs within your niche. Here are five ways to keep involved and be aware of changes that affect your business:

1. Know your local newspaper and radio and television stations. Offer to provide information or technical expertise on nutrition-related topics. As long as people continue to eat, food and nutrition will always be popular topics

in the media. To help establish yourself as a professional resource, send your business card to media contacts, offer to respond to the latest food fad, and send your own press releases on newsworthy events and projects.

2. Interact with local business leaders. Be involved with professional business groups, offer to do a presentation to the Chamber of Commerce, and attend or exhibit at such groups' events.

3. Expand your network to other professional groups. If your niche is cardiovascular health, become involved with professional organizations for nurses and exercise physiologists. Because my business focuses on wellness, I joined regional groups to expand my service area and to become known to more possible referral agents for new corporate opportunities.

4. Do not forget past satisfied customers. Make phone calls, send brief notes about an upcoming event, or clip and photocopy an interesting article and send it to them. In the rapidly changing field of nutrition, there are many opportunities to stay in touch with your past customers. Send a free quarterly newsletter that highlights new services and clearly signals your technical competency.

5. Be involved in your own professional group. Registered dietitians and technicians can network on local, state, and national levels. Join and become actively involved in the dietetic practice groups. Peer interaction provides support, mentoring, validation, and opportunities to show leadership. By becoming involved, you will gain valuable insight into how other practitioners reach their target markets.

Marketing a service is a continuous process that presents daily challenges for any professional. To be more successful, take the time to define your services, identify your niche, send the right signals, and build your network.

References

1. Spence AM. *Market Signaling: Information Structure of Job Markets and Related Phenomena.* Cambridge, MA: Harvard University Press; 1974.

2. Herbig P, Milewicz J. Market signaling in the professional services. *Journal of Professional Services Marketing.* 1993; 8: 2.

3. Bloom PN, Reve T. The role of strategic information transmission in a bargaining model. *Economic Journal* (UK), 1990; 98 (390): 50-57.

Bibliography

Aguiar A. Part two: applications to specific professional service sectors. Marketing in the public sector is easy . . . (getting the contract is something else!), *Journal of Professional Services Marketing.* 1993; 8: 2.

Lovelock C. *Services Marketing.* 2nd ed. Englewood Cliffs, NJ: Prentice Hall; 1991.

Onkvisit S, Shaw J. Part one: marketing theories, models and general issues. Is services marketing "really" different? *Journal of Professional Services Marketing.* 1991; 7: 2.

Nancy Clark, MS, RD, Director of Nutrition Services, SportsMedicine Brookline, Brookline, Massachusetts, and Author of The Athlete's Kitchen *and* Nancy Clark's Sports Nutrition Guidebook

Any dietitian who has ventured into private practice well knows the feeling of an empty office. In my first years at SportsMedicine Brookline (one of the largest athletic injury clinics in New England), I can remember pacing back and forth in that emptiness and repeatedly asking myself, "Just how can I get (paying) clients to come into my office — especially healthy, active, sports-minded people?"

Although labeling myself as a specialist in sports nutrition originally sounded great, the reality was that specialization eliminated many potential clients, such as inactive people in need of low-sodium, low-cholesterol, and diabetic diets. I was faced with the challenge of convincing healthy people, who were already well-read and well-versed in nutrition, that they could benefit from paying money to listen to my song and dance.

What did I have to offer to marathoners, fitness exercisers, and other recreational and competitive athletes? They could learn all about carbo-loading and pregame eating simply by reading books and magazines. But they couldn't find success with weight control from reading yet another diet book. That's where they were "in pain" and would pay for help.

I recalled the words of wisdom of the busines consultant Dr. Jeffrey Lant, who said, "Tell them what benefits they'll get *now*." After all, people spend money for help only when they are in pain and looking for solutions to problems they can't solve by themselves. I could help solve their problems and offer them such benefits as having more energy, strength, and stamina; performing better and setting personal records; feeling great both today and in the future; and losing weight while maintaining energy to exercise.

Such benefits are attractive to people active in sports, many of whom are struggling with food. Sad but true, eating disorders and weight concerns prevail among the athletic population, particularly active women. In fact, 40 percent of my new clients come looking for help with weight reduction. They want to know how to maintain enough energy to exercise while ridding themselves of those final few pounds. Another 30 percent of my clients come with disordered eating patterns or eating disorders and want to know how they can be lean, fit, healthy, *and* eat normally.

These well-read fitness buffs have already devoured the popular nutrition books, been to every other well-marketed weight-control center, or found comfort at numerous Overeaters Anonymous meetings. Because their pain and struggling continue, they finally come into my office as their last hope, after having procrastinated at least six to twelve months before gathering enough courage to make an appointment. They feel depressed, inadequate, ashamed, and embarrassed. "Why can't I do something as simple as eat normally? . . . as lose weight successfully? . . . as enjoy one cookie and leave the rest for another day?"

To ease the embarrassment and erase the feelings of inadequacy that surround the decision to get nutrition help, we have to offer an invitation that is easy for people to accept. One gentle approach is to offer a nutrition checkup.

I've put fliers titled "Do You Need a Nutrition Checkup?" in SportsMedicine Brookline's central waiting room and each examining room. The nutrition-concerned athletes who flow through our office generally read this flier and tuck it into their pockets. Then, one day, in a moment of pain, they acknowledge their need for help for something as simple as "eating right" and call to make an appointment. The gentle nutrition checkup approach seems to take the edge off the embarrassment felt by these athletic, seemingly healthy, definitely well-read, intelligent people.

Doctors recommend a yearly medical checkup. People think nothing about going to the dentist twice a year for a dental checkup. Why can't RDs market the importance of a nutrition checkup, not only for the active person who struggles with food, but also for people in the varied seasons of life: growing teenagers involved in school sports, college students, eat-on-the-run adults, solo cooks, pregnant athletes, active families, and master athletes? I welcome all ADA members to add a Nutrition Checkup to their list of offerings. With 62,000 members promoting the same message, we'll have a far stronger voice than my one whisper in Boston, and we'll all reap the benefits. Without question, power comes in numbers.

Who needs a nutrition check-up? You do if you

• Eat on the run and survive on hit-or-miss meals
• Struggle with creeping obesity and dislike your body image
• Routinely go on and off diets, only to regain the weight you lost
• Limit your intake of red meat or dairy products
• Take vitamin pills . . . or wonder if you should
• Constantly cope with a stressful lifestyle
• Exercise rigorously, compulsively, or excessively
• Feel chronically fatigued or routinely lack energy to train at your best
• Obsess about food and have undesired binges that seem out of control
• Are discontent with your current eating patterns
• Have a slow metabolism and seem to maintain your weight on very little food
• Have high cholesterol, diabetes, or hypertension — or have relatives with these conditions
• Want to invest in your health and future well-being — as well as those of your family

Chapter 8

How to Market a Product

Kathy King Helm, RD, Private Practitioner,
Lake Dallas, Texas

Volumes are written on the different strategies for marketing a product. Obviously, you market broccoli differently than you market a book. But it is not so obvious that you market a new natural sports drink differently than you market Gatorade. The pricing, packaging, distribution, and advertising mix will be different because the natural sports drink is intended to appeal to a different target market.

The revenue from a product is sometimes called *passive income,* because once the product is manufactured, you do not have to be there to make the sale. But anyone who has tried to sell homemade cookies while they are still fresh, or pack and transport glass jars of gourmet fruit jam, or negotiate with a bookstore to sell a new cookbook, or market a software program by direct mail will tell you that you cannot be passive if you want to be successful. It takes everything you have to make it all work.

If you look at the financial success stories in the dietetic profession, you will see that selling a product is a promising way to make money. Using the same philosophy, a clinical department or nutrition therapist in private practice can develop and sell low-fat cooking videotapes (see the case study "Pursuing the Public Market Through Videos" in Chapter 19) and a hospital food service can add catering, contract bulk feeding, or off-hours wholesale pastry production. But, unlike selling a service, selling a product often requires a larger financial investment and, some believe, higher risk.

FIVE KEYS TO SUCCESSFUL PRODUCT MARKETING

Five very important keys to success in marketing a product are:

The Characteristics of the Product. Don't introduce a new product unless it has proprietary (patented, copyrighted, trademarked) competitive advantages. If it's not unique, don't spend your time and money on it. If there is no barrier to a competitor's entering the market with a product that is just as good or better than yours, you'll quickly be competing on price. You could have a marketing success, but you'll have a business failure if you can't sell it at a profit. (1)

The Timing in the Marketplace. If your target market is not ready for your product, it usually will not sell well. With our fast-paced communication and lifestyles, it may not be long before the market is ready – or it may take years. For example, until the popcorn market matured, Orville Redenbacher was unable to attract enough interest in his high-priced, high-quality popcorn.

In 1977, when I tried to sell a natural sports drink product to Coca-Cola of New York, the new products manager said, "I don't know if 'natural' is where the market is going. If we're first in the market with a natural drink, it will cost us millions of dollars to educate the public, and then everyone else will come along and say, 'me too.'" Timing can make or break a product. That is why it's so important to watch nutrition and health trends when you want to be one of the first in the market to take advantage of them.

The Competitive Positioning of the Product. Look at and evaluate the competition to your product (see Chapter 5). Then decide how you will make your product more attractive to potential buyers. You may choose a different niche of buyers than the strongest competitors pursue, or you may decide to change the message. If there is a strong, well-financed leader in the market, as the follower, you must capitalize on what you can do better and different. You might change the packaging or name to appeal to a more elite group. Or you might decide that you will keep your overhead very low, change the packaging to lively colors, reduce the price slightly, and go for volume sales in the youth market.

Whatever your strategy, make your advertising, image, and messages unique and appealing to your target market. If you can't attract attention and solicit the response that you intend, it doesn't matter if the product is wonderful.

The Marketing Mix (4 P's) You Choose for the Product. As mentioned earlier, your *product* should have proprietary competitive advantages that will keep your competitors from copying it exactly. You can patent the function or design; copyright any written booklets, artwork, or music score; and trademark the name or logo.

There are exceptions, such as A&W Root Beer, which is not patented. It owns the majority of the root beer market because of its good taste and people-pleasing frosty mug. Sometimes being first pays off. Another business strategy used years ago by the first commercial manufacturer of granola was to hit the market, make a big splash and lots of money, and then sell out to a big cereal company before being put out of business by Kellogg or Quaker Oats.

Many markets today are so saturated with new products that very few will actually make it big. Consider hiring a university entrepreneurial department to assess the market potential for your product. Check with your state universities, government libraries, and invention groups for referrals.

Place, or *distribution*, will be another major hurdle in selling your product. Distribution-related factors should be thoroughly checked out before you manufacture your product, because you don't want it to be the wrong size to fit on a typical retail shelf, or in a carton to ship by UPS, and the like. If your buyers want your children's drink in a plastic bottle to avoid breakage, you want to know that before you have a warehouse full of product packed in glass.

You may think that it would be great to sell your gizmo in big discount stores, but suppliers say that the largest chain requires that you have 2 million gizmos in inventory. And you must be willing to take every piece back if customers return them for any reason. Moreover, you will usually negotiate away most of your profit to make such a big sale in the first place. In the grocery industry, budgets for new cereals must include $5 million more than they did five years ago to cover the slotting fees grocery stores charge food manufacturers for shelf space. So distribution can be tricky and expensive. (For an example of successful distribution, see the case study in this chapter on R.W. Frookies, a company started by Randye Worth, MA, RD, and her entrepreneurial husband, Richard Worth.)

Price is important in creating the perceived value of a product in customers' minds. Price is not much of an issue if the function, design, and physical packaging or persons involved (as in a video) meet or exceed the customers' expectations. Price will be a barrier to sales if expectations are not met. Usually, the price of a product is higher when it is first introduced on the market (before competitors hit and underprice it), so you recoup some of your initial investment. (See Chapter 21 for more information on pricing strategies.)

Promotion lets the target market know what the product is, what it does, how wonderful it is, how it fits their needs, and where to get it. A product should have a distinctive brand name and a short, easy-to-remember slogan or subtitle that quickly explains important information to the consumer. The right colors in packaging or product design can easily distinguish a product from its competition and be a strong marketing tool.

As mentioned in this book many times, advertising is changing to include more direct contact and individualized marketing. Direct mail, TV home shopping, catalogues, cable TV, and trade shows that promote closer contact with customers and their needs are growing in popularity. Developing and selling a product to the dietetic market is not as risky as selling to the public because we know our needs better. However, potential sales volume is greatly reduced. (See Chapter 12 for detailed information on promotion.)

Adequate Funding. Adequate funding must be allocated to promoting your product or you shouldn't spend your time and energy manufacturing it. You will face many expenses, such as product inventory, legal and accounting fees, engineering designs, models and molds, import fees (on products or components made overseas), telephone and office expenses, transportation of inventory, warehousing, packaging, labels, advertising copy or taped commercials, air time, and so on.

John Luther and Jim McManus, marketing consultants from Westport, Connecticut, offer two additional suggestions: (1)

- Don't bet the ranch. Always hold some assets in reserve.

- Test market your product by getting into business. There is nothing theoretical about it. Just do focus groups in at least two geographic regions to get a reality check that you are on target. The old thinking was that if you test marketed a product in a "representative" city, like Denver, and consumers liked it, it would sell nationwide. That did not prove to be true. (See Chapter 32 for details on how to create and use focus groups.)

BUNDLING AND UNBUNDLING

Bundling and unbundling can be successful marketing strategies, especially when you sell several lower-cost items. For example, if you have a $9.95 weight-loss tape and a new low-fat cookbook that retails for $12.95, you could offer them both for $19.95 (the price of all great deals)! That's bundling, or grouping products together. Unbundling is just the opposite. (For an example of unbundling, see Leni Reed's case study in this chapter.)

INTERESTING READING

Two very interesting books on product marketing are *How To Create Your Own Fad and Make a Million Dollars,* by Ken Hakuta, (2) and *Toyland: The High-Stakes Game of the Toy Industry,* by Stern and Schoenhaus. (3) Although these two books talk about the toy industry, the manufacturing trials, competition, retail problems, and the like, are often similar to those in other markets.

A third book that offers very entertaining reading is *The Rejects,* by Nathan Aaseng. (4) It explores the difficulties and negative feedback that inventors of well-known, highly successful products or services had to endure to make their ideas successful.

To organize a venture to sell a product, you should always research and fill out a business and a marketing plan (see Chapter 20). These plans will help you organize and check the feasibility of your venture.

References

1. Richman T. How to grow a product-based business. *Inc.* April 1990.

2. Hakuta K. *How To Create Your Own Fad and Make a Million Dollars.* New York, NY: Avon Books; 1987.

3. Stern S, Schoenhaus T. *Toyland: The High-Stakes Game of the Toy Industry.* Chicago, IL: Contemporary Books; 1990.

4. Aaseng N. *The Rejects.* Minneapolis, MN: Lerner Publications; 1989.

Case Study: **R.W. FROOKIE: THE GOOD-FOR-YOU COOKIE**

Kathy King Helm, RD, Private Practitioner, Lake Dallas, Texas

Randye Worth, MS, RD, co-founder of R.W. Frookies, Inc., along with her husband, Richard Worth, has been cooking all her life, and she's even made a career out of it. Today she is Executive Vice President and Director of Research and Development for R.W. Frookies, Inc., the multimillion dollar New York-based "good-for-you" cookie company.

After receiving her master's degree in food and nutrition from New York University, Randye began working as a nutritionist for the American Health Foundation, and then worked as Test Kitchen Director for Irena Chalmers Cookbooks, Inc.; an account executive for Burson-Marsteller, Inc., a public relations firm; and as a private practitioner. She is the author of the cookbook *Cooking with Steamers.*

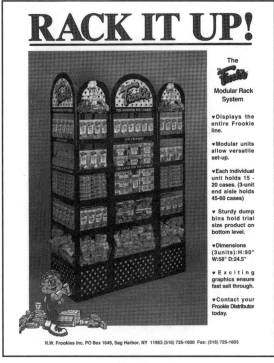

Frookies Product and Display Flyer.
(Copyright Randye Worth. Reprinted with permission.)

A DIETITIAN'S ANSWER TO MRS. FIELD'S COOKIES

In 1982 Randye met Richard, an entrepreneur who owned Sorrell Ridge® fruit-juice-sweetened jams, at the New York Fancy Food Show. A few years later, he sold Sorrell Ridge,® and was anxious to try something new. Using the same concept, Randye and Richard decided to develop fruit-sweetened cookies that are good for you. With Randye's cooking expertise and Richard's marketing and business expertise, R.W. Frookies (fruit + cookies) was born in 1988, after three years of business planning and baking cookies in Randye's tiny Manhattan apartment.

The success of the Frookie product line is fantastic by anyone's standards. In the first nine months of business, the company's sales surpassed estimates for year five. By the end of the first fifteen months in business, revenues topped $17.5 million.

INNOVATIVE MARKETING ON A BUDGET

One of the biggest hurdles Richard Worth had to overcome in getting their new products into grocery stores was the newly emerging policy of charging slotting allowances. These are fees that grocers charge manufacturers for shelf space. To sidestep the issue, Richard created his own free-standing, colorful, end-of-the-aisle display cases. His new point-of-purchase displays attracted consumers' attention, as did coupons in newspapers and some radio advertising. In the first three months, Worth sold 70,000 cases of cookies, and grocers began to perceive R.W. Frookies as a low-risk, steady-selling product line.

THE FUTURE

As more and more major players in the national cookie market respond to the competitive threat from R.W. Frookies by marketing fat-free or low-fat cookies of their own, Worth feels they have several things in their favor: (1) they enjoy a nine-month lead into the marketplace, (2) consumers tend to be loyal to the people who create a category, (3) large companies with high-fat cookies have the problem of marketing a new, healthier line without competing against or discrediting their own top-selling, high-fat products, and (4) as the big companies take over the market, it may expand the category instead of making a Frookie crumble.

The point is well taken when Worth states, "If slotting fees were as powerful a decade ago as they are today, Haagen Dazs, Sorrell Ridge Farms, Celestial Seasonings Tea, Near East Pilaf, Ben & Jerry's Ice Cream, and a host of other products would have perished in infancy. Deep pockets, not a superior mousetrap, has become the key to success in this treacherous market."

Bibliography

Brown PB. Cookie Monsters. *Inc.* February 1989: 55-58.

R.W. Frookies. Nutritionist's talents add up to one smart Frookie! 1992. Company release.

Worth R. Slotting fees are crippling the food industry. *Food Distribution Magazine*; January 1992: 74.

Case Study: SELL MORE PRODUCTS BY UNBUNDLING THEM

Leni Reed, MPH, RD, President, SUPERMARKET SAVVY,®
and Editor/Publisher of SUPERMARKET SCOOP™

The MBAs may call it unbundling; I call it common sense, and I'd say it works. Here's how unbundling worked for my company, SUPERMARKET SAVVY.®

Years ago, I created the first instructional package called SUPERMARKET SAVVY® Tour Training Kit, a high-ticket item to teach dietitians and others how to give supermarket tours. To improve communication with the people giving tours and to keep them better up-to-date, I created a newsletter with a brand-name shopping guide of healthy foods. When I first offered the *SUPERMARKET SCOOP*™ newsletter, only people who had purchased my kit could subscribe. In other words, you had to be a "member of the club" before you could sign up for the newsletter. That kept the newsletter pretty exclusive, but it also helped to sell kits, and that was the main goal at the time.

When sales of the kit started to slow down, I concluded that demand had peaked. At that time, I decided to unbundle the newsletter from the package and make it stand alone. Accordingly, someone could subscribe to the newsletter (a medium-priced item) whether or not they owned the kit.

This past year, I unbundled the SUPERMARKET SAVVY® Brand-Name Shopping List, ten-page, ready-to-copy, client-education fact sheet on healthy foods, from the newsletter. Now, I have three items to sell at a variety of prices instead of just one high-ticket one. (Newsletter subscribers still receive the list as part of their subscription.)

Selling the list separately was profitable in itself, but more importantly, it dramatically improved newsletter sales to new markets — and that was the real goal. With every sale of the shopping list, I sent a sample newsletter and an order form that offers a price break specifically for new subscribers. By selling the less-expensive item to a more varied market, I was able to introduce my newsletter to people who did not conduct tours but could use the information.

Looking back on the process of unbundling, here are my conclusions and recommendations:

- Think big first. Offer the total package. Don't offer bits and pieces right away. Bundle products that have similar purposes or offer complementary benefits to the target market. Market the completeness and uniqueness of the package.

- Start by pitching to the high end of the target market. There's always a high end, and you can count on these customers to pay the price of a big package as long as your product delivers what you promise. Also, the high end of the market tends to be made up of successful and capable people. It's an added plus to have your product in their hands.

- After you've given the high end of the market time to develop, start thinking about how you can break up your package and appeal to the mass market.

- When you break up your package, be sure at least one of the parts is a lower-cost entry product — one that will appeal to the mass market. Think of this product as the one to get your foot in the door. Map out a plan to market your other products to everyone who buys your entry product.

Marketing the big package helps to create an aura of exclusivity and quality that can only help your sales in the long run. If the individual products are unique and of high quality, unbundling the package at the right time and in the right way helps to keep your sales growing.

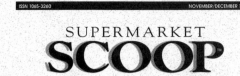

Chapter 9

Marketing Yourself: Growing a Career

Evelyn Tribole, MS, RD, Nutrition Therapist and Author, Beverly Hills, California

It's never to soon to write "marketing myself" into your job description. (1)

Personal marketing is not the exclusive domain of entrepreneurial dietitians. The average person will change careers eight times within a lifetime.(2) While you may still remain in dietetics, it is quite possible that you will make several career changes within the field. Growing a career is much like growing any business, and the tools used for business growth, especially marketing, can help you get where you want to be. Marketing has become an essential element in the success of any product or person.

Whether you're in a nine-to-five job or self-employed, personal marketing is the key to growing your career, whether up the corporate ladder or into a solo business. The author and business consultant D.A. Benton *(Lions Don't Need to Roar)* concludes from her work that competence alone does not lead to professional success. (3) It's like the author who has written a stunning and elegant book – unless others know about it, there's little chance of its making the bestseller list. As an outpatient hospital dietitian, you may offer the world's best nutrition counseling service, but if no one knows about it, success becomes illusive. You need to be able to communicate what value you add and what you have to contribute, whether it's to your own employer or your clients.

The advantage of using strategic marketing for your career growth is that not only are you more likely to arrive where you want to be, but you'll also be more apt to find satisfaction working at something you enjoy. The career direction you choose will drive the process of determining where you should concentrate your marketing efforts.

CHOOSING YOUR CAREER DIRECTION

Successful careers usually just don't happen to people. Satisfying career growth requires active planning. You need to assess where you're at and the trends that affect where you want to go.

Create a Personal Vision and Mission Statement

A personal mission statement can help you clarify your career direction, focus your energy on the professional/business activities you want to engage in, and identify the philosophies and values that will guide your major career decisions. Your mission statement, by laying out your personal vision, becomes a living document to navigate your career by and should be consulted periodically.

Begin by analyzing several issues, including the purpose of your career endeavor and the career path you are in. Where would you like to see yourself professionally, in one, five, or ten years? What kind of skills will take you there? What are your current strengths?

Pursue Your Passions
Barbara Williams, MS, RD, Executive Dietitian, ARA Healthcare Nutrition Services, Danbury, Connecticut

As the business climate changes and corporations right-size to save on overhead, some dietitians will be challenged to keep their jobs. No longer are businesses feeling obligated to carry employees who just make do. The person and the position must be essential, or both will go with the next budget cut.

Nutrition is one of the hottest topics in the public arena today, and new educational programs and job opportunities are flourishing as never before. There is no excuse for remaining in a job that doesn't excite you or where you have nothing to offer.

If our profession is to grow and continue to flourish, each of us must have a strong sense of commitment to hold dietetics to a higher standard. We must have the zeal to examine with microscopic vision the dynamics of the changing events in our environment and seize the opportunities to make a difference.

Take the time to visualize what impact you can have. Ask yourself what aspect of dietetics you feel passionate about. Do you feel enough passion that you are willing to pursue solutions, no matter what? Are you visionary enough to see trends and directions in the environment that, if pursued, would greatly enhance yourself and the

Continued on page 61

To help shape your career path, describe your area of interest and your ideal work setting. For example, you may want to be a nutrition communications executive in a public relations firm or a nutrition counselor in a private practice.

Next, identify at least ten tasks or responsibilities that you really enjoy doing and ten tasks that you dislike. Keep in mind the process of these tasks, not just the outcome. The key to productivity and career satisfaction is to do what you love to do. For example, there is a difference between enjoying the process of writing and enjoying the sight of your name in the byline of an article. If you don't enjoy the process of writing, the glamour of the byline wears off very quickly. Figure 9-1 can help you assess your true preferences. It's devastating to arrive at your career goal only to discover you don't like it!

Continued from page 60

dietetic profession? Have you thought about the additional skills you will need to take on new responsibilities or upgrade and continue to hold your current position? Do you know the needs of your present employer, your community, and the city?

Dietitians must avoid becoming victims of the paradigm shift, which suggests that you can become extinct if you permit others to do the things you should be doing. For example, why let nursing screen patients when you can creatively devise a screening plan yourself? Why not actively become

Figure 9-1. Are You in Love with the Image or the Process?

CAREER PATH	IMAGE	REALITY . . . THE PROCESS
Private counseling practice	Independent, successful, lots of clients	1. Do you enjoy the process of counseling? 2. Do you enjoy counseling over and over again each day? (Billable hours are usually hours counseling.) 3. Do you enjoy administrative work?
Nutrition writer for magazine, newspaper, or public relations company	National recognition, creative, authoritative	1. Do you enjoy writing? 2. Do you enjoy tracking down information, researching, and interviewing people? 3. Do you enjoy and work well under deadline pressure?
Corporate executive	Manage projects and people, high levels of respect and responsibility	1. Do you enjoy being responsible for projects and people? 2. Do you enjoy being a team player, or do you get frustrated by red tape and bureaucratic delays?
Entrepreneur	Create and manage diverse projects or a business, risk taker, autonomous	1. Do you enjoy taking risks? Are you good at follow-up? 2. Can you picture yourself preparing project proposals for which you may not get paid or rewarded? 3. Can you handle down times without panic?

BUILD YOUR SKILLS: DEVELOP YOUR UNIQUE PRODUCTS AND SERVICES

Based on your skills assessment, identify the steps you need to take to strengthen or develop your skills. To help you decide the best career steps for you, consider developing your own personal board of advisers. Creating a team of personal advisers could be the single most important career strategy, according to the career consultant Jack Falvey. Ideally, this team would consist of five or six people who are willing to provide advice, leads, ideas, and a career overview from a perspective you couldn't take on your own. Team members might include a favorite mentor, a businessperson skilled in the work you presently do, a practitioner who already does what you want to do, your banker or accountant, a trusted dietitian friend, and a business or career adviser.

involved in seeking clinical privileges that allow you to determine patients' diets as well as provide total care for monitoring patients nutritionally? If we can be easily replaced by a nurse, a floppy disk, or a person with less training, it may be that our job description needs to be updated and upgraded to a higher level of skills.

Edna Langholz, a past ADA president and Copher Award recipient, stated in her election statement, "Unless we strive for the very best in ourselves, we will never know how good we could have been." So, what are we waiting for?

Minicase: I had already published a few national magazine articles and one book when I decided to shift my career path to focus on writing. I consulted four writers with whom I had ongoing relationships (from being interviewed for their food and nutrition stories) and posed some key questions: Should I pursue a degree in journalism? Would it be advantageous? And would it make a difference? I was surprised to learn that three of the four writers already thought I had the advantage of being an expert, a dietitian. They thought such expertise, when combined with my published articles and book, demonstrated my ability to write and follow through with assignments. My informal advisory group (three of the four) did not think a journalism degree was necessary, but encouraged me to attend local journalism and writing workshops and classes. Their advice proved to be not only prudent, but (dozens of articles later) time saving.

BECOMING KNOWN PROFESSIONALLY AND PUBLICLY: PROMOTING YOURSELF IN THE INTERNAL AND EXTERNAL MARKETPLACES

You don't need to become a household name to everyone in your organization or profession. As you begin to focus on promoting your personal assets (based on your career goals), choose target markets in which it's important for you to be known. A critical task in successfully promoting yourself is to be visible to the people you want to be known by.

Minicase: Visibility needs to be focused. Being visible just for the sake of being visible will do little to accomplish your personal objectives. A successful dietitian in a major metropolitan city decided that she wanted to make a career change to get away from counseling patients in a busy doctors' office. She thought her first step in personal marketing was to become visible, so she began giving a lot of community-based talks. She had a general idea of what she wanted to do, consult to area restaurants. She had little experience in restaurant consulting, but had contacts in the industry who thought highly of her as a nutrition professional. Her community talks were doing little to get her closer to her actual target, the local restaurant industry.

Her best chance for visibility was to explore opportunities with her existing restaurant contacts. Through one contact, she was able to land a semi-regular nutrition column in a regional restaurant trade journal. This offered her visibility to her potential target customers while keeping her abreast of restaurant trends. She also joined local restaurant organizations to increase her local visibility.

MARKET TO YOUR PEERS

Peer contacts, especially outside your current employment, can be a valuable asset that is often overlooked. Getting to know peers who are engaged in the type of work you wish to be doing (or doing more of) is a great way to begin carving your niche. For example, one dietitian wanted to do more eating-disorders counseling as part of her private practice. She began to contact dietitians specializing in that area to let them know of her current experience with eating disorders and desire to expand. It soon paid off. One of the dietitians she had contacted was too busy to give a local talk on nutrition to eating-disorder therapists and recommended her. While she did not get paid for her talk, she met valuable referral contacts and demonstrated her knowledge and ability to work with patients. Soon her patient referrals had significantly risen. The critical link – a dietitian peer.

BEYOND JOINING PROFESSIONAL GROUPS

Joining a professional group, such as a local chapter of The American Dietetic Association or a dietetic practice group, is a great way to meet peers. Too often, however, an individual joins a group and nothing happens. The key to benefit from organizations is to become an active participant. Consider joining committees that you have a real interest in and that can develop your skills. For example, if you have a desire to grow into a management position with budgeting responsibility, taking a leadership role or a treasurer position can help enhance compatible managerial skills. Specialty practice groups, such as in the Dietetic Practice Groups of ADA, are a good way to meet peers with similar interests. Participating in committee work or taking a leadership role in a national group will also increase your visibility in your area of interest.

Keep in mind, however, that committee work is not a substitute for one-on-one meetings. Your time and money might be best spent if you invest in just a few organizations and save what you would have paid in extra dues for a personal networking budget. Then use that money to take a special contact or referral source to lunch, for example, to help solidify your business relationship.

MARKET TO YOUR CURRENT EMPLOYER

You cannot assume that just because you are holding a job, your career will automatically move ahead. Personal marketing within your own organization is important for your growth. Consider

- Joining cross-department committees
- Writing a column for your company or hospital newsletter
- Taking a member of another department out to lunch (One hospital-based outpatient dietitian began to take physicians out to lunch and built a personal network. It's no surprise that her referrals increased.)
- Giving presentations to other departments on a nutrition topic of interest
- Identifying the movers and shakers in your company and seeking them out as mentors (Cultivate those relationships by being a valuable resource and keeping in touch.)
- Recruiting your boss to help align your career-development plans with the company's strategic plan

MARKET TO YOUR COMMUNITY

First, identify the members of your community and what their needs are. Then match their needs with one of your strengths, whether it's speaking, writing, or other personal assets.

The Power of Speech

Giving a presentation, whether to your peers or to the local community, is an effective way to demonstrate your abilities. There can come a time, however, of diminishing returns, when a decision needs to be made about the value of fees versus exposure. It makes sense to offer pro bono work as a community service, but after awhile, it may not be costeffective to speak for little pay. Establish a speaking fee. If the group is unable to pay your fee, be prepared to refer a couple of other effective nutrition speakers. It helps both the organization and a peer.

One cautionary note: People who speak at conferences for the sole purpose of selling their product or service turn off their audiences. The marketing consultant Frank Sonneberg advises that a speaker must begin by giving value without expecting to receive benefits (although there will eventually be a payoff).

The Power of the Pen

While writing may not always be monetarily rewarding, you can reap dividends from the personal exposure. Always negotiate the space for a bionote, a brief one or two-sentence description of who you are and what you do, such as, "John Doe is a registered dietitian and private nutrition counselor in Bigtown, USA." Most publications offer this opportunity, especially if you are getting little to no writing fee. Consider these readily available writing opportunities for career exposure:

- Corporate wellness newsletters
- Hospital newsletters
- Professional organization newsletters, such as ADA *Courier* and DPG newsletters
- Menus that provide space for nutrition tips
- Weekly newspapers
- Trade journals and newsletters

BUILD CREDIBILITY AND CAREER EQUITY

Be prepared to pay your professional dues and build equity in your career. This usually means working pro bono on selected projects in the initial phases of career building or career shifting. It's important to distinguish, however, which pro bono projects will pay off in such nonfinancial dividends as meeting worthwhile new contacts, gaining exposure, building experience and skills, and so forth. If you will benefit in any of these areas, it's most likely worth your time and effort. Don't take on projects, however, that make you resent the lack of pay or underpayment: you're not likely to be fully committed, and both you and the organization will lose. Also take care not to overextend yourself and take on too many projects. While promising career growth, accepting too many projects could stretch you too thin and interfere with your ability to shine.

Credibility is a valuable asset that makes you a desirable employee or consultant. You don't earn credibility overnight; it's a slow investment process. Four key components of professional credibility are honesty, responsiveness, consistency or reliability, and forethought. Here are some steps to solidify and enhance your credibility:

Continued on page 65

Q: How Can I Make Sure Corporate Clients Remember Me for Future Business?

Mona Boyd Browne, RD, Owner, Nutrition Communication Services, New York, New York

A: It's easy. Just remember service, service, service . . . and quality! Marketing yourself and your services is essential to obtain repeat business from corporate clients in today's marketplace. Use these simple techniques to keep clients coming back for more.

Eye Appeal Is Buy Appeal

Image is more than what you see in the mirror — a good image makes people want to enlist your services. All clients want to feel their consultant is the cream of the crop, the most sought after, the most qualified, and the most successful. A successful professional image says to clients, "This consultant is just what we need."

As everyone knows, a professional image means "dress for success," but for women, that doesn't mean a navy blue suit with a bow at the neck. Both men and women should wear suitable business attire when making business calls. Carry materials in a briefcase or folder to avoid damaging corners and edges of papers. Written proposals and presentations should be bound or offered in a folder. Any written material should be clearly typed and well-written, and all photocopies should be of the highest quality you can get.

- *Be accessible*. You don't have to be glued to your phone, but having voice mail or an answering machine allows people to reach you.

- *Be responsive*. Try to return phone calls within 24 hours. Let people know the best times to reach you. Be an active listener.

- *Be a resource*. If you can't help, know who can. Provide names of a few competent colleagues whom a prospective client or organization can seek out. Your ability to provide excellent referrals will reinforce your professional value even if you are unable to get personally involved in a project. You also reinforce your value to the colleague who accepts the project.

- *Be gracious*. Don't forget important details, such as thank-you notes for referrals or special efforts by colleagues. Remember to acknowledge the contributions of others. Share the glory.

- *Be sensitive to other people's time constraints*. When following up on a referral or lead, take care not to use someone's name without first obtaining permission.

EVALUATE YOUR PERSONAL MARKETABILITY

One key to success is always to be prepared for every opportunity that comes your way. Developing a professional portfolio is one way to keep ready. Samples of projects, clips of articles about you, and letters of recommendation can enhance your professional presence. Of course, you should have an updated résumé that is accurate and concise. Other printed material, such as a brochure, business card, Rolodex card, and brief biography could be useful, but you need to be careful not to overwhelm people with too much information. Pick and choose carefully. Customize your portfolio according to the position or project you are seeking. Portfolio folders are an easy way to present information without a lot of clutter. Be sure to tuck your business card inside – there are usually spots for this.

Videotapes of presentations or television appearances can also effectively showcase your abilities. If you are seeking writing opportunities, be sure to include a sample of your work, whether it's a newsletter, column, or magazine article.

Develop an ongoing way to get and utilize feedback about your job performance, whether it's from your boss, your clients, or a peer.

Use the checklist in Figure 9-2 to help assess your career marketability, and you'll be on your way to shaping a career that you enjoy.

References

1. McDermott LC. Marketing yourself as "Me, Inc." *Training & Development Journal*. September 1992: 77.

2. Bolles R. *What Color Is Your Parachute?* Berkeley, CA: Ten Speed Press; 1991.

3. Benton DA. *Lions Don't Need to Roar*. New York, NY: Warner Books; 1992.

Continued from page 64

Quality of Work = Your Reputation
The consultant who consistently produces high-quality work and delivers on time is highly valued. The chance to do something bigger and better often arises because of the reputation you have earned for doing a job well. Build your reputation on each project by being creative, dependable, and credible.

Packaging Makes Perfect
Your product and services are judged in part by how you present yourself: your physical appearance, dress, manner, preparedness, presentation, attitude, and reputation. Arrive for meetings on time, be prepared, ask intelligent questions, and provide timely follow-up. Setting and maintaining high standards tells your client that you offer high quality.

The Power of the Pen
Appreciate the contribution that impressive correspondence makes. A well-written memo to a client, an organized, comprehensive proposal or report – these make a lasting positive impression. Content is important, but so are neatness, timeliness, and grammatical correctness. Remember, your correspondence is an extension of your professional image.

It's in the Extras
Go the extra mile for your clients. Consistently point out opportunities for future projects, clip and mail relevant research articles, send prompt follow-up and thank-you notes, and remember appropriate personal dates, anniversaries, and holidays. It's the little things that make a client remember *you* and your services.

Motto: Go for the Three E's!
A consultant who is excited, enthusiastic, and eager can create job opportunities through hard work and innovation. Work together with your clients for a better bottom line!

Figure 9-2. Your Personal Marketability: A Checklist

1. Identify Personal Vision and Assess Needs.
- ❑ I have long-range goals and a career vision for my professional life.
- ❑ I know what skills or new knowledge will be required to progress in my career.
- ❑ I have explored ways of applying my current skills to enhance career options.
- ❑ I am able to identify tasks or responsibilities that I enjoy performing.

2. Develop Your Unique Products and Services.
- ❑ I have a role model, mentor, or personal advisory board whom I can learn from and who support my professional goals.
- ❑ I read journals regularly and am aware of key issues in the nutrition field.
- ❑ I take care of myself physically and am described as a person with a lot of energy.
- ❑ I understand the power sources in my organization (or referral base) and ways to develop my own.
- ❑ I take classes or workshops to help develop or refine skills.
- ❑ I participate in professional organization committees to help develop my skills.

3. Promote Yourself in the Internal and External Marketplace.
- ❑ My boss (or referral sources) know who I am.
- ❑ I am visible in a professional organization, preferably in a leadership role.
- ❑ I keep in contact with colleagues I have met at professional meetings.
- ❑ I keep in contact with people I have worked with in the past.
- ❑ I have a network I can call on for problem-solving assistance.
- ❑ I am involved in cross-department committees or problem-solving groups.

4. Build Credibility by Providing High-Quality Services.
- ❑ I have a good relationship with my superiors.
- ❑ I have a good relationship with my peers.
- ❑ I have a good relationship with my subordinates.
- ❑ I speak out and listen to my customers (internal and external) to understand their needs.
- ❑ Other people seek out my opinion on work-related subjects.
- ❑ I am accessible and responsive to requests.
- ❑ I am seen as a problem-solver and committed to action.

5. Evaluate Your Personal Marketability.
- ❑ I seek out feedback (external and internal, at all levels) regarding my performance.
- ❑ I use feedback to improve my performance.
- ❑ I maintain contact with professionals in my field to help determine my marketplace value and future trends in the field.
- ❑ My resume is current, well-organized, concise, and ready-to-go.
- ❑ I have engaged my boss in the process of aligning my career development plans with the company's strategic goals.

Adapted from Lynda McDermott, Marketing Yourself as Me, Inc., Training & Development, Sept. 1992: 84. Copyright Lynda McDermott. Reprinted with permission.

Bibliography

Egles L. Are you invisible? Get noticed and get promoted. *Women in Business*. March–April 1993: 6.

Falvey J. Career navigation: learn to plot your own destiny rather than let it drift. *Training & Development Journal*. February 1988: 32.

Helm KK. *The Entrepreneurial Nutritionist*. 2nd ed. Lake Dallas, TX: Helm Seminars; 1991.

Morrisey GL. Your personal mission statement: a foundation for your future. *Training & Development Journal*. November 1992: 71.

Overman S. Weighing career anchors. *HR Magazine*. March 1993: 56.

Peterson CD. Your entrepreneurial career. *Success*. November 1992: 16.

Rhodes NJ. Learn to build equity in your career. *Marketing News*. May 1986; 23: 9.

Roane S. *The Secrets of Savvy Networking*. New York, NY: Warner Books; 1993.

Sonneberg FK. The professional and personal profits of networking. *Training & Development Journal*. September 1990: 55.

Marketing of Dietetic Technicians

Gary Desbiens, DTR, Director of Nutrition Services, Parkview Memorial Hospital, Brunswick, Maine

Traditionally, dietetic technicians worked either in acute or extended care facilities. This no longer holds true. A new breed of dietetic technicians is emerging – one that isn't content merely to sit in a diet office processing menus. Today's dietetic technicians wish to be creative in seeking the best ways to utilize their acquired knowledge and skills. They hunger for one-on-one patient-client interaction in a wellness or disease-prevention setting, where they can provide counseling on proper nutrition for optimum health.

Today's dietetic technicians seek employment opportunities that enhance their abilities while staying within their legal scope of practice. They work in varied settings with very diverse responsibilities, such as public health nutrition programs, child nutrition, school lunch and elderly feeding programs, and food-service-management firms, to name only a few.

How did the following dietetic technicians market themselves to obtain their positions? All felt the need to be more challenged. They were willing to take a risk and be persistent. Once they made the decision to further their careers, the next step was to network with other dietetic professionals and community leaders. They pursued their goals by volunteering to different agencies in their communities, such as the American Heart Association, the American Cancer Society, and the AIDS Support Services. Volunteer work can open many doors to opportunity. Interviewees also identified education and involvement in district, state, or national dietetic associations as prime areas for career advancement.

PROFILE 1

Debra Mardenborough, DTR, works at the Clement Center's KAP (Knowledge, Attitude, and Practice) Wellness Center Program in Cleveland, Ohio. The grant-funded program targets inner-city African-American and Hispanic populations. Debra's role as a dietetic technician in this program is to promote wellness in the community. Her presentations in supermarkets, hunger sites, and grade schools teach individuals how to reduce the consumption of sodium, fat, and sugar in their daily diets. Debra also provides nutrition counseling for clients identified through a community outreach program as having hypertension, hypercholesterolemia, or diabetes mellitus.

Debra has held this position for two years. She feels that she won the position because she "wasn't afraid of taking risks, was willing to work in the community to build positive relationships, was a people person, and had the ability to be creative and generate new ideas."

PROFILE 2

Susan Ayres, DTR, began her career in dietetics working as a menu clerk in a local hospital. In just a short period of time, she realized that she wanted more in life and enrolled in a dietetic technician program. Following her graduation, Sue's first position was as a management dietetic technician. Her job included supervising tray-service personnel, developing procedures for in-service training, upholding sanitation standards, and assisting with catering.

After two years, Sue moved to the clinical arena, where her main focus was the cardiac patient. For a period of twelve years, Sue educated patients on the Prudent, or low-cholesterol diet, and became an active member of the local American Heart Association Nutrition Task Force Committee and the York County Nutrition Education Committee.

In 1980, a new door opened for Sue. She was appointed to serve on The American Dietetic Association's Council on Practice Quality Assurance Committee, where she assisted with the developing of the Standards of Practice. This was followed by her appointment to the Commission on Dietetic Registration as the first dietetic technician registered member.

By 1989, after fifteen years of being employed as a hospital dietetic technician, Sue wanted a new challenge, so she interviewed and won a position as Food Service Director of the Dallastown Area School District in Pennsylvania. In this position, Sue feeds approximately 4,200 students at the elementary- and secondary-school levels. She manages a staff of 70 employees at seven different schools. Her knowledge of nutrition and her skills as a manager complement her ability to provide nutritious lunches at minimal cost, while ensuring compliance with both government regulations and dietary guidelines. As director, Sue also purchases all food and supplies needed by the schools and assists in the financial policy, planning, and administering of accounting procedures for fiscal control.

Sue feels that she acquired this position simply by doing her homework. She states it is important to "contact someone who has a similar position and be prepared to ask questions; research the history of the facility; know your potential customers and products; and lastly, stage a mock interview to help reduce anxiety and increase self-confidence."

PROFILE 3

Ann Murdock, DTR, is Director of Nutrition Services at HCA Denton Community Hospital in Denton, Texas, a 104-bed acute care facility. Her responsibilities as director are many and varied. She oversees the complete operations of food production, patient tray service, cafeteria, and catering. She is responsible for developing departmental policies and procedures, as well as fiscal and capital budgets; procuring all food and supplies needed in the department; hiring, training, and evaluating all employees; and maintaining the physical environment to meet the required sanitation standards.

Ann began her career by working as an unskilled relief cook, dishwasher, and stocker in an extended care facility. As she learned about therapeutic diets, her interest in food service and nutrition emerged. To further herself in the field, Ann enrolled in a dietary managers training program. Upon completion of this program, she received a certificate qualifying her to manage a food-service department. This, however, did not completely satisfy Ann's thirst for knowledge. She decided that if she were to go any further in the field, she would have to enroll in the dietetic technician program.

During the time Ann pursued her education, she became Food Service Supervisor for an extended care facility that was in the process of enlarging. This immediately thrust Ann into the middle of a construction project. Not only did she have to contend with the retraining of staff to meet the increased needs of the department, but she found herself spending a large part of her day meeting with construction workers, plumbers, and electricians.

After seven years of employment at this facility, Ann was ready for a new challenge. She took a position as Nutrition Service Supervisor at a newly built hospital, where she assumed the purchasing functions, revised the cafeteria menu to offer more selections, and upgraded internal catering, while investigating ways to provide outside catering. As time progressed, Ann became Associate Director, with full management responsibility of the department. Unfortunately, the facility's lack of growth forced the downsizing of services and staff, and Ann didn't find the position as appealing as it once was.

Ann then moved to her current position as Director of Nutrition Services. She states that one of the things she enjoys most about her job is the use of computers. Ann's department was the first to go live on the order-entry system that communicates admissions, discharges, and diet orders. Ann feels that the dietetic technician program gave her a good knowledge base on which to build and develop her skills. She says, "The combination of nutrition and management classes was good, but I feel the benefit of classes in personnel management, psychology, and sociology are often not realized until you are out there on the job and find yourself in situations that you can relate directly back to a class."

PROFILE 4

Lynne Feher, DTR, has been employed for three and one-half years as a Nutrition Consultant at Hazelwood Farms Bakeries in Missouri. Upon hiring, it was her responsibility to collect nutrition information on all ingredients used in the bakery products. This data, when entered into the computer, produced a nutritional analysis on all Hazelwood Farms products. Lynne also baked and tested products.

As Lynne's term of employment increased, so did her responsibilities. Her position expanded to include labeling of products and ensuring their conformance to governmental regulations, including the Nutrition Labeling and Education Act. Lynne's other duties include sensory evaluation or taste testing during product development, the approval of all raw ingredients used at Hazelwood Farms, and the providing of nutrition information to staff, customers, and consumers. Lynne also helps market products. She just developed a brochure to help the sales force sell a new line of pies and completed a product-photography session for new packaging.

Lynne finds her position very rewarding and challenging. She feels that if the local hospital had had a dietetic technician position open when she graduated, her career would have taken the usual path. Says Lynne, "I learned to accept new challenges and overcome the fear that sometimes accompanies them. I have always volunteered to do whatever needs doing, even if it is outside my general job description. I try to give a little more than what is asked for in order to prove myself capable and willing."

PROFILE 5

Bob Wilson is truly a nontraditional dietetic technician. He graduated with honors with a four-year bachelor of science degree in biology, earned a two-year degree at an accredited dietetic technician program, and also has extensive personal experience and expertise in weight management. He works as a Nutrition Specialist at Kaiser

Permanente, under dietitians' supervision at the Department of Health Education, where he teaches the "Freedom from Fat" program and other health-related classes, and serves as a dietary interviewer for two of their research studies – one for children, the other for adults. In his own wellness practice, he guides clients toward a discovery of a "healthy eating/lifestyle plan" that works for them, while focusing on "self-acceptance and self-love."

What special qualifications does Bob have to be an expert in the field of weight management? Bob's interest in weight management originated out of personal experience. He relates that at an early age he "started using food as a comfort due to family problems," and by age sixteen, he weighed about 400 pounds. In 1972, Bob started to take control of his life. He joined Weight Watchers and lost 118 pounds in seven months. To help overcome his compulsive eating, Bob worked with a twelve-step program. He now maintains his weight at about 154 pounds.

Through these programs, Bob first experienced the concept of nutrition. His success in losing weight inspired him so much that he wanted to work in the community helping overweight people to make lifestyle changes. Aware of his goal, but feeling unprepared, he chose to pursue studies in the field of nutrition at a local community college. On completion of his degree, he was ready to take up the challenge of his dream and offer a more highly educated option to the public than those found at most weight-loss centers.

Bob began to co-instruct the Body Shop Program for overweight children, and developed and taught a series of weight-management classes. His talents did not go unnoticed. In 1987, Bob was offered a position under dietitians' supervision at the West Metro Food Compulsions Clinic and then at the Oregon Dietitians' Clinic. Later, he became a behavioral educator for a medically supervised fasting program. Because of his entertaining speaking skills and empathetic personality, Bob is a big hit with people who want to lose weight.

All of Bob's knowledge and experience culminated in his writing a self-help book to aid individuals in identifying workable options for permanent lifestyle changes, and producing and marketing of a series of videotapes.

SUMMARY

The preceding sampling of dietetic technicians is just that – only a sampling. The two-year dietetic technician programs across the country have provided students with a solid knowledge base that can be utilized in the various practice settings. Today's dietetic technician, however, is an entrepreneur, willing to take that knowledge and creatively expand on it, moving from traditional to nontraditional roles.

Dietetic technicians need to take the risks of charting their own courses. Boundless opportunities are available. The challenge is to recognize your talents and skills, have faith in yourself, and, in the words of Henry David Thoreau, "Go confidently in the direction of your dreams."

Marketing Social Programs

Chapter 11

Bettye Nowlin, MPH, RD, Dairy Council of California, Calabasas, California

Social Marketing is the design, implementation and control of programs seeking to increase the acceptability of a social idea, cause or practice in a targeted group, utilizing market segmentation, consumer research, concept development, communications, facilitation, incentives and exchange theory to maximize target group response. – Philip Kotler (1)

Social marketing was first introduced in the early 1970s as an effort to apply commercial marketing methods to help "sell" ideas, behaviors, and social programs instead of products. The opportunity for social marketing is timely because it offers a systems approach for public health promotion and communication efforts. Although everyone has access to the media, their use has to be strategically planned.

SUCCESSFUL SOCIAL MARKETING PROGRAMS

Most successful public health campaigns are community-based, multistrategy, and audience-centered. Social marketing campaigns that have emerged in the last decade promoting dietary behavior change have incorporated these elements.

Two case studies and a sidebar in this chapter show the exciting breadth of social marketing efforts. "Reclaiming Quality Leftovers to Feed the Hungry" tells about a program in Tarrant County, Texas, where volunteers work telephones each day and transport donated, prepared, but unsold food from hotels, restaurants, and hospitals to homeless feeding programs. A core of volunteers manage the program, organize civic support, and promote media coverage to keep the interest and program growing.

Two bold innovative national campaigns are Project LEAN (Low-Fat Eating for America Now) and the 5-A-Day program. These campaigns will serve as valuable models for future social marketing efforts in nutrition and other preventive health behaviors.

Project LEAN is the first national social marketing campaign developed and funded by a private foundation, the Henry J. Kaiser Family Foundation. The campaign was designed to encourage people to reduce the intake of fat in their diets.

The 5-A-Day program is the first national collaborative effort between public and private organizations to develop a social marketing program promoting the importance of eating at least five servings of fruits and vegetables each day as a way to improve health and reduce the risk of disease.

HOW TO SET UP A SOCIAL MARKETING PROGRAM

The social marketing process consists of four phases: strategy development, formulation, implementation, and assessment. The components of each phase are not always essential to every program, that is, a national campaign may use them all, while a local campaign may not. An analysis of individual situations will offer an opportunity to examine all the possibilities of the social marketing process. Then you can assess and apply the components that are appropriate to your program. The four phases can be briefly outlined as follows:

Phase I   Develop Strategies: Identify your objectives and the components of your strategy.

Problem	Identify health problems, needed marketing, and message points.
Objective	Develop realistic and measurable objectives for the communications program.
Target Groups	Identify your primary, secondary, and tertiary audiences.
Proposed Behavior Change	Define the exact desired outcome.
Resistant Points	Uncover the resistant points, or barriers, that appear to work against the adoption of desired behaviors.
Media	Assess media accessibility and which media reach your target groups best. Identify any contacts that you may already know.

Phase II   Strategy Formulation: Develop specific strategies for messages, target groups, media, and research.

Messages	Identify the points you want to communicate to your audience.
Target Groups	Divide your intended audience into target groups.
Media	Select the media that are the most appropriate delivery channels.
Research	Identify how you will evaluate the performance of each component and the impact of the complete program.

Phase III   Implementation: Design and test prototype materials. Then produce and implement the program.

Pretest	Pretest all materials to ensure that messages are clear, culturally relevant, practical, motivational, appealing, memorable, and free of negatives.
Media	Prepare a media plan to coordinate the scheduling of media activities; specify media mix, desired reach, frequency, and continuity.
Promotion Plan	Begin media plan, train field personnel, and develop your presentation to community-based groups whose support will enhance and strengthen the impact of the campaign.

Project LEAN – Lessons Learned from a National Social Marketing Campaign
Sarah Samuels, DrPH, Health Program and Policy Consultant, Oakland, California, and Former Program Officer, Henry J. Kaiser Family Foundation, Menlo Park, California

The Henry J. Kaiser Family Foundation initiated a social marketing campaign in 1987 to reduce the nation's risk for heart disease and some cancers. Consensus on recommendations for dietary change has stimulated the development of a variety of social marketing campaigns to promote behavior change. Project LEAN is a national campaign with the goal of reducing dietary fat consumption to 30 percent of total calories through public service advertising, publicity, and point-of-purchase programs in restaurants, supermarkets, and school and employee cafeterias.

The public service advertising reached 50 percent of the television-viewing audience, and the print publicity reached more than 35 million readers. The toll-free telephone hot line received more than 300,000 calls.

Continued on page 73

Phase IV   Assess Strategies: Evaluate the program's effectiveness and determine needed modifications. The final phase of managing a social marketing program involves evaluation. Two major concerns are whether the program brought about the intended changes, and whether the changes are societally and ethically desirable.

Process Evaluation	Determine the strengths and weakness of each component while the program is in operation and adjust as necessary.
Summary	Evaluate program over an extended period. Is it meeting objectives? Is it cost-effective?

BENEFITS AND PITFALLS OF SOCIAL MARKETING

Social marketing makes it possible to:

1. Maximize awareness of health and nutrition messages through the mass media

2. Educate the target population on how to deal with specific health and nutrition problems

3. Reach the largest number of people with a well-planned nutrition program at the least cost

4. Engage in partnerships and coalition building with key opinion leaders from the health and nutrition community

5. Engage in message development through collaboration in a consensus-building atmosphere

A number of problems may arise. For example:

1. There will be little or no immediate feedback or reinforcement for the health behaviors being promoted.

2. The targeted audiences may not be motivated to change their behavior.

3. Differences in cultural, religious, and individual beliefs and practices may present stumbling blocks.

4. It may be difficult to achieve broad consensus on concepts and messages.

5. Distribution channels may be harder to control.

6. Adequate time may not be allowed to ensure smooth implementation of activities and technical review of messages.

7. The project may be costly and time-consuming for staff and volunteers.

8. The target population may be hard to analyze.

SUMMARY

Social marketing is a relatively new approach to changing behavior in socially desirable ways. Although it is not simple to creatively apply marketing techniques to change health behavior, it can be done. Being involved in a campaign that ultimately improves the overall health of the public can be very rewarding.

Continued from page 72

Thirty-four organizations joined the foundation partnership and raised $350,000 for collaborative activities. Thirteen states implemented local campaigns. Lessons have been learned about the use of the media, market segmentation, effective spokespersons, and successful partnerships.

All campaign activities were carried out with the support of a national coalition of participating organizations called Partners for Better Health. Public service announcements (PSAs) were produced in partnership with the Advertising Council. The foundation has selected the National Center for Nutrition and Dietetics, the public education initiative of ADA, to continue Project LEAN, plus the project has continued in many states and communities across the country.

Adapted from Samuels, SE, Project LEAN – lessons learned from a national social marketing campaign, Public Health Rep. 1993; 108:45-53.

REFERENCES

1. Kotler P. *Social Marketing, Strategies for Changing Public Behavior* New York: The Free Press; 1989.

BIBLIOGRAPHY

American Dietetic Association. *1993 Survey of American Dietary Habits*. The Wirthlin Group; 1993. Sponsored by Kraft General Foods.

Kotler P. *Marketing Management*. Englewood Cliffs, NJ: PrenticeHall; 1976.

Manoff R. *Social Marketing, a New Imperative for Public Health*. Westport, CT: Praeger Publishers; 1985.

Case Study: RECLAIMING QUALITY LEFTOVERS TO FEED THE HUNGRY

Janet Hendrix, MS, RD, Health Care Specialist, Ben E. Keith (Food Broker), Fort Worth, Texas

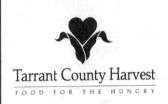

(817) 589-REAP

**6540 Boca Raton Boulevard
Suite 152
Fort Worth, Texas 76112**

Tarrant County Harvest, Inc., founded in 1991, is an all-volunteer, non-profit organization w̲... is to help feed hung... Tarrant County. The lo... U.S.A. Harvest, Tarrant C... serves as a link betw... industry and organizati... for needy people.

To some people, the food you throw away is not just a lot of garbage! Tarrant County Harvest was organized by a group of dietitians to address the problem of hunger and malnutrition in their metropolitan county in the Fort Worth, Texas area. The concept is simple: local restaurants, hotels, hospitals, caterers, and others are asked to donate unserved food that they would otherwise throw away. Volunteers transport the donated food to agencies licensed to feed the hungry. Food is not stored, since it is taken directly from a donor to a recipient organization charged with feeding the hungry.

Tarrant County Harvest, a local chapter of USA Harvest, was organized in 1991 with fewer than six volunteers. Since that time, 350 volunteers have solicited and transported one million pounds of food to 64 recipient agencies. Nutritious, high-quality, prepared foods from feeding establishments and grocery stores are delivered frozen or chilled within 30 minutes to maintain food safety.

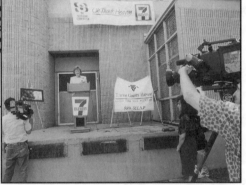

MARKETING MAKES US SUCCESSFUL

We owe much of our success to a strong, carefully planned, and continuous marketing campaign. For example:

- Media coverage is solicited through press releases for Harvest events. The 1992 Fall Harvest Banquet was a newsworthy occasion with a good message and many civic leaders in attendance. It was covered on the late news by the local ABC-TV station, which resulted in more community awareness, more volunteers, and more food sources.

- A speakers' bureau provides information to local groups in an effort to attract volunteers and in-kind donations of goods and services, since the entire program functions without funds.

- A local answering service volunteers its time to answer calls for our program 24 hours a day. The number to their service is used in all our marketing.

- A four-color brochure for food establishments contains a pre-addressed postcard to mail for follow-up contact.

- A local university created a video for public education.

- Networking among chefs, dietitians, the local dietetic association, local businesses, and owners of restaurants and fast-food outlets results in increased contributions.

- Donations of food by weight are recorded and summarized monthly. Potential tax benefits from donating the food enable businesses to see their affiliation with Tarrant County Harvest as a positive financial decision.
- Car phones, beepers, telephone answering machines, the answering service, computers and word processors, and organized scheduling help keep communication and information current.

USA Harvest is spreading to all parts of the United States, Canada, and Europe. For more information on local chapters, call 1-800-USA-4-FOOD.

Case Study: **DEVELOPING A NATIONWIDE, PUBLIC-PRIVATE PARTNERSHIP TO PROMOTE FRUITS AND VEGETABLES: THE 5-A-DAY PROGRAM**

Elizabeth Pivonka, PhD, RD, Director of Nutrition and Services, Produce for Better Health Foundation, Newark, Delaware

Most nutrition professionals are somewhat familiar with the 5-A-Day program. It is the largest ever industry and government joint nutrition education program, and the first nationwide health promotion program focusing specifically on the importance of fruits and vegetables in Americans' diets. The message is simple: eat five servings of fruits and vegetables every day for better health. 5-A-Day is jointly sponsored by the National Cancer Institute (NCI) and the Produce for Better Health Education (PBH). The goal of the program is to increase fruit and vegetable consumption to five or more servings a day by the year 2000.

5-A-Day was started in 1988 by the California Department of Health Services through a grant from NCI. This campaign focused mainly on retail, media, and government channels to inform consumers about 5-A-Day. The California effort was the springboard for the national program in 1991.

CHALLENGES OF THIS TYPE OF PROGRAM

To understand the 5-A-Day program and to use it as a model for other public-private partnerships, one must understand the general prevailing issues, which include message support, competition, credibility, and the active interest of key participants.

Message Support

Because the fruit and vegetable industry is so diverse, with several hundred different fruit and vegetable items, many different commodity boards have been organized to meet the marketing needs of each commodity. Partly because of this diversity, there has never been a promotion to increase the consumption of fruits and vegetables as a total food group. Developing a message like 5-A-Day, which the whole fruit and vegetable industry was willing to help fund and support, has been essential for the success of the program.

Competition

Another big step to overcome was competition among those wanting to promote their own messages. Retail organizations, for example, didn't want to promote the same message as their competition in the same market area. Also, each commodity group wants to be sure that its product is featured prominently in 5-A-Day materials. While efforts are undertaken to be equitable at the national level, it is difficult to make everyone happy all of the time.

Convincing the industry that the success of the program hinged on all parties promoting the same message was essential. Only then would the 5-A-Day message appear credible, not just a self-serving promotion. Industry members understand that 5-A-Day is a long-term investment that will benefit everybody's business and that nothing will change overnight. Nutrition professionals need to understand business motives if they want to work successfully with the private sector in promoting nutrition-marketing programs.

Credibility

The support from the National Cancer Institute significantly advanced the credibility of the 5-A-Day message in the eyes of consumers. While some industry members were hesitant to link their product with cancer (thinking that cancer produced a negative image with consumers), they recognize the benefits of having the message come from a credible health authority.

Produce Growers', Shippers', and Retailers' Interest

Enjoying support from a credible health authority and having a great program are not enough, however. The fruit and vegetable industry also had to be interested. 5-A-Day has been successful not because of tremendous marketing efforts, but because there was a groundswell of interest from within the fruit and vegetable industry. Interest came from the bottom up instead of from the top down.

START-UP ACTIVITIES

Once the fruit and vegetable industry and NCI determined they could develop a win-win strategy that could help consumers protect their health while eating more of food they liked, the next step was to establish an infrastructure to house the project and obtain start-up funding. The Produce for Better Health Foundation, a not-for-profit education organization, was incorporated to coordinate 5-A-Day efforts for the industry and to work as a partner with NCI. Other start-up activities included:

- Development of a strategic plan (a component critical to any effective program)
- Conducting a baseline survey of fruit and vegetable consumption and attitudes about fruits and vegetables so we could later determine the effectiveness of our marketing efforts
- Setting up license agreements (Since the logo is the property of NCI, license agreements were developed between the Foundation and NCI, and between the Foundation and its industry members to protect the use of the logo.)
- Development of the first program materials and messages to distribute through industry participants to consumers nationwide
- Development of a Program Guidebook to set guidelines for implementing the program

MARKETING PROJECTS

The following are examples of what various groups are asked to do when participating in 5-A-Day efforts:

- *Grocery retailers* are asked to mount two promotions each year, such as placing the logo and message on plastic bags and paper sacks, purchasing and hanging posters and distributing brochures at point of sale, conducting in-store taste-testing or tours, and advertising in newspapers and on the radio.
- *Suppliers and merchandisers* are asked to put the logo on their produce packages, place 5-A-Day stickers on their bananas or other produce, promote the message in their advertising, and offer new promotional materials to retailers.
- *Noncommercial food-service operators* are asked to conduct two theme-related program events per year, including placement of signs, brochures, table tents, and menu boards at point of sale. They are encouraged to hold contests, wear buttons, and advertise the program.
- *State health authorities (health departments)* are asked to coordinate 5-A-Day activities in their state. They may sublicense state-community coalitions, develop new 5-A-Day program materials, conduct state and local promotional activities and media events at least once a year, and conduct statewide 5-A-Day evaluations.

RESULTS AFTER TWO YEARS

Program materials developed to date include four different brochures, corresponding posters and point-of-sale artwork, recipes, advertising copy, radio public service announcements (PSAs), video PSAs, food-demonstration guidelines, training videos, in-store point-of-sale videos, tip cards, hats, aprons, and T-shirts. Various promotional themes have been used since the start of the program, including "Eat More Fruits and Vegetables," "Eat More Salads," "Easy Entertaining," "Fast and East," "Eat More Salads II," "5-A-Day Week," and "Healthy Gift Baskets."

Media activities in 1992 included an NCI press conference to release 5-A-Day baseline-survey consumption results; PBH's World's Largest Cornucopia, and PBH's survey of gubernatorial candidates. Media activities in 1993 include PBH's survey of National Football League fruit- and vegetable-eating habits; a five-minute meals media tour; state proclamations from governors proclaiming 5-A-Day weeks, and the World's Largest Gift Basket. Media impressions generated since the start of the national program in October 1991 through March 1993 total more than 1.6 billion.

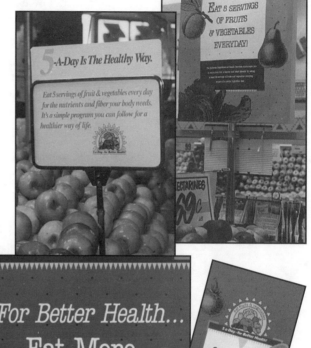

Currently the program is being implemented in all 50 states by almost 300 different grocery retail organizations (representing more than 30,000 supermarkets), more than 300 merchandiser and supplier companies (commodity boards and other retail suppliers), more than 20 food-service distributors, and 18 state health departments. Industry members spent more than $18,000,000 on the program in 1992. Nine grants were awarded by NCI in 1993, worth approximately $400,000 each per year. NCI is conducting message development and message testing.

FUTURE PROGRAMS

Areas of future expansion include working in the commercial food-service area, developing materials for ethnic and vulnerable populations, working more with children, continuing to expand retail and non-commercial food-service activities, and expanding media coverage and consumer awareness of the program and its messages.

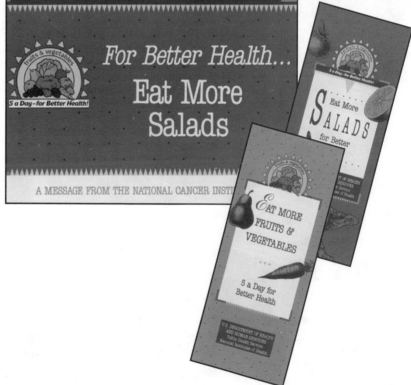

5-A-Day Marketing Tools

Promotion: Public Relations, Advertising, Direct Mail, Trade Shows, and Other Strategies

Kathy King Helm, RD, Private Practitioner, Lake Dallas, Texas

Promotion is a component of marketing; marketing encompasses all the planning and strategizing, while promotion's purpose is to attract attention. Tooting our own horn is the best way to lead the parade to our doorstep. That means promotion – from distributing business cards and advertising in the *Yellow Pages*, to writing newspaper columns, appearing on TV talk shows, and giving speeches to civic groups. Promotion is all the communication used to familiarize others with us and our products. It's more important now than ever, because the competition – frequently well-funded – is becoming slick and sophisticated.

PROMOTIONAL STRATEGIES

We often naively assume that promotion is not necessary if, as professionals, we possess the right credentials and our products or services are good. We often neglect to include an adequate budget for promoting our programs, not realizing that an excellent program may fail, despite meticulous attention to its development, because of insufficient or poor-quality promotion.

Promotion will attract far more clients to our doors than will any form of legislation. The focus of health care has shifted toward health promotion and the well individual, and we dietitians must accept that our services are only one of many nutrition-information options available to the consumer. To stand above the crowd, we must offer excellence with flair.

Because of the nature of our business – health care and service – our product is usually intangible (except, of course, in food service). An intangible product cannot be held or visually evaluated like a new coat. Weight-loss programs or consultation services cannot be experienced in advance. Therefore, surrogates that represent and promote dietetic services (business cards, brochures, résumés, proposals, letters of reference, portfolios, and the like) are extremely important, especially to those who have not yet sampled our programs and skills. The provider of an intangible service is inseparable from that service in the minds of most clients.

Self-Packaging

You may have an excellent message to deliver and an outstanding product for the consumer. But if you as the messenger, salesperson, agent, and provider of service are not well packaged, the venture may not succeed. Time and effort, and usually money, must be spent on preparing yourself for the job. This packaging includes not only expertise and appearance, but also communication skills and how you sell your ideas.

If you look closely at professionals and businesspeople you consider successful, you will notice they promote themselves well. Self-promotion is a skill that can be learned. It creates greater awareness of you and your expertise, engenders professional and personal opportunities, improves your effectiveness as a service provider, and creates demand for your services.

You may often overlook or ignore opportunities to promote yourself for fear of looking too aggressive or self-serving. In today's competitive and fast-paced marketplace, no one can afford to let opportunity pass by so easily. If you do not distinguish yourself and your expertise, others will quickly take your place.

After promotion attracts business, quality performance engenders loyalty and respect and keeps clients coming back. Word-of-mouth advertising can be your best form of promotion. Third-party endorsement carries great weight.

Negative publicity travels as fast as the positive form. Day-to-day encounters and off-the-cuff statements overheard in elevators may be as important to your professional image as presentations.

Planning Your Promotion

When trying to evaluate which forms of promotion to use, review a list of promotional options, such as the one in Figure 12-1, and hypothetically try to fit each form to your product, budget, and audience. Look for ideas that are creative, unique, affordable, and in good taste. Promotion is most successful when designed for multiple exposures of the name, logo, and message to the target market over an extended period.

Of course, advertising and public relations firms and individual consultants can create promotional campaigns for a fee. You can expect to pay anywhere from $50 to $200 per hour plus out-of-pocket expenses and the cost of materials. If you are seeking the advice of outside public relations counsel, consult your *Yellow Pages* and call colleagues who have used public relations firms. There also are some solo operators who do freelance promotion at a more modest rate. Dietitians who work for others may have access to in-house public relations and advertising departments or consultants that could make a program or department sparkle, if given adequate time, guidance, and budget.

Promotion costs should be seen as part of the investment necessary to create demand for nutrition services. You certainly will be using your time or someone else's to implement the plan, and you may also spend money on brochures, news releases, flyers, and other materials. The challenge is to choose wisely so that promotional programs are cost-effective.

THE PIECES OF THE PROMOTION PUZZLE

There are six potential pieces of a promotional plan:

1. Public Relations
2. Advertising
3. Direct Mail
4. Trade Shows
5. Personal Promotion
6. Graphic and Print Materials

Figure 12-1. Promotional Tools

Public Relations	
❏ Publicity	❏ News Releases
❏ Press Kits	❏ Media Interviews
❏ News Conferences	❏ Press Briefings
❏ Cosponsorship	❏ Special Events
❏ Celebrities	

Advertising

Direct Mail

Trade Shows

Personal Promotion Aids	
❏ One-to-One	❏ Communication
❏ Networking	❏ Business Cards
❏ Letters	❏ Résumés
❏ Letters of Reference	❏ Use of a Name
❏ Public Speaking	❏ Writing

Graphic and Print Materials	
❏ Logos	❏ Brochures
❏ Portfolios	❏ Proposals
❏ Posters	❏ Banners
❏ Computer Graphics	❏ Giveaways

Each piece is important to the whole because each piece works to reinforce the others. The more pieces you use, the stronger the image that you present to your customers and to your potential customers and referral agents.

How the Pieces Work

Public relations provides low-cost or no-cost publicity about you, your service or product, and your company; advertising elicits a response from the customer; direct mail provides your customers with the means to take immediate action; trade shows offer you the opportunity to meet with a large number of high-potential new prospects in one setting; and personal promotion keeps you and your message in front of your customers on a daily basis (1).

Begin your comprehensive promotional plan by looking at the pieces. Use press releases to create a positive impression about your company and staff. Then do a direct mailing to tell your target audience a little more about your service or product. Enter a trade show and run an ad in trade publications inviting attendees to stop by your booth for a free demonstration or gift. If you leave pieces out along the way, the picture you're trying to paint may not make as much sense to your customers, or its impact may be diminished (1).

PUBLIC RELATIONS

Public relations (PR) is an organized effort to promote a favorable image of an individual, an organization, or a product in the marketplace. PR can be internal or external. Internal PR focuses on employees and their families. External PR is aimed at outside target audiences, such as customers, clients, suppliers, the press, the government (local, state, or federal officials), local business leaders, stockholders, security analysts, the consumer public, or the local community.

Public relations can involve many different activities, such as increasing exposure by staging major media events; producing brochures, newsletters, or other promotional materials; sponsoring a community event; or adopting new customer programs to promote goodwill. Today, most health organizations and many private-practice professionals hire public relations consultants or have an in-house PR staff. Other national companies and associations have a network of spokespersons in the field. In the case of The American Dietetic Association, ambassadors and state media representatives are interviewed by print and broadcast media during periodic media blitzes focusing on nutrition topics of national interest.

Five Keys to a Successful PR Campaign

As you plan, ask yourself about the following five keys to a successful PR campaign:

1. *Purpose.* Why are you promoting yourself?
2. *Product.* Are you promoting yourself, your product, or a service?
3. *Plan.* Who are you trying to reach and what do you want them to do or think?
4. *Packaging.* How can you differentiate yourself in a way that will grab attention?
5. *Promotion.* What's the vehicle? A feature story? A blurb? An article?

Publicity is planned news. You can easily recognize prearranged publicity when you see media coverage of a company-sponsored 10K race or a hospital's new OB class.

Ideally, your publicity will include both an announcement of your coming event and coverage of the event itself. When planning a special event, you may want to include a local celebrity or consider cosponsorship with a philanthropic organization to improve the possibility of media coverage and attract a larger attendance. You can also mail news releases prior to the event to the newspapers and radio and television stations in your area. There is no charge for publicity (other than the cost of your time and materials), but there's no guarantee of coverage, either. (For more specific advice on publicity, see Chapter 22.)

News releases or press releases are the staple of the public relations business. Releases are used by dietitians for many purposes: to announce an appointment or the opening of a practice; to give details of a special event; to announce an upcoming appearance before a local group; and to announce the introduction of a new product, the publication of a book, or the release of an association's position paper. (For suggestions on how to write a press release, see Chapter 23.)

News releases are also an inexpensive format for direct mail. Corporations, health professionals, and members of associations or community organizations may be appropriate targets. Keep your colleagues as well as the press informed of your activities so they can pass on the information to their constituencies.

Press kits are used to interest the broadcast and print media in a story on your service, product, book, or speaking engagement (see Chapter 25). The kit may include a variety of items:

- A press release or pitch letter describing the product you wish to publicize (see Chapters 23 and 24)
- A sample of the product, or copies of newspaper articles, advertisements, brochures, or critical reviews
- A résumé or short biographical sketch (see Chapter 26)
- Backgrounders describing related studies, endorsements, historical information, and the like
- 5" x 7" black-and-white glossy photos of you and of the product

Press kits should be descriptive, attractive, and to the point. They should provide solid information and explain why the public should be interested in the topic. Although press kits can be very elaborate, with printed covers and numerous photos, they can also be as simple as several of the above items placed in a large pocket folder.

Media interviews expose the local area – or, sometimes, the nation – to a dietitian's views and influence. You can reach more people in five minutes on the radio or in one newspaper article than you can in ten years of one-to-one counseling and public speaking combined. Being introduced on a television program or quoted in the newspaper as an expert in nutrition quickly establishes you as a credible professional in the eyes of the public. Always mention the ADA, your RD or DTR credentials, and the fact that more than 64,000 ADA member dietitians nationwide can answer the public's nutrition questions. The Association can provide clout and backup that extend your own personal influence as a dietitian. (See Chapter 13 for more information on gaining media exposure.)

News conferences are called to announce to the media an important event, scientific discovery, product, or the like. For example, The American Dietetic Association and other organizations called a joint press conference in Washington, D.C., to announce their support for FDA's proposed labeling regulations on dietary supplements. Usually, a formal statement is made, followed by a question-and-answer session.

Press briefings – one-on-one desk-side interviews or more formal editorial board briefings – are used to provide the media in-depth background information on a specific subject.

Cosponsorship of events and activities has proven to be a very successful promotional method for many ventures. Cosponsorship can cut costs. It also increases your visibility and extends your reach through exposure to and potential support from your cosponsor's mailing list. When considering potential cosponsors, evaluate what skills, resources, and public image are required to complement what you have to offer. For example, a hospital could cosponsor a city health-promotion campaign with a local newspaper or television station. The media-related sponsor could offer publicity and celebrities, while the hospital could provide the project development, management, and personnel.

In any partnership, all participants should contribute to and benefit from the relationship, or problems will arise. A project plan clearly identifying all participants' contributions, assignments, and deadlines will help cosponsored activities run more smoothly and equitably.

Special events and rewards can generate excitement for your program and good media coverage. Staging such events at times that permit live, on-site TV coverage often increases publicity tremendously. The noon or later-afternoon news programs are often interested in covering local events with their live mobile camera units. Consider a dedication, an anniversary celebration, a milestone occurrence, a groundbreaking, a fun run or race, a bike race or other athletic event, a nutrition day or health fair, a food tasting, a free assessment or screening, a testimonial dinner or roast, or an event that ties in with a civic celebration, a holiday, or a seasonal theme. Award presentations offer an opportunity to thank those who have made special contributions of time, money, or resources to your project. A tip: high-quality, engraved or beautifully designed invitations make a strong impression on those invited to your event and help put them in a festive frame of mind.

Celebrities attract attention. The media want to interview them and the public wants to see and mingle with them. Hiring a media or sports celebrity, or persuading such a person to become involved as an act of charity, may help assure success for your venture. It certainly helps your advance publicity. Just be sure that the celebrity's public image matches the one you want to create for your program or event.

ADVERTISING

Advertising is purchased promotion in print or on broadcast media. It is used to draw potential buyers' attention, teach your customers something new about your product, change customers' attitudes, or remind them of past satisfaction with your product or company. Advertising exposes a large number of people to your message. You can better control the timing and quality of the exposure because you are a paying customer.

The choice of media depends on your target market, budget, and goals. Potential buyers must be exposed to an ad several times before they remember it, so advertising campaigns must optimize frequency and reach (the approximate number of people who see or hear the ad). Some practitioners have been very successful in using advertising for their private practices; others have not. The approaches that have worked best are *Yellow Pages* advertising and ongoing ads in newspapers and on the radio. Continually evaluate the effectiveness of different forms of advertising by asking every client how he or she heard of your services or product.

To evaluate the cost of advertising, divide the average fee for an initial consultation or whatever you are selling into the total cost for the advertising. For example, if a radio campaign costs $300 per month and you charge $60 for an initial consultation, you will pay for the ad, or break even, with five new patients per month, which is reasonable. In contrast, if the advertising costs $800 per month and you charge only $40 for your instruction, it will take twenty new patients per month to break even and cover your advertising costs!

First decide what you want your ad to do. There are then four keys to successful advertising (1, 2, 3):

1. *Stimulus/Response.* What response do you want from your audience? Select the appropriate stimulus to evoke that response.

2. *Surprise.* Never underestimate the element of surprise in an ad. Surprise grabs attention and makes a lasting impression.

3. *Emotion.* Love, fear, sadness, and humor involve the audience and make your point with impact. Remember "Where's the beef?" See how easily you recalled that ad?

4. *Relevance.* Make sure your ad leaves your audience thinking, "They're talking about me!" If it doesn't, you've lost an opportunity, and perhaps a sale.

SELECTING THE APPROPRIATE MEDIA

Television delivers visual movement and impact, but the cost is high, and 15- or 30-second spots offer only limited time to convey your information. Radio airtime is a cost-effective way to get your message heard frequently, but radio does not always have its listeners' full attention because it often just plays in the background. Newspapers don't offer glossy four-color photo opportunities, and the competition for the readers' attention can be fierce among advertisements, but you can reach a lot of people in a timely fashion. *Yellow Pages* advertising can be very effective in that surveys show 77 percent of adults consult their directory every month – at the time they are looking for something to buy. The most common errors people make in *Yellow Pages* advertising is placing ads so small that they contain too little information or are not competitive in their category, or placing their ads under the wrong category, so they see little response. Figure 12-2 shows some examples of effective *Yellow Pages* ads.

Figure 12-2. Yellow Pages Ads

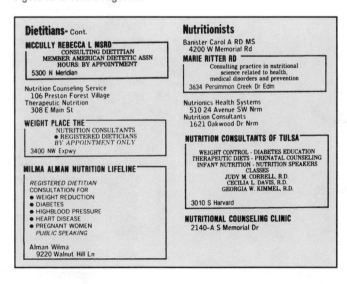

Television

Network TV is expensive for the small business owner. As mentioned in an earlier chapter, the marketing experts Rapp and Collins, authors of *The Great Marketing Turnaround*, (3) believe that mass marketing on network TV is not particularly effective at stimulating customers to buy products, especially considering the relative cost. If you use network TV, check into buying one of these less-expensive options (1):

- *Preemptible time.* You pay for a certain time slot and your commercial will air then, unless someone else pays a higher price for the same spot, thus preempting you.
- *Run-of-station time.* You pay a certain price for the week, and the station places your spots in unsold time.
- *Distress time.* You wait until the last possible minute and buy unsold airtime at a lower price.

Buyer beware! If you purchase bargain airtime, monitor it carefully to make sure it delivers an audience worth your investment. For example, if you buy distress time on the late movie, be sure your ad runs in the first hour, not during the last ten minutes (1).

Cable

Sometimes referred to as *narrowcasting* (as opposed to network TV, which is *broadcasting*), cable is a good alternative for many small businesses that rely on local or neighborhood customers. Cable is less expensive, and many cable operators help you produce simple, low-cost commercials. However, your purchasing options will vary, depending on the age and sophistication of the cable operator's equipment, and you may find yourself relegated to one specific time slot for an entire week (1).

Radio

When you advertise on the radio, if you choose the appropriate type of music or talk format, you can reach a specific demographic group and achieve frequency fairly easily. Ads must be particularly attention-grabbing to be remembered. With radio, as with TV time, the more popular stations and time slots are the most expensive because more people are listening or viewing at that time.

Print

The number of specialty magazines and journals has been steadily on the rise, meaning there's a newspaper, magazine, or journal for just about any group you'd like to target, whether it's business-to-business or consumer-oriented. And people who buy those publications are actively looking for information. (1) Consult the *Gale Directory of Publications and Broadcast Media* or other trade resources in your local library for rates, circulations, and ad specifications for consumer magazines, trade journals, and radio and television stations.

One possible disadvantage of print advertising is long lead times, which means that ads do not come out for two or three months and can't be changed quickly. It also takes longer to build an audience when a publication comes out only once a month or once a quarter. Also, some publications may be cluttered with competitive advertising, making it more difficult for your message to stand out.

When choosing between newspapers and magazines, remember that magazines allow for more efficient targeting, but have longer lead times. Newspapers reach a broad audience quickly, but may not reach the people you're looking for when they're making buying decisions.

Six Key Media Concepts

Price is always an issue, but spending more money will not necessarily make your ads more successful. You can make your ad campaign work for you if you keep these six key media concepts in mind (1, 2, 3):

1. *Concentration.* It is usually more productive to concentrate limited funds instead of spreading them over a variety of media. Customers are more likely to remember you or your product when they see your message multiple times. Twenty-five radio spots are more effective than one radio spot, one TV spot, and one newspaper ad.

2. *Reach.* Reach is the number of people exposed at least once to the vehicle carrying your ad. For example, you may be able to reach 25,000 people through your local weekly newspaper. Reach accumulates as you add media, concentration, or frequency.

3. *Frequency and continuity.* One of the jobs of your ad is to teach people, and people learn through repetition. That means frequent exposure to your message. So if you have to choose between one glossy four-color image or ten black-and-white ads, go for the black-and-white ones. The fact that your ad will run ten times increases the chance that a prospect will see it more than once.

4. *Visibility and impact.* If your ad is not memorable, it will not matter how many times you run it. It must grab your audience and get their attention! Don't throw your money away. Just remember the four essential considerations: stimulus/response, emotion, surprise, and relevance.

5. *Awareness of your competition.* Don't copy your competitors, but know what they are doing. If they have more money for advertising, look for a new message or target a different market niche. For example, if they are going after large catered affairs, go after small parties for people with incomes over $70,000. Know your competitors' strengths and weaknesses – why what they are doing works, or does not work.

6. *Testing what you're doing.* The owner of a large department-store chain once said, "I'm wasting my money on 50 percent of my advertising budget – I just don't know which 50 percent." Test your advertising strategy. It can be as simple as asking callers how they heard of your service; running the same ad in two different media, each with a different telephone number; or using coded order forms.

When you advertise, just remember the basics – first determine the response you want from your audience, choose a message that will stimulate that response, find the medium that enhances your message, and keep the message consistent.

DIRECT MAIL

Use direct mail when you know specifically whom you want to contact (usually either potential clients or referral agents). The average response rate to direct mail is usually 1 percent to 2 percent – higher than that for most other forms of advertising. When dietitians are known in the community, their response rate from direct mail to physicians and clinics has been as high as 30 percent.

Direct mail can be used to conduct marketing surveys, to announce a new office location or new services, to acquaint potential clients or referral agents with your services, or to generate leads and sell your product or service. Mailings should be personally addressed, whenever possible, instead of "To whom it may concern" or "Occupant." Membership lists of your local medical society or national dietetic practice groups, the *Yellow Pages,* and shared business cards are good sources of names and addresses. Many organizations charge a fee and require an explanation of how their membership lists will be used. Other lists of potential clients or subscribers can be purchased, often as mailing labels. (See Chapter 27 for more information on direct mail.)

TRADE SHOWS

Trade shows are a one-on-one sales medium that can produce very attractive sales figures. According to the Small Business Administration, 54 percent of the *qualified* prospects who hear your pitch at a national trade show will turn into sales. The keys to success at trade shows are careful selection of the shows and sales staff, attractive booth and location, a good sales pitch and system to qualify leads, and excellent follow-up. (See Chapter 28 for specific hints on how to market at trade shows.)

PERSONAL PROMOTION AIDS

One-to-one communication can be your most effective form of promotion. It affords the opportunity to speak, hear, see, and exchange viewpoints face to face. And with this direct approach, people are more likely to remember your message. As the promoter, you can read the body language and expressions of each listener and then adjust your presentation to maximize its impact.

Satisfied customers are invaluable walking promoters. Potential clients are often influenced to try a dietitian's service by a satisfied former client who receives no profit or gain from the referral and therefore has high credibility.

Networking with other individuals in and out of the dietetic profession is an important promotional tool that may change your perspective and offer new insights and professional opportunities. When you start a new job or join a business or professional organization, it is especially crucial that you introduce yourself to peers, supervisors, and officers (executives) alike. Offering support and showing eagerness to become involved may increase your

Figure 12-3. Business Cards

Copyright Carol Banister, Nancy Gelbard, Leslie D. Grant, Kathy King Helm, and Andrea Stark. Reprinted with permission.

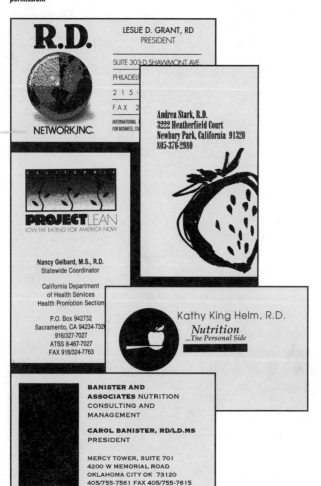

personal influence and power (see Chapter 38).

Business cards are the most common communication tool used by business and professional people to promote services, facilitate networking, and provide a handy reminder of a phone number or appointment date. The typical card includes your name, RD or DTR credential, title, place of business, mailing address with zip code, and phone number with area code. Colors, print styles, logos, layouts, and other design elements may be used creatively. Figure 12-3 shows examples of actual business cards, and Figure 12-4 shows letterheads; generally, the two are coordinated. These examples of business cards and letterheads used by dietitians in various areas of practice may stimulate your creative thinking. However, the designs of others may not be copied directly.

Letters or notes are excellent ways to improve communication and thus promote referrals and client loyalty. Practitioners who send frequent letters, such as follow-up letters to physicians or notes to clients and colleagues, show their concern and involvement. Telephone calls also serve this function. Increased communication may produce positive outcomes.

More frequent communication can also strengthen your ties with community or professional organizations. Letters to editors of newspapers, magazines, and journals give you a chance to air your views and educate others. Opportunities abound to present a sound interpretation of the latest nutrition "discovery," fad diet, or other published form of misinformation. Personal letters to community leaders, authors, and other individuals may help you identify allies and expand your network.

Ask one or more people to proofread and evaluate all of your important and potentially controversial written communication. All typed or handwritten correspondence should look as professional as possible. It represents you and should convey the image you want to project. Attractively printed letterheads and envelopes enhance the professional appearance of your correspondence.

Résumés can be powerful tools of self-promotion. A well-thought-out résumé may give you a competitive edge in job negotiations. It may be used, along with a letter of introduction, to acquaint potential clients with you and your services. It may be sent to sponsors of speaking engagements or media interviewers to assist in introducing you, or included with a publishing or business proposal. You may want to write several different résumés representing your varied areas of expertise. A résumé may be either chronological, listing your experience in reverse chronological order, or functional, highlighting your skills and responsibilities. Variations include the curriculum vitae or vita, an expanded version of a résumé that includes published books and papers, and the biographical sketch, which is written in paragraph form. All of these should be updated on a regular basis to fit new markets and reflect new skills and accomplishments. (For more on résumés, see Chapter 26.)

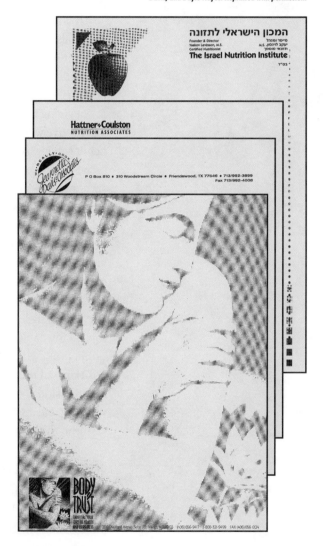

Figure 12-4. Letterheads
Copyright Yaakov Levinson, Ann M. Coulston, Jeanetta Davis, and Dayle Hayes. Reprinted with permission.

Letters of reference or introduction can lend credibility to you and your services. They are most effective when written by someone who knows your recent work but is also objective – perhaps a satisfied client or the head of clinical services. Such letters may be included with résumés to introduce yourself to potential clients or to offer new programs to established markets. They document your success with past ventures.

Use of a trade name to identify a specific program, event, activity, or business helps you and others differentiate between programs and increases recognition in the minds of your target market. If you are in business for yourself, choose a name that is descriptive and easy to remember. You can use your personal name; a straightforward name, such as Baltimore Nutrition Services; or a catchy name, like Nutrition Thyme for a culinary class on good nutrition.

It is important to use your name and RD or DTR credential on all promotional materials. Go beyond the generic title Dietetics Department, and begin seeking recognition for yourself and others in your department.

Public speaking is a promotional opportunity of great value to dietitians. The public is willing and eager to hear information and guidance about nutrition. Speaking or giving workshops to community, church, school, and professional groups is an effective way to teach, influence, and motivate others, and to introduce a product or service. A good way to get your name known around town is to speak before some of your key target audiences, such as physicians or senior citizens. But public speaking, like media interviewing, requires special skills and training. (For more information, see Chapter 35.)

Writing is a significant way for a dietitian to reach a particular audience with pertinent information and at the same time enhance credibility and increase name awareness. Assume, for example, that you would like to counsel some of the employees at a large manufacturing corporation in town. One way to reach them might be through their employee newsletter. To find out, contact the newsletter's editor and suggest a column on nutrition or a guest article on one of today's hot topics. You could make the same suggestion to a local newspaper editor. By positioning yourself as a civic-minded expert on nutrition, you will again enhance your position and the possibilities for more work in your chosen field. Publishing articles in professional journals and newsletters is another way to establish yourself. The visibility and credibility gained from these experiences will reinforce your name and status in the eyes of peers and present and potential clients.

GRAPHIC AND PRINT MATERIAL

Logos are pictorial symbols or names in stylized letters that stand for a product, service, event, or business. A logo can add visual interest and create a distinctive professional identity. It is used to improve audience recall or recognition by providing a cohesive, consistent look to all printed materials.

Use of your logo provides you with trademark rights in the United States. Federal registration, although not mandatory, is evidence of your exclusive right to use the logo. You can formally document your claim to your logo by registering it with the U.S. Patent and Trademark Office, Washington, DC 20231. A logo that is used on a product, such as food or a software program, can be registered as a trademark; if a logo is used for a service, such as nutrition counseling, it can be registered as a service mark. A logo will not be registered if another logo design in the same basic category (such as health associations) is too similar. It is not difficult to register a logo. An application must be filed along with a fee and samples of the logo. A lawyer can conduct a trademark search and consult on the filing of the application. You can also request an application form and information booklet from the Patent and Trademark Office. It is the responsibility of the owner to defend the right to the logo and to pay for any legal action. Some sample logos are shown in Figure 12-3.

Brochures are used to describe and promote your products, services, and programs. Brochures may be handed out at speaking engagements, included in materials given to clients, mailed to target markets or the press, or left in waiting rooms. Brochures are surrogates of you and your services. They should be attractive, well written, and easy to read. A public relations expert might help you improve the wording; a graphic artist, the presentation. It is usually worth the extra money to enhance the brochure's appearance with color, a photo or drawing, and good-quality paper, since the quality of your work will be judged by the quality of your promotion. The importance of a professional look in all communications cannot be overstressed. (See Chapter 29 for specific tips on how to write a brochure.)

Portfolios are visual presentations of the services you offer. They may be simple, such as a three-ring binder with color photos of your catering selections or samples of creative projects completed for clients, or sophisticated, such as a professionally created flip chart with graphs and sales projections. Using a portfolio in interviews helps potential clients better understand and visualize your services.

Proposals are comprehensive promotional and sales tools used to interest a client, administrator, or financial backer in your service or new program. Proposals can range from a simple one-page typewritten information sheet to a slide show or tasting session accompanied by a typeset, bound, multipage document – the higher the stakes, the more elaborate the presentation. Proposals should be only long enough to interest the potential client and make the sale. Care should be exercised to ensure that good ideas and explanations are not so detailed that clients can carry out the projects without you. (See Chapter 34 for more information on proposals.)

Posters and signs are potentially effective promotion tools, especially when used in hallways, storefronts, or cafeterias where the target market must pass them several times each day. They generally are not as effective in drawing business when placed randomly in public places, although libraries, supermarkets, and local businesses are often willing to accommodate you with space in their windows or on their bulletin boards.

Posters should be designed to be eye-catching, to provide pertinent information (date, place, time), and, most important, to entice the reader to respond or to attend the program. A phone number or tear-off mail-in card may be included for those who want more information.

Banners draw attention and create name recognition. They create a festive mood and are a great promotional tool for large areas where crowds gather. They can be used at the finish line of a fun run, in a lobby during a wellness festival, or over the cafeteria door to promote a new line of light and natural foods, for example. Banners can be made with paper and paint; however, they can be reused many times if they are made from cloth. Lettering, layout, and graphics all demand careful attention, perhaps from a graphics arts professional. Remember that a program is often prejudged by the quality of the items that promote it.

OTHER AUDIOVISUAL AIDS

Other audiovisual aids that can be used for promotional as well as educational purposes include slides and slide tapes, multi-image slide shows, videotapes, and multimedia presentations. For instance, if you take a booth at a local health fair to promote your coordinated exercise and nutrition program, a five-minute videotape that automatically repeats would be a good way to stop traffic on the aisle. If you are attempting to sell your kitchen-design skills to a new client, a slide show might be the most impressive way to present what you have done in the past.

Computer graphics can enhance many forms of visual promotion. They need not be elaborate. You might use a graphics imaging program on your personal computer to give a simple flyer a more professional appearance. Another program could produce colorful bar and pie charts for your sales presentation. You might hire a computer graphics house to create impressive three-dimensional effects for the title of your videotape. Computer-generated slides are an inexpensive way to add a graphic element and color to a slide presentation and can be purchased from most slide houses. Computers can save you time and money in creating visuals, and computer graphics used appropriately can help convey a high-tech, up-to-the-minute image.

Giveaways, such as T-shirts, clipboards, notebooks, mugs, bumper stickers, gym bags, sweatbands, posters, and refrigerator magnets with program or company names or logos are popular promotion items. The more useful and practical an item is, the more it will be used and the more the name or logo will be displayed. Such items are sometimes sold as fund raisers rather than given away.

Promotion is essential for every dietitian in carrying out marketing plans. But beyond that, it is an exciting challenge to your initiative and creativity.

References

1. *Promotion: Solving the Puzzle.* Arlington, VA: Small Business Video Library; 1990.

2. Caples J. *Tested Advertising Methods.* Englewood Cliffs, NJ: Prentice-Hall; 1974.

3. Rapp S, Collins T. *The Great Marketing Turnaround.* Englewood Cliffs, NJ: Prentice-Hall; 1990.

Bibliography

Public Relations

Harris T. *Choosing and Working with Your Public Relations Firm.* Lincolnwood, IL: NTC Business Books; 1992.

Lant J. *The Unabashed Self-Promoter's Guide: What Every Man, Woman, Child, and Organization in America Needs to Know About Getting Ahead by Exploiting the Media.* New York, NY: JLA Publications; 1980.

Saffir L, Tarrant J. *Power Public Relations.* Lincolnwood, IL: NTC Business Books; 1993.

Advertising

Business Publication Advertising Source. Wilmette, IL: Standard Rate & Data Service. Published monthly.

Caples J. *Tested Advertising Methods.* Englewood Cliffs, NJ: Prentice-Hall; 1974.

Consumer Publication Advertising Source. Wilmette, IL: Standard Rate & Data Service. Published monthly.

Gale Directory of Publications and Broadcast Media. Detroit, MI: Gale Research. Published yearly. Also on software.

Rapp S, Collins T. *The Great Marketing Turnaround.* Englewood Cliffs, NJ: Prentice-Hall; 1990.

Direct Mail

Burnett E. *The Complete Direct Mail List Book.* Englewood Cliffs, NJ: Prentice-Hall; 1988.

Nash E. *Direct Marketing Strategy, Planning & Execution.* New York, NY: McGraw-Hill; 1984.

Simon J. *How to Start and Operate a Mail-Order Business.* 5th ed. New York, NY: McGraw-Hill; 1993

Stone R. *Successful Direct Mail Methods.* Chicago, IL: Crain Publishing Co.; 1975.

Trade Shows

Miller S. *How to Get the Most out of Trade Shows.* Lincolnwood, IL: NTC Business Books; 1992.

Trade Shows and Professional Exhibits Directory. Detroit, MI: Gale Research. Published yearly.

International Exhibitors Association, 5103-B Backlick Road, Annadale, VA 22003, 703-941-3725.

Case Study: **WRITING A NEWSPAPER COLUMN TO BUILD YOUR IMAGE**

Celia Topping, MNS, RD, Vice President of Clinical Services, NutriSmart, Inc., Rochester, New York

As an owner of a health education and promotion corporation, I sought ways to provide visibility for my company. Since September 1991, I have written a biweekly newspaper column called "Nutrition Know-How" in the Rochester, New York, Gannett newspapers. The column has successfully helped me to:

- Provide a community service

- Reinforce the role of the RD as the nutrition expert

- Increase readers' food and nutrition awareness

- Illustrate my expertise and knowledge

- Enhance the visibility and image of my company

As a result of the column, other reporters often contact me for comments on nutrition topics, which provides further opportunities for media visibility.

GETTING STARTED

Do Your Homework!

- Become familiar with local newspapers, reporters, and their beats.

- First contact the paper with the greatest potential. Keep trying if the first isn't interested.

- Know your competition. Generally, editors prefer local sources.

- Consider targeting the health, food, or lifestyle editor. The health column may offer the widest readership.

- Develop and nurture a good working relationship with the editors. Put them on your mailing list, invite them to district nutrition seminars, send monthly clippings and nutrition notes, and send "I liked your article on..." letters.

- Be current. Be sure you are receiving press releases, new product information, news clippings, and health news. In addition to the lay press, I use a computer information service.

Showcase Your Style

- Prepare three sample columns on timely, seasonal topics. Make them sizzle. Pass them by a colleague for review.

- List ten other potential topics to show your creativity and range.

- I opted for the question-and-answer format, which seems more personal and connected with the reader.

Do Lunch

- Over lunch, dialogue with your prospective editor.

- Explain why the editor's audience would be interested in your column. Don't overly flatter the editor or ask favors.

- Meet the editor's needs, not your needs.

- Suggest a trial period.

- Find out about the editor's budget. Don't be afraid to ask for a fee, but don't be surprised if you're not offered more than $25 to $50 per column, unless you have a well-known reputation. Payment may or may not be offered. Knowing there was no budget, I volunteered to write a column, but requested that a trailer listing my company and credentials be included with each column. The column provides tremendous visibility. That kind of advertising is very expensive. However, when asked to write a feature article for the paper, I request and receive payment.

WRITING THE COLUMN

Content

- Choose the topic from the reader's perspective. Then think of the reader as you write. This has been the most valuable tip for me to keep in mind.

- Translate the science of nutrition into real-life activities or behaviors. I write about the art of healthy eating, such as how to select from a school cafeteria menu or pack a picnic cooler.

- Be practical. I often include toll-free 800 numbers, such as the USDA Food and Poultry Hotline or the NCND Consumer Nutrition Hotline, or recommend a free brochure.

- Use bullets to ensure the information is easy to scan.

- Be accurate. I often check with a product's corporate public relations department, the USDA, and trade associations, and try to include quotes with my sources' names to add interest and even more credibility.

- Stress the positive — the do's, not the don'ts.

- Make the column easy-to-read, conversational, and entertaining as well as informative. For example, I related the origins of granola cereal to a health movement over 100 years ago that had a local connection. I also reviewed the nutritional value of all the local pizza and frozen yogurt establishments. Such an approach adds to the uniqueness and appeal of the column.

Procedures

- Encourage readers' questions, but be prepared to create your own questions. In my column, the questions are typeset in bold and end with the sender's initials and the town in which he or she resides.

- Answer two or three questions per column, choosing one of the topics for expanded treatment.

- Make every word count. Keep your column tight and bright, brief and easy-to-understand. Don't be afraid to use bullets.

- Keep the column to the editor's specified length. My column is 400 to 450 words. My editor rarely changes my column, except to delete a line or two if it runs too long.

- End each column with a trailer about who you are. My trailer reads: *Celia Topping, a registered dietitian, is Vice President of Clinical Services for NutriSmart, Inc.,* a food and nutrition consulting firm in Rochester. Her column runs every other week.

Newspaper column written by dietitian

A royal pain responds to a simple treatment

- With each column appears: *Got a question? Get your nutrition answers by writing to Celia Topping, c/o Eating In, 55 Exchange Blvd., Rochester, NY 14614.*

- Submit two or three suggested titles for each column, and let the editor make the final selection or contribute her own. This gives the editor some control and input and usually works well.

- Respect deadlines. I set my deadline 24 hours ahead of what is required.

- Check regularly with the editor. Be prepared with fresh ideas and suggestions.

Postscripts

- I ask that questions be sent to me in care of the newspaper, rather than to my own business address, so my editor knows how popular the column is.

- I send my column by modem directly to the newspaper so it is automatically on their computers. As backup, I send a hard copy in the mail.

- Since I volunteer to write the columns for no charge, the paper does not own them. Therefore, I can offer the same columns, or modified columns, to another smaller newspaper if I choose. Discuss this with your editor. Be alert for publication dates so columns do not appear simultaneously.

- Inquire about liability. In my case, the newspaper is responsible for what appears in print. Insurance for writers is available, but costly. Professional liability insurance does not usually cover writing.

- Potentially, any column can be syndicated, which means that other newspapers may reprint the column, usually for a fee to you or to the service that represents your column, which will then pay you.

SUMMARY

Writing a newspaper column in your local market helps establish your reputation and credibility with your readers. If you are published in regional or national publications, it can open the door for speaking engagements and promote sales of your products. If you don't mind deadlines and have a knack for communicating through the written word, consider writing a newspaper column.

Pursuing the Potential of the Media

Mary Lee Chin, MS, RD, Denver, and Joan Horbiak, MS, RD, Philadelphia, Media Consultants

Themes prospects that you or a member of your organization will be called upon for an interview – print or electronic – are skyrocketing. We live in a media age, surrounded by 11,500 newspapers, a quarter billion billboards, and 162 million television sets and radios. And rarely a day goes by without nutrition making front-page news. As the public's interest in nutrition grows, the media's search for dietitians with stories and reports also grows. According to Jane Kirby, the food editor of *Glamour* magazine, "We're always on the lookout for new nutrition experts and resources. We just don't want to quote the same people all the time." You might think that nutrition experts would be in frequent contact with someone like Jane. Instead, Jane and a wide variety of reporters and producers agree, "We need to see more dietitians with specific areas of expertise on our Rolodexes." The media want to talk to you! But don't wait for the media to come knocking at your door. The success stories will come from dietitians who create rather than wait for media opportunities. The keys are to learn how the media work, what they want, and when they want it, and to build media relationships. Learning the rules of the game can help you meet the Media Age head on and win.

THE RULES OF THE GAME

The rules of the game are based on years of doing, not theory. The rules are simple and may sound like common sense. But according to media producers, reporters, editors, and correspondents, there is a big difference between common sense and common practice when interviewing health professionals!

Know the Types of Media

Your press strategies must take into account the kinds of media available and the diverse ways in which different media organizations formulate news stories. Be prepared to capitalize on the opportunities offered by these differences:

- Local television stations offer news shows with special health reports and community affairs programs.

- Community cable stations can offer local news programming, community access channels, and public affairs programming.

- Public affairs television stations can provide local news programming as well as a diverse mix of locally produced public affairs programming.

- Newspapers have various beat reporters covering specialized issues for the hard news section, plus business, food, lifestyle, consumer, environment, and style sections offering soft news.

Most issues can be marketed from a variety of angles, or points of view. For example, a story could be covered as a business topic, a lifestyle matter, a consumer concern, a legal question, an editorial opinion, or a local or national issue, depending on how it is framed. You may want to shop around for a reporter who has a good understanding of your issue. In the end, an editor or news director will make the final decision on who covers your story for the media outlet. However, if you are actively promoting a story, as opposed to just reacting to a reporter's request for information, you are in a better position to approach a specific reporter with your idea.

Be sure your information is in a format suited to the medium you've selected. Types of news formats include hard news, soft news, face-to-face interviews, panel discussions, and news conferences. Understanding the media will enable you to provide information in the format that best meets each medium's needs.

Determine whether your story is hard or soft news. *Hard news* follows the format of who, what, where, when and how. Such news is timely and affects a great number of people.

Soft news is treated as a feature story as long as it has value. Such information is less urgent, but must still have a "news hook" related to a timely topic. You may suggest a feature story by writing or phoning an editor and presenting a summary that will grab attention and demonstrate the significance of the story. Or you may provide the editor with a backgrounder as a feature sample. You must maintain exclusivity when pitching a soft news feature.

Know What's Newsworthy

The key to getting positive coverage from the media is to have a story that is really newsworthy and to tell the media about it. Every hour of every day the media need to fill "news holes" with stories. Nanci Hellmich, the health reporter for *USA Today*, points out that dietitians need to look at what they do with a new perspective. "I'm always looking for the new and interesting, but 'new' can simply mean a different twist on an old idea," she explains. "Dietitians work with creative approaches to what may seem like old, worn-out topics such as weight reduction, and they don't even recognize it. They routinely deal with the angst that we want to capture and write about." Fresh tips and tactics you have developed for your patients will also be new and beneficial for the public.

The media are interested in what you are doing, and they are even more interested in what you are seeing. Dietitians are in a unique position to spot and evaluate emerging trends, such as changes in the foods people eat and buy. Also breaking nutrition news can have immediate impact: the Alar scare, a hurricane's effect on water safety, or a new study on cholesterol, for example. The media cannot always wait until top health authorities issue recommendations. Because you are a nutrition expert, your rapid response to breaking news is newsworthy. The media are hungry for stories filled with energy, grace, and humor. To appeal to the media, a good story should be both newsworthy and entertaining. Also keep in mind that simplicity counts more than wisdom. If you pitch a story in the style of a professional journal article, it will be rejected. Finally, a story must be timely and of current interest. Stories that follow a trend or buck a current way of thinking are attention getting.

Become a Media Tracker

Keep your eyes and ears open and your antennae out. New ideas and policies are often reported in small in-house publications or presented in speeches and academic papers to limited audiences. Professional journals, newsletters, magazines, and articles are also launching pads for new developments or ideas. Stay in touch by subscribing to nutrition journals and newsletters. Beat reporters, especially health reporters, subscribe to the *New England Journal of Medicine* and *Science* magazine.

Monitor the popular press to assess what is important to the public. "Piggyback" and focus your story on what is happening locally. Read your local newspaper and at least one national newspaper daily, such as *USA Today*, the *Wall Street Journal*, the *New York Times*, or the *Los Angeles Times*.

Become a television media monitor. Television news follows and reports on consumer trends. If an issue is in the national news, think about its local impact. Local news outlets are always looking for sidebars to national stories. The trick is to stay ahead of your local station on story ideas.

Some of your best press coverage will come from your watching, listening, and reading the media and applying the principles of other stories to your issues.

Develop a News Hook

A newsworthy story should have an interesting "news hook," or "peg." Hooks can be humorous, seasonal, of human interest, or scientific, but they must also be practical. Delia Hammock, the director and editor of the diet and fitness section of *Good Housekeeping* magazine emphasizes, "I want dietitians to bowl my readers over with practicality and positive messages. I'm tired of health professionals who take the joy out of eating." Can the reader or the listener use your information? Talk about lifestyle changes, not diets. In the past, magazines could present a different diet every month. Today, readership polls show that diets are out and practical tips, recipes, and how-to's are in.

Hammock identifies three key ingredients every successful story must include:

- Taste – taste still outranks nutrition in food choices

- Fast and fit – eating on the run and fast nutrition are key

- Value – gourmet and high-end food take a back seat to value meals, especially during these tough economic times

Put a "face" in your story. Articles in most daily newspapers describe national and local problems in human terms. To humanize a story, the lead paragraph often presents a victim or a beneficiary. Personal stories are also essential elements in television and radio news stories.

Any approach to the media that does not have a good story to tell is not likely to be of much interest to the reporters.

Know Your Audience

Once you have developed your story, it's time to shape your examples to meet the needs of your audience. Who are you going to reach with your information? What do you know about them? Nothing angers the media more than a "one size fits all" approach. Each publication, newspaper, and television or radio station has a different focus and needs. As Jane Kirby of *Glamour* notes, "If you're talking about sodium, my readers want to hear about weight gain, puffiness, and PMS, not hypertension. Hypertension may work for *Family Circle*, but not *Glamour*. I like a dietitian who has examples that are right for my readers." Glenn Ruppa of CNBC adds, "Nothing is more annoying than a guest who doesn't understand our audience."

Do your homework – analyze and tailor the details of your story to meet the needs and interests of your medium's audience. And never pitch a story or give an interview without first reading the publication or watching or listening to the show. Remember, amateurs think of the story while professionals think of the audience.

Keep It Simple!

An important fact to remember when giving interviews is that people don't remember much. One classic research study showed that audiences will forget 75 percent or more of what you say in 24 hours or less.

To be most effective, develop a clear, simple speaking style. Plan to express one quality message. Have no more than two or three key points to convey. Write them down. Take out the jargon. Use conversational language and put some zip into your delivery. Work to make your material simple, direct, fresh, quotable, and easy to understand.

If you really want to make your point, you had better make it short, and you had better make it simple. In fact, complex messages are trashed by the media. Dr. David Hnida, the medical correspondent for NBC Television News, frankly points out, "Viewers today want extremely practical information – it needs to be of service in their lives. Stories or reports that are presented as too complicated or research-oriented, I just blow off!" And Carolyn O'Neil of CNN News adds, "It's important not to come off as the ivory-tower expert. The RD's strength is the ability to relate to the public as a knowledgeable friend, to share and understand the problems, and to give advice and information on a personal level."

And "just say no" to nutritionese. The use of technical words causes confusion. The truth is that most people aren't as comfortable with science as we are. We speak of the RDAs and RDIs. What does this mean to average women struggling through the supermarket jungle? Mention antioxidants, and they'll reach for the dictionary. Say biotechnology, and they think artificial, manufactured, or engineered. People shop for food, not nutrients, and they crave easy-to-digest information. The fastest way to put your audience to sleep is to speak in a language they don't understand. Be concise. Crystallize your thoughts into a few hard-hitting, quotable sentences. Don't be an information dump. With the media, less is more.

Make Your Messages Snap, Crackle, and Pop

If you want your words to have impact, give your audience something they can see. People remember 50 percent more of what they see *and* hear than what they hear only. Marty Young of CNN insists, "If you can't tell a story with pictures, then it won't work for television."

You can also paint a picture with words. For example, describe a serving of meat as the size of a deck of cards, rather than saying it weighs three ounces. Draw attention to the flavor and texture delights of a vegetable medley rather than its relative fiber content. Don't bore your audience with the statistic that 37 percent of the average American's calories come from fat. Shock them with the fact that a client consumes the equivalent of a can of Crisco per week!

Don't overlook the power of sound. Sizzle burgers, stir-fry seafood, chop vegetables, blend drinks, pop corn, crack eggs, and whip egg whites.

And remember, you are your own best visual aid in interviews. Look good and use winning moves to accent your message. Pound your fists, point your fingers, lean forward, raise your eyebrows, and smile like the actors in toothpaste commercials! But please don't rock back and forth – such movement is distracting and a sign of nervousness. Molly Gee, the nutrition reporter for KTRK TV in Houston advises, "Be animated, energetic, and believable. I hate entertaining talking heads. In this day of the remote control, people zap you by. Use a visual to make the story come alive."

Sound, visual images, and action are the spices that add pizzazz to your messages.

Practice the Pleasure Principle

People have received more than the recommended allowance of bad news about food. According to members of the media, consumers are fed up and ready to throw in their napkins. Eating isn't fun anymore! This trend is supported by a 1993 ADA Gallup survey which revealed that many people frequently just don't find eating pleasurable. Keep in mind the Food Marketing Institute's 1994 survey, in which nine out of ten shoppers reported that taste was the most important factor when they shopped for food.

When developing a story or being interviewed, your job is to bring back the joy of eating. When giving advice, don't insist on perfection. Take words like *never, must, always, should,* and *shouldn't* out of your vocabulary.

Build Good Media Relations

Review past media coverage of the issues you target. Spend some time in the public library or the reference room of your local newspaper. Review how the national and local media have covered the story. "Be familiar with the publication," insists Marti Meitus, the food editor of the *Denver Rocky Mountain News.* "It's irritating," she continues, "to get a pitch from someone who obviously has not read the paper, hasn't a clue about the objective of the section, and offers me a story that I wrote about last week."

Find out if the local media have covered your topic. If so, track bylines to see who wrote the articles. If not, suggest stories when you approach reporters with ideas. And find a local angle that will make local readers more interested.

Select the media that will best reach your audience. If your information is aimed at a broad audience, select television, daily or weekly newspapers, or popular radio. For targeted audiences, contact specialty journals, trade publications, or special sections of the newspaper. If your sphere of influence is local, select local media. If it is statewide, select regional media. Community-based, African-American, Asian-American, and Hispanic newspapers, radio, and television can be used to reach ethnic markets. If your influence is national in scope, select a national publication, wire service, or broadcast medium.

Know Lead Times

Be sure your information is timely and meets the deadline of the selected medium. For newspapers and television, check with the receptionist who answers the phone to find out deadline times. Do not call during the few hours before deadline.

Think ahead when working with magazines. Most magazines work six months in advance. "Don't pitch a story on ice cream in August. We're working on Christmas cookies," informs Jane Kirby, the food editor of *Glamour.*

Pitch the Media: Proactive Story Placement

The media are constantly on the look-out for good stories and credible people to quote. If you want to get their attention, send a notched Rolodex card with your name and area of expertise in bold letters across the top. Members of the media live by their Rolodexes.

Success in pitching stories with local media depends upon building strong relationships with reporters and editors. Assignment editors and city editors usually have the final word on doing a story. If you have cultivated a reporter who can make a strong pitch to the editor in favor of your story, success is more likely.

Briefly outline your story, starting with a strong attention-getting lead and supporting bullet points. Send it to the appropriate print reporter or assignment editor. Follow up with a telephone call a few days later. Identify yourself and ask if it is a good time to talk or if you can make arrangements to contact them at a more convenient time. Make sure you have all your information at hand, know what you are going to say, and get to the point quickly. Busy reporters will appreciate your succinctness.

Figure 13-1. Contacting Broadcast Media

FORMAT	CONTACT	LEAD TIME
Television		
News		
studio interview	Associate Producer Assignment Editor	6 weeks - 2 months
on location in a city	Assignment Editor	48 - 72 hours a.m. reminder
on location in a small town	Special Representative	5 days - 48 hours reminder call
Women's Programs	Associate Producer	6 weeks - 2 months
Talk Shows	Associate Producer	6 weeks - 2 months
Consumer Interest Spots	Associate Producer	6 weeks - 2 months
Public Service Announcements (PSAs)	Director of Public Service or Community Affairs	1 month
Radio		
News		
studio interview	Program Director	6 weeks
events announcement	Program Director	2 - 3 weeks mail 1 - 2 week call 2 - 3 days reminder
Talk Shows	Show Host or Producer	1 month - 6 weeks
Call-In Shows	Show Host or Producer	1 month - 6 weeks
Public Affairs Programs	Show Host or Producer	1 month - 6 weeks
Public Service Announcements (PSAs) events announcement	Director of Public Service or Community Affairs	2 - 3 weeks

If you do not know which reporter to contact, send your story idea to the newspaper's city desk or the television station's assignment editor. For radio, direct your letter to the producer of the show you are targeting. Reporters are inundated with faxes. Skip this avenue of approach unless you have already spoken with a reporter who has asked you to fax the information. Generally, do not use the phone to make your first contact with a reporter unless you have a breaking news story.

When a reporter expresses interest, send your information, making sure to spell names and addresses correctly. Allow time for the information to arrive. Then follow up with a phone call to arrange the interview and the story.

When reporters express no interest in your story, thank them for their time and ask if they would be interested in being contacted in the future about significant nutrition stories.

If a reporter is vague about doing your story and asks you to call back later, make arrangements to call back once. If the reporter is still vague, express polite thanks and say that you plan to take the story to another media outlet. If it is a good story, this may be just enough to heighten the reporter's interest in taking action.

Don't be discouraged by initial rejection of story ideas. Persistence and, above all, good stories pay off. Work to establish personal contacts with the journalists who are most likely to place your stories. Some information that will be useful in selecting and contacting broadcast and print media is presented in Figures 13-1 and 13-2.

Figure 13-2. Contacting Print Media

FORMAT	CONTACT	LEAD TIME
Newspapers		
Dailies		
General release	Editor, Feature Editor or a specific editor, i.e., Food, Fitness, Lifestyle, Health, Science, Medical, etc.	1 month
Holiday release	"	2 months
Weeklies		
General release	"	6 weeks
Holiday release	"	8 - 10 weeks
Consumer Magazines		
General release	"	6 months
Holiday release	"	7 - 8 months
Trade Publications		
Small Publications		
General release	"	3 months
Large Publications		
General release	"	4 - 6 months

MAINTAINING GOOD PRESS RELATIONS

Understand how the media work. Paper overload, telephone tag, and breaking news events are all the daily realities of a reporter's life.

Never ask to have a story read or sent to you for approval before publication.

After a story is completed, leave a short message or send a note letting the reporter know the positive response you have received to the story. This is not a thank-you note, but a "job-well-done" note. "Send love letters to us when we do a good job. Most of the time we get attack letters from readers when they don't like what we wrote," says Delia Hammock of *Good Housekeeping* magazine. Also keep in touch with the media, and not just when you want something.

The most successful press coverage does not just happen. Know what you want the coverage to be, and work with reporters so they will understand your position. In the end, the article or newscast will be the responsibility of the reporter. Unless you are a journalist, you will not be able to write the article, headline, or script, but, the more you know about what you want, the better your chances of achieving it.

RELAX, HAVE FUN, AND ENJOY

We've saved the most important advice for the last. That is, relax and enjoy yourself. And please don't take things personally. Once, after I stayed up all night making Healthy Halloween Treats for the five o'clock news, my story was cut for a segment on Spam. Anything goes!

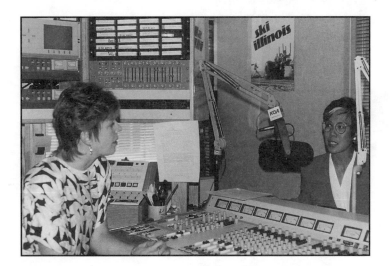

Dietitian Being Interviewed

You will see a return on the energy and resources you expend in your media effort. A media appearance confers a professional credibility that advertising cannot buy. More importantly, it is your opportunity to touch and change the lives of hundreds, or even thousands, of people with sound, credible, useful, and interesting nutrition news.

See working with the media as an exciting challenge. And even if you pitch a story and it doesn't get picked up, you will learn something that you can use the next time. You have nothing to lose and everything to gain.

Marketing and Business Ethics

Mindy G. Hermann, MBA, RD, President, Hermann Communications, Inc., Mount Kisco, New York

Recent growth in the visibility of and respect for dietitians has opened up tremendous opportunities in the business world. It is no longer unusual for dietitians to work in public relations firms, food companies, Fortune 500 corporations, and entrepreneurial ventures. Additionally, more and more dietitians consult for companies that market nutrition-related products or services. Yet as these and other nutrition-business links continue to strengthen, dietitians will be forced to make more decisions regarding the ethics of their affiliations with business and its use of marketing.

One school of thought holds that medical and health-care fields cannot be both professions and businesses since the morals and economics of the two appear to be incompatible (1). A fundamental moral tenet of health care is to care for the masses. In fact, the mission of The American Dietetic Association (ADA) includes "the promotion of optimal health and nutritional status of the population" (2). However, once financial considerations enter into health-care delivery, the public may no longer able to receive consistent information or levels of care; affordability, rather than quality, may become a major influence on health-care decisions.

In marketing a product or service to the public, it is imperative that the dietetic professional represent the facts accurately and fairly. The professional must avoid conflicts of interest, especially of creating the impression that a personal opinion is objective and free from outside influences when in fact there is potential bias. This can occur when a dietetics professional works for or owns a company, or in some other way would benefit from downgrading the competition or promoting a product.

It is common today for companies to want to hire dietitians to represent them. The practitioner's credibility can lend support to the claims made by the product's marketing team. The ethical concern arises when the practitioner's credibility is used to bolster an otherwise lacking product or service.

When articles or books are written, credit should be given to the original sources of quotes and information. Copyrighted materials (videos, booklets, educational materials, and so on) should not be reprinted without the copyright holder's (publisher's or author's) consent.

To assist in ethical decision making, many health-care professions, including dietetics, have developed codes of ethics, the principles of which can and should be used to make business decisions.

PERSONAL AND PROFESSIONAL ETHICS

The following selected principles from the "Code of Ethics for the Profession of Dietetics" are particularly relevant for dietitians and diet technicians in business (3):

1. *The dietetic practitioner provides professional services with objectivity and with respect for the unique needs and values of individuals.*

The dietitian is called on to be client-oriented instead of self-oriented.

Adapted from Hermann M, Ethics in the business of nutrition, Topics in Clinical Nutrition, 7:3; 1-5, with permission of Aspen Publishers, Inc., © 1992.

4. *The dietetic practitioner conducts herself/himself with honesty, integrity, and fairness.*

This professional standard should take precedence over business practice and behavior; if the two are in conflict, ADA's standard should be held in higher regard.

5. *The dietetic practitioner remains free of conflict of interest while fulfilling the objectives and maintaining the integrity of the dietetic profession.*

Conflict of interest is serious enough to warrant its own section in ADA's procedure manual.

10. *The dietetic practitioner provides sufficient information to enable clients to make their own informed decisions.*

This includes full disclosure of the benefits, risks, and cost of service, treatment, or products.

12. *The dietetic practitioner promotes or endorses products in a manner that is neither false nor misleading.*

Once again, the professional standard supersedes business policy.

13. *The dietetic practitioner permits use of her/his name for the purpose of certifying that dietetic services have been rendered only if she/he has provided or supervised the provision of those services.*

This clause recognizes the value to business of being affiliated with a credentialed practitioner with the requisite education and assurance of competence.

16. *The dietetic practitioner makes all reasonable effort to avoid bias in any kind of professional evaluation.*

This standard requires that a practitioner base opinions on valid research and objective reasoning.

CAN YOU CONSULT FOR A COMPANY AND REMAIN UNBIASED?

The following hypothetical situation offers one example of how ADA's Code of Ethics can be used to make business decisions about a nutrition product:

Dietitian 1 is approached by Company W to speak at a conference sponsored by Company W and to serve on its medical advisory board. Company W also plans to use Dietitian 1's name in its publications and in a listing on its letterhead of advisory board members. Dietitian 1's acceptance of this offer will constitute an implied endorsement of Company W's product (Product W).

According to the Code of Ethics, Dietitian 1 should be able to (1) avoid conflict of interest between Product W and her existing work, (2) disclose any implied or explicit endorsement, and (3) remain neutral in her present and future decisions, evaluations, or actions regarding Product W and its competitors. The principles mentioned earlier from the Code of Ethics can help Dietitian 1 to make a sound decision regarding whether or not to affiliate with Company W.

If Dietitian 1 decides to work with Company W, she can remain ethical by being totally objective and honest when asked to render a professional opinion on the category of products to which Product W belongs, for example, predigested enteral formulas or high-fiber cereals, or on specific products. Be careful when you are choosing your alliances because they will reflect on your clinical and professional judgment.

CAN YOU BE A SPOKESPERSON FOR A FOOD COMPANY THAT SELLS A VARIETY OF FOODS — SOME LOW-FAT AND OTHERS NOT?

A second scenario involves Company X, the manufacturer of a line of luncheon meats (Product X), some of which are relatively low in fat and others of which are quite high in fat. Dietitian 2 is approached to act as Product X's spokesperson, representing Product X to the media and to other dietitians. Dietitian 2 feels that all aspects of this potential business arrangement adhere to the Code of Ethics. However, he has reservations about promoting luncheon meats to his colleagues, even though he subscribes to the maxim that foods are neither good nor bad.

In making his decision, Dietitian 2 must realize that his reputation will be closely aligned with all of Company X's products unless he clearly promotes only the lower-fat items, which could be the case. Then he must decide whether Product X's message can fit into his concept of a healthy diet and take the job, or whether the message is false or misleading and turn down the job. Again, ADA's ethical principles can facilitate Dietitian 2's decision making.

Other health professions are faced with similar challenges to remain ethical once ties with industry have been forged. The ethical standards of pharmacists, for example, are at risk when drug companies pay pharmacists for research or presentations (4). A heightened awareness of ethics is creating an environment in which pharmacists, physicians, and other medical professionals routinely disclose to colleagues their financial relationships with industry. ADA fully supports this practice. As of January 1992, the *Journal of the American Dietetic Association* requires that authors reveal any financial support of research or other work that is related to a journal article's authorship.

CAN YOU BE EMPLOYED, SERVE ON ADA, AND CONSULT FOR A FOOD COMPANY?

Ethical decisions that affect one's employer or employers are more complex. The most important step is to evaluate who one's employers are and what the potential impact of one's business action is on each of them. Dietitian 3 is a full-time employee of a world-renowned medical center and also serves on several important ADA committees. Company Y, whose products are used by the medical center, invites Dietitian 3 to serve on its medical advisory board, receive financial remuneration for consulting time, and have her name appear in Company Y's publications.

In this case, Dietitian 3 has three "employers": the medical center, ADA, and Company Y. The medical center should be approached first for approval. The use of Dietitian 3's affiliation is valuable to Company Y because it lends credibility to Product Y and suggests product endorsement by the medical center. For this reason, Dietitian 3's appropriate ethical action is to first ask her employer for approval. Depending upon the will of the decision makers and their regard for the product, the employer may do one of three things: (1) allow the dietitian to consult and use the employer's name, (2) allow the dietitian to consult but not mention the employer, or (3) refuse to allow the dietitian to consult.

The dietitian should contact ADA next. ADA spells out standards of behavior not only for employees but also for volunteers, officers, committee and council members, and their immediate families. Its conflict of interest statement prohibits a volunteer from disclosing "information relating to the business of the Association that can be used by another entity that does business or seeks to do business with the Association" (5). Dietitian 3 cannot reveal any information about the inner workings or business plans of ADA to Company Y. Furthermore, any mention by Company Y of Dietitian 3's position in ADA must be cleared by ADA.

The primary ethical question pertaining to Company Y is whether Dietitian 3 can work for Company Y while upholding her professional standards and those of the medical center and ADA. The dietitian does that by first gaining permission to work with the company, then by representing her affliations as agreed with the employer and ADA, and by keeping the proprietary information of each business separate and confidential.

CAN YOU REMAIN UNBIASED?

Dietitian 4 works full-time in a public relations firm and does freelance writing outside the scope of her regular job. A magazine asks Dietitian 4 to write an article on fat-free salad dressings. Dietitian 4's full-time employer represents a salad dressing manufacturer (Company Z). The ethically correct decision is to turn down the magazine assignment because of conflict of interest. It is virtually impossible for Dietitian 4 to write an article without the appearance of bias, given her prior relationship with Company Z and her employer's objective to have Company Z's products mentioned in the media. However, in this case, the dietitian can tell the magazine editor about the apparent conflict and let the editor decide whether to go forward, or she can turn down the assignment without mentioning it.

CLIENT CONSIDERATIONS

As illustrated previously, ADA's Code of Ethics spells out guidelines for ethical decision making as it pertains to clients (3). Unfortunately, these guidelines become harder to uphold as economic considerations cause dietitians to run their practices based as much on finances as on services. A recent survey of patients being followed by physicians found that patients considered it unethical for physicians to charge as much as they did for services (6). Dietitians may find it difficult to price their services to be both profitable and fair, since their fees often are not reimbursed by third-party payers and are borne instead by the client. The loser in this ethics-economics tug-of-war is the client.

CONCLUSION

Dietitians can use the Positions and Ethical Code of ADA to help them make decisions regarding the ethics of their professional-business behaviors and practices. Additionally, guidelines and guidance must be culled from one's own standards of conduct and the policies of one's employer. It is helpful to break ethical decision making into at least two steps: (1) determining what one's personal rules of conduct are, and (2) thinking through who will be affected by the decision and how to weigh their interest in it (7).

Dietitians can ask themselves, "What, if any, aspects of this situation might have ethical consequences for me personally, for my superior, for the members of my work group, for my organization, and for society as a whole?" (8)

References

1. Agich GJ. Medicine as business and profession. *Theor Med.* 1990; 11: 311-324.

2. The American Dietetic Association. *Bylaws.* 1990.

3. Code of ethics for the profession of dietetics. *J Am Diet Assoc.* 1988; 88:1592-1596.

4. Zilz DA. Interdependence in pharmacy: risks, rewards, and responsibilities. *Am J Hosp Pharm.* 1990; 47(8):1759-1765.

5. The American Dietetic Association. *Policy and Procedure Manual.* Conflict of interest/general. August 1989.

6. Connelly JE, DalleMura S. Ethical problems in the medical office. *JAMA.* 1988; 259:812-815.

7. Cadbury A. Ethical managers make their own rules. *Harvard Business Review.* 1987; 65(5):69-73.

8. Rice D, Dreilinger C. Rights and wrongs of ethics training. *Training & Development Journal.* 1990; 44:103.

Chapter 15

Negotiating Agreements

Felicia Busch, MPH, RD, and Julie Mattson Ostrow, MS, RD,
Felicia Busch and Associates, St. Paul, Minnesota

Your ability to negotiate may be key to the success or failure of your business or department. In today's business climate, negotiations can and should be conducted so that both parties win. The ultimate goal in the negotiation process is to reach an agreement that is satisfying to all. For many, the idea of negotiating a contract with a potential client may seem intimidating. Actually, it is a skill often used in our daily lives. We negotiate chores with our families, project assignments with co-workers, and entertainment schedules with friends. Entrepreneurial and intrapreneurial dietitians need to develop and practice their negotiation skills to attain the appropriate compensation for their work. To enhance your effectiveness in negotiating, try this eight-step approach.

Step 1: Prepare. Learn all that you can about the company and key contacts before any sales efforts are begun. Read the business section of the newspaper, community business papers and magazines, and research in the library. Find out who your competitors are and how to differentiate your services from what they offer. Determine what has to be done and develop alternatives. Focus on the value that you can bring.

Step 2: Discuss. During the discussion, listen. Listening is a skill you may need to work on because it is often easy to talk too much. Not only is talking too much unprofessional, but it could also lead you into making too many concessions.

Step 3: Signal. Signaling is a method of moving negotiations forward by testing the other side's willingness to modify their position. Asking a potential client to consider a particular option or feature of your service is a signal. For example, you might ask, "If enough employees sign up for the weight-loss class to fill two groups, can we schedule two groups?"

Step 4: Propose. Once your signal is read, it is time to discuss the proposition. Offer a position that has some room for compromise. It might be advantageous to offer several levels of service instead of a fixed proposal. Consider asking for more than you will settle for so you will have items or fees to bargain away. For example, you might say, "We can offer your corporation a group weight-loss program, a healthy lifestyle seminar, individual nutrition consultations for employees with heart disease and diabetes, and healthy food selections for your vending machines and cafeteria. Our most comprehensive plan offers all four services."

Step 5: Respond. Now is the time for you to respond to any new objections. Carefully consider any concession that the other side may offer as an opportunity for compromise. Determine what they really want and what you require in return. Consider options that may be new to the discussion and will better satisfy both parties.

Step 6: Bargain. You may have to bargain to get what you want. Be sure to keep your offer conditional by making comments such as, "If I agree to this, then you agree to . . ."

Step 7: Close. The key to a final agreement is the close. Restate the final decision so that all parties understand what the proposal is. To bring the other party to closure, consider asking, "What will it take for you to come to an agreement?" or

"How soon can we start if we agree today?" or "So if you get . . . and I get . . . , do we have an agreement?"

Step 8: Agree. The goal of every negotiation should be to agree. When an agreement is reached, write it down before anyone leaves.

CONTRACTS

Contracts are one of the tools of a successful businessperson. Today's business environment demands that dietitians use clear and meaningful documents to outline their services. Contracts also form the basis for negotiations.

A contract is an agreement that creates an obligation. To be considered legal, a contract must include these basic parts: an offer and acceptance, consideration of who gets what, parties who are capable of entering into a contract, and subject matter or a purpose that is legal.

While some verbal agreements may be legally enforced, written contracts are far preferable. A written contract may take various forms, ranging from a simple letter of agreement to a detailed formal document drafted by an attorney. A written contract can spell out the terms of your proposed work and help avert misunderstandings. If necessary, a written contract can also be used as evidence in a court of law.

Generally, a letter of agreement is a contract written in simple language that spells out the details of a work proposal. Such agreements may be written on your own company stationery and typically run no longer than three pages. Included at the end of the letter is space for both parties' signatures. See Figure 15-1 for an example of a letter of agreement.

More formal contracts may be required when financial risk is greater, when intellectual property is involved, or when you are working with a large corporation, many different people, or over a long period of time (see Figure 15-2). Since contracts contain more legal language and include many more details, they are best drafted by lawyers. At the very least, you should have an attorney review a contract before you sign it. You should never verbally agree to a contract's provisions if you intend to have your attorney review the contract before you sign it. Voicing premature agreement can create significant misunderstanding if you later decide to renegotiate something.

When writing a letter of agreement or other contract, ask yourself these questions:

1. *Who* is your client? Are you contracting with an individual for one-time services or with a corporation for ongoing work? Who is the key decision maker who will authorize work? Who will own the copyright or legal right to your work?

2. *What* exact services are you to perform? What is needed from your client for you to carry out your work in the manner described? What products are included in the agreement? What can you hope to gain from this work in addition to fees?

Figure 15-1. Letter of Agreement (enlarged in Appendix)

AGREEMENT FOR NUTRITION CONSULTING SERVICES

This document shall serve as a Letter of Agreement between Nutrition Consultants, Inc., 1234 Apple, Saint Paul, Minnesota, and HealthSystems, Inc., 0000 Avenue South, Minneapolis, Minnesota. The contract period is from October 15, 1995 through October 14, 1996.

Nutrition Consultants, Inc., shall be compensated for services in developing a registered dietitian referral system in the amount of $3,500.00. Reimbursable expenses in addition to the fixed fee shall include long-distance telephone calls, photocopying, postage, fax services, mailing lists, incentive awards, and other incidentals directly related to provision of services.

In addition, Nutrition Consultants, Inc., agrees to seek out promotional opportunities for HealthSystems, Inc., to assist in increasing its client base. These activities will focus on RDs, the local media, and corporations. For this ongoing service, Nutrition Consultants, Inc., will be compensated by a monthly retainer of $500.00 for the duration of this agreement.

Requested services outside the scope of this agreement will be billed at the rate of $75.00 per hour. All additional services will require advance authorization from the designated HealthSystems, Inc., representative.

A monthly activity report will be submitted, along with an invoice for direct and other authorized expenses, by the first of each month. Invoices are to be paid by the fifteenth of the month in which they are submitted. Interest in the amount of 8 percent per annum will be added to all late payments.

Nutrition Consultants, Inc., agrees to maintain current registrations, licenses, malpractice insurance, and all other requirements necessary to practice as registered dietitians in the state of Minnesota.

Both Nutrition Consultants, Inc., and HealthSystems, Inc., acknowledge that the relationship entered into by this agreement is that of independent parties and not that of employer and employee. Both parties enter into this temporary relationship for the purpose of affecting the provisions of this Letter of Agreement, and do not deem or construe to create a relationship as agents, employees, or representatives of each other.

Either party may terminate this agreement, with or without cause, at any time upon giving the other party sixty (60) days' written notice.

HealthSystems, Inc.   Nutrition Consultants, Inc.

By_____   By_____

Its_____   Its_____
    Designated Representative   Designated Representative

Date_____   Date_____

Figure 15-2. Formal Contract (enlarged in Appendix)

AGREEMENT BETWEEN
CORPORATE HEALTH-CARE CORPORATION
AND
NUTRITION CONSULTANTS, INC.

THIS AGREEMENT, effective January 1, 1995, between Corporate Health-Care Corporation ("CHC") and Nutrition Consultants, Inc. ("NCI").

WHEREAS, CHC is a for-profit corporation organized and operated for the purposes of developing and marketing alternative health-care delivery systems and related products and services; and

WHEREAS, CHC desires to arrange for the development and implementation of health-promotion programs and NCI are duly registered dietitians and health educators who desire to develop and implement health-promotion programs for CHC;

THEREFORE, in consideration of the mutual covenants herein contained, the parties hereby agree as follows:

SECTION 1. NUTRITION CONSULTANTS, INC., OBLIGATIONS:

1.01. Food for Health Program. NCI shall develop, implement, and maintain the Food for Health Program for CHC. The Food for Health Program shall consist of, but not be limited to: (a) presentations on good nutrition; (b) the development of guidelines for healthy eating; (c) demonstrations of practical and healthy food preparation; and (d) the development of brochures and other literature on the subject of good nutrition. See Attachment A for details.

1.02. Health-Promotion Program Articles and Publications. NCI shall research, develop, and write health-promotion articles for the magazines, brochures, and other written media published by CHC. NCI shall develop and provide health-related scientific data for the magazines, brochures, and other written media published by CHC. The publication of such articles and scientific data shall be subject to the final approval of CHC.

1.03. Media Placements. NCI shall develop, implement, and coordinate media placements for the promotion of the Food for Health Program and other health-promotion programs developed by NCI or CHC. NCI shall also develop, implement, and coordinate media placements concerning general health information as a public service to local communities. NCI shall obtain final approval on all media placements prior to scheduling a media placement or committing CHC in any manner.

1.04. Liability Insurance. NCI shall procure and maintain, at their sole expense, professional liability insurance with remaining coverage satisfactory to CHC. Upon request by CHC, NCI shall provide evidence of insurance coverage. NCI shall notify CHC, in writing, to the attention of the Chief Executive Officer, within ten (10) days of changes in carriers, changes in remaining coverage, or notification to NCI of any claims against, denials of, restriction on, termination of, or changes in NCI professional liability insurance.

1.05. Laws, Regulations, and Licenses. NCI shall maintain all federal, state, and local licenses, permits, and association memberships, without restriction, required to practice as registered dietitians or health educators. NCI shall notify CHC in writing, to the attention of the Chief Executive Officer, within ten (10) days of any suspension, revocation, limitation, qualification, or other restriction on NCI's licenses, permits, and/or association memberships by any state in which NCI is licensed as dietitians, health educators, or other health-care professionals.

SECTION 2. CHC OBLIGATIONS

2.01. Payment for Services. CHC shall reimburse NCI for services rendered under the Agreement ("Contract Fee") an amount equal to thirty-three thousand and six hundred dollars ($33,600) in the contract year January 1, 1995, through December 31, 1996. The contract year thereafter shall be the calendar year from January 1 through December 31. CHC shall pay NCI in monthly payments of two thousand eight hundred ($2,800.00) the first business day of each month beginning with January 1, 1995, made payable to NCI.

2.02. Payment of Out-of-Pocket Expenses. CHC shall reimburse NCI for all reasonable out-of-pocket expenses, including, but not limited to, supplies, subscriptions, educational resources, travel expenses, and mileage that are incurred in connection with the provision of services under this Agreement. Said out-of-pocket expenses shall be limited to $1800.00 per annum for supplies and travel, and to $350.00 per annum for subscriptions and educational resources as determined by the budget. Said out-of-pocket expenses shall not include normal travel and mileage between NCI's place of business and CHC's corporate headquarters.

2.03. Office Space. CHC shall provide adequate work space and support staff to NCI at CHC's corporate headquarters as detailed in Attachment B.

2.04. Copyrights and Trademarks. Any health-promotion data, information, articles, publications, brochures, or programs, and any specific information connected therewith, uniquely developed or implemented by NCI for CHC shall be considered the property of CHC. CHC shall have the rights to all copyrights and trademarks for all uniquely developed health-promotion data, information, articles, publications, and programs, and the specific information connected therewith.

SECTION 3. TERM AND TERMINATION

3.01. Term. The term of this agreement shall commence on January 1, 1995 and shall continue and remain in effect through the remainder of the calendar year 1995, and for each calendar year thereafter until such time as this Agreement is terminated as hereinafter provided.

3.02. Termination. This agreement may be terminated by CHC, with or without cause, or by NCI, with or without cause, upon sixty (60) days written notice to the other party.

SECTION 4. MISCELLANEOUS

4.01. Independent Contractors. The relationship between CHC and NCI is that of independent contractors only and NCI is not an employee or agent of CHC. Nothing contained in this Agreement shall constitute or be construed to be or create a partnership, joint venture, or an association between CHC and NCI, nor shall either party, or its employees, agents, and representatives be considered employees, agents, or representatives of the other party.

4.02. Amendment. Any amendment to this Agreement proposed by CHC at least thirty (30) days prior to the effective date of such amendment is incorporated herein; provided, however, that in the event any change or modification to this Agreement is requested by any State or Federal regulatory authority as a result of a filing of this Agreement with such authority, such change or modification shall be incorporated into this Agreement from the effective date of this Agreement.

4.03. Assignment. CHC shall have the absolute right, in its sole discretion, to assign all or any of its rights or responsibilities hereunder to any corporation that is a subsidiary or affiliate of CHC. In the event of assignment, this Agreement shall be binding upon and inure to the benefit of CHC's successors and assigns. NCI shall not have the right to assign any of their rights without the prior written consent of CHC, which consent shall not be unreasonably withheld.

4.04. No Waiver of Rights. The failure of any party to insist upon the strict observation or performance of any provision of this Agreement or to exercise any right or remedy shall not impair or waive any such right or remedy. Every right and remedy given by this Agreement to the parties may be exercised from time to time and as often as appropriate.

4.05. Entire Agreement. This Agreement is the entire Agreement between the parties. No representations or agreements between the parties, oral or otherwise, has any force or effect.

4.06. Impossibility of Performance. Neither CHC nor NCI shall be deemed to be in default of this Agreement if prevented from performing for reasons beyond its control, including without limitation, governmental laws and regulation, acts of God, wars, and strikes. In such case, the parties shall negotiate in good faith with the goal and intent of preserving this Agreement and the respective rights and obligations of the parties.

4.07. Governing Law. This Agreement shall be construed in accordance with the laws of the state of Minnesota.

IN WITNESS HEREOF, the parties hereto have caused this Agreement to be executed.

CORPORATE HEALTH PLAN CORPORATION
0000 Eagle Drive
St. Paul, Minnesota XXXXX
By _____
Its _____
Date _____

NUTRITION CONSULTANTS, INC.
1234 Apple St.
St. Paul, Minnesota XXXXX
By _____
Its _____
Date _____

3. *When* does the work start? When is the expected completion date of the project? Is there a final deadline or a series of deadline dates prior to completion? When will you be paid?

4. *Where* will meetings be held and services performed? Are travel expenses included in the fee or paid as an additional reimbursable expense?

5. *What* are the client's expectations in this agreement? Can you show the client a sample of your work that is similar to what's expected?

FEES

A contract should also spell out the method in which you will be paid. Two of the most commonly used methods are fixed fee (by the project) and cost per hour or day. (For a detailed explanation of how to determine your fees, see Chapter 21.)

Fixed, or Project, Fee

When charging a fixed fee, you must accurately estimate the number of hours you will spend on the project, plus make allowances for additional expenses you may incur. Most clients like a fixed-fee arrangement because it enables them to budget the entire project up front. Under this method, you assume all the risk if the project goes over the budgeted number of hours, so it is wise to estimate a range of hours to give yourself some leeway. Be sure to ask for separate payment for reimbursable expenses, such as mileage, long-distance phone calls, and supplies purchased on behalf of the project. Your client may want to place a limit on such expenses.

Cost

Under the cost method of payment, you simply charge your hourly or daily rate, which should include overhead for the duration of the project and other expenses. Many clients prefer to limit the total number of hours allowed. You can include a "not to exceed" clause in such cases.

SUMMARY

The purpose of negotiation is to identify, discuss, and reach agreement about the expectations of each party involved in a business situation. The clearer the parties can be in describing their needs and expectations, the more likely they are to reach an agreement that satisfies all. Jim Rose, MS, RD, a former consultant and food-service director, used to write a list and description or show a sample of what the client would own at the end of his contract, such as a new staffing schedule, a new employee policy manual, or a new patient trayline layout, so there were no miscommunicated expectations.

Bibliography

Hartman GM. *Making the Deal – Quick Tips for Successful Negotiating.* New York, NY: John Wiley and Sons; 1992.

Hisrich RD, Brush CG. *The Woman Entrepreneur.* Lexington, KY: DC Heath and Company; 1986.

Kishel G, Kishel P. *Cashing in on the Consulting Boom.* New York, NY: John Wiley and Sons; 1985.

Marketing Within Primary Market Segments

Creating Opportunities,

Rather than Waiting

for Opportunities to

Present Themselves,

Is the Essence of Achieving

Competitive Advantage.

The Challenge, Then,

Is Identifying Markets

and Trends Where the

Greatest Opportunity Lies.

That, essentially, is the thinking that spurred The American Dietetic Association to begin revising its strategic plan and led to the creation of the Strategic Thinking Initiative (STI), a blueprint for helping the dietetics profession achieve competitive advantage in a rapidly changing environment. Four key market segments were identified as markets of the future:

- Acute and long-term health care,
- Prevention and wellness,
- Food service, and
- Consumer education.

From: Achieving Competitive Advantage. The American Dietetic Association Annual Report, Chicago, IL: 1991-1993;2.

Chapter 16

Clinical Markets: Acute and Long-Term Care

*Chris Biesemeier, MS, RD, Administrative Clinical Dietitian,
St. Luke's Hospital, Kansas City, Missouri*

Health care has entered an era of reform and cost containment. Services are being evaluated for their relevance to health outcomes. Third-party payers are hesitant to cover additional services, including nutrition, unless it can be shown that there is a definite payoff in saving health-care dollars.

In the acute setting, reimbursement depends on payer mix (who is paying the bill) and the provisions in each person's policy. Many insurance companies have followed the lead of the Health Care Financing Administration (HCFA) and initiated reimbursement systems similar to the Medicare system of fixed rates based on primary diagnosis (Diagnosis Related Groups, or DRGs).

With cost containment has come a reduction in the length of stay, together with an increase in the severity of illness, or acuity, of persons being admitted. To help cut costs, nonacute services are being shifted to other settings – the outpatient area, the home, skilled-nursing facilities, and long-term care facilities. These shifts have created a demand for new services and new skills.

As reimbursement in the acute setting has been reduced or limited, hospitals have downsized their staffs. Remaining staff feel pressure to do more and more, while the expectations for the quality of care have increased. Computers are being incorporated into daily routines to streamline activities and provide both data and data evaluation.

Hospitals are embracing long overdue initiatives for improvement. Total Quality Management (TQM) and Continuous Quality Improvement (CQI) initiatives are underway. Staff are being empowered to make decisions affecting the delivery of health care. Other initiatives, such as patient-focused care, collaborative care, and primary nursing, are being undertaken as well. Each of these initiatives presents opportunities for improved care and at the same time challenges staff to learn new strategies and remain informed about the activities of other units or departments.

In addition to the changes in the health-care environment, there have been shifts in the demographics of the population. These shifts affect nutrition care and provide opportunities for additional services. The number of older Americans is increasing and will continue to increase for some time to come. There is a focus on the health-care needs of women and a recognition of the role that women play in making health-care decisions for themselves and their families.

Hospitals and long-term care facilities have responded to the challenges in health care. Individual hospitals have evolved into health-care systems that provide care in a variety of settings. Affiliating with physicians, especially primary-care physicians, has become a priority for hospitals because such practitioners may become the primary gatekeepers (referral agents) for medical care.

There is vigorous competition for health-care business. Hospital marketing departments are focusing on the promotion of positive images and the differentiation of their services from those of other institutions. All of this is taking place in an environment of increased public awareness about health issues and heightened expectations for cost control and quality. In addition to these larger health-care concerns, dietitians have to contend with issues that are unique to their profession.

For example:

- Reimbursement for nutrition services is limited.

- Other health-care providers are willing, and sometimes anxious, to provide nutrition services.

- Access to patients can be limited by the need for physician referrals in some instances and by a limited staff size in others.

- The image and role of dietitians may not be fully appreciated.

WHY MARKET NUTRITION SERVICES?

Carefully designed marketing strategies and valid cost-benefit statistics are the keys to opening doors and removing barriers to initiating nutrition programs and justifying present positions. This is especially relevant in the acute-care setting, where over the past few years, the number of dietitian and dietetic technician positions has continued to decline.

With all the initiatives that are taking place, it is an exciting time for registered dietitians and dietetic technicians to be working in health care. You have the opportunity to be part of the change process as it is occurring and to demonstrate that you possess survival skills. Increased revenue, reduction in the cost of care, and the achievement of organizational goals are outcomes you can achieve.

WHO ARE YOUR CUSTOMERS?

Nutrition services can be marketed to many potential targets in health care. At times, it can be tempting to develop marketing plans and nutrition programs for all the potential targets. However, in reality, there is neither time nor energy to do this. As a result, it is necessary to evaluate potential targets and select those with the maximum payoff.

This is the approach that the leadership of The American Dietetic Association used when they identified *key linkages* as part of the evaluation and goal-setting process in the Strategic Thinking Initiative (STI). STI identified physicians as the first key linkage in the acute and long-term care settings. Health-care payers were identified as the second key linkage. Additional primary linkages are patients, administrators, and members of nursing administration and staff. There are many more secondary linkages.

The specifics of marketing plans for each target group will differ. However, your overall approach should be to form partnerships with the members of your target group to meet mutual goals. Physicians care about the quality of service patients receive. However, in an acute-care setting, physicians are often sensitive to anyone they perceive as intruding in their relationships with their patients, including dietitians and nurses. By developing credibility and trust and showing dedication, you can help your working relationships with physicians grow into team efforts.

Health-care payers and administrators are concerned about financial issues as well as quality of care. Increasingly, with the growth of capitated reimbursement, the cost savings achieved are as important to individuals in these two target groups as the amount of additional revenue a service can generate. Keep records that show your cost-benefit figures and use them in your marketing.

Insurance case managers are also interested in reducing the cost of care, but they are more focused on decreasing hospital admissions and the length of stay of inpatients. They may be willing to consider reimbursement for nutrition services that can affect either factor. Care provided in the home setting is by design less costly than care provided in the acute setting. This is a selling point to use in marketing home nutrition services.

HOSPITAL MARKETING STRATEGIES

Hospital marketing departments with larger promotional budgets are always looking for ways to promote hospitals and their services to both existing and potential customers. Nutrition is hot news that capitalizes on the public's interest in food and the prevention and treatment of disease by diet. Check to see if your hospital's marketing department will collaborate on campaigns that will promote your activities and brochures.

Hospital clinical departments use a variety of promotion strategies to market themselves or generate revenue, such as:

- Writing columns for local newspapers
- Supplying medical experts to the media
- Participating in health fairs
- Developing cookbooks
- Conducting cooking classes and grocery store tours
- Writing articles and patient-education materials

Each of these activities opens the door to marketing nutrition within the organization and to spreading the message of good nutrition to the community.

Internally, you can market nutrition and nutrition care by changing how you do business:

- As a strategy to improve patient satisfaction, streamline the guidelines for modified diets for inpatients and present the changes to your hospital nursing and medical staffs.

- Expand your diet manual into a broader nutritional care manual with prenatal, breastfeeding, pre- and postsurgical at-home feeding guidelines, grocery store shopping, and healthy cooking tips. Sell it to the public, your referring medical staff, and your patients. Provide in-services to demonstrate its use in patient care. Enter the manual into the hospital computer system as a quick reference on diets and nutrition guidelines for all staff.

- Clinical nutrition staff members can collaborate on research activities or serve as primary investigators. Research reinforces the importance of nutrition and positions the dietetics professional as an expert in the field.

- Position your staff dietitians as experts by sponsoring nutritional presentations and symposia for the medical and nursing staffs, the community, and local dietitians.

Marketing Nutrition in Managed Care
Lauren McNabb, MA, RD, LD, Owner, Nutrition Consultants of Dallas, and former Internship Director, Baylor University Medical Center, Dallas, Texas

To survive in health care, dietitians must work within the growing framework of managed systems of patient care (pre-admission through postdischarge) and managed care programs like Health Maintenance Organizations (HMOs) and Preferred Provider Organizations (PPOs). The focuses of managed care are to save money and improve the quality of the services provided.

The keys to working within managed care in institutions are
• Preadmission or inpatient screening to identify patients who are at risk for aggressive nutrition intervention
• Documentation and tracking of intervention outcomes to show the effectiveness of nutrition intervention
• Collaboration with case managers and other health professionals for the good of the patient

Continued page 117

HOW TO GET STARTED

Laying the Groundwork

To be successful in the hospital setting, you need both organizational awareness and a network of influence. Organizational awareness can be accomplished by attending management and other meetings, reading the newsletters of other departments, attending bedside and patient-care rounds and case conferences, participating on quality-assurance teams, and volunteering for advisory boards.

Sometimes, a request to attend meetings is all that is needed to get your foot in the door. If your request is not immediately accepted, you might try another approach, such as sending the committee chair an article illustrating the relevance of nutrition to the issues dealt with by the committee. For instance, send a copy of The American Dietetic Association's position on the ethics of feeding and the withdrawal of feedings to the chair of the Ethics Committee, with a note stating your willingness to serve as a resource to the committee whenever decisions related to nutrition are being made.

Once on a committee, your active participation reinforces the vital role played by a dietetics professional. Also, identify key players on the committee and develop relationships with them. The times before and after meetings provide an excellent opportunity for networking. Discussions about pending decisions are more informal at such times than during actual meetings.

Another useful strategy is to schedule meetings with institutional decision makers and decision influencers to discuss how nutrition affects the work they do. Examples of these individuals are the directors of nursing, quality assurance, utilization review, home health, medical records, collaborative care, social work services, and managed care. Meetings should be scheduled at intervals to maintain a good information network.

Charting the Course

It is important to select two or three target groups and develop marketing strategies for each one. During the planning process, include members of your staff – not only the registered dietitians, but also the dietetic technicians, diet clerks, and foodservice supervisors. Input from different perspectives will enhance the quality of the end product.

The Next Step – Making a Proposal

A plan or proposal must be presented in a simple and easy-to-understand manner. Others do not necessarily understand nutrition terms and concepts, although the ideas may seem logical and obvious to dietitians. A helpful norm used in business is to limit a proposal to the amount of information that will fit in a one-page typed memo (see Chapter 34).

In health-care organizations, many layers of approval must be worked through prior to implementing any program. This complexity in decision making increases the likelihood that multiple changes will be made in the original proposal. However, as noted earlier, by including people in the planning phase who are affected by a program, you increase the likelihood of their buying in when implementation occurs. In your proposal, suggest a trial or test period to give yourself a chance to observe and refine systems before committing all your allocated resources. A proposal

In private practice, dietitians must create alliances – for example, with insurers, case-management companies, and physicians – to provide good nutrition therapy for their patients. They must also work with individuals outside the field of nutrition to let them know that good nutrition saves money. In such cases, it is useful to cite the numerous studies that link nutrition with enhanced immunocompetence and decreased complications from diabetes, lowered risk of cardiovascular disease, and the like, all of which lead to lower costs and improved quality of life.

Suggestions for alliances within managed care:

• *Case managers* are quickly becoming the gatekeepers to most medical services. Case managers rely on other health professionals to implement care plans in a cost-effective manner. Let them know how dietitians can affect the bottom line of a patient's care by decreasing expensive drug usage (in the case of high cholesterol or diabetes), or decreasing the risk of repeat hospitalizations (such as with AIDS patients).

• *Insurers* still hold the key to payment for services rendered. Using real case studies to illustrate cost savings is an excellent way to begin discussions with insurance companies.

• *Physicians,* in the future of health care, will make decisions and direct patient care based on practice guidelines and outcome data. In addition, under capitation, physicians will receive a flat dollar amount to take care of all patients in a particular plan. Dietitians can actually save physicians money by keeping patients out of physicians' offices with effective nutrition therapies that help control blood glucose, cholesterol, and the like.

• *Patients* are the end users of all health care that is delivered. They decide which insurance plan to subscribe to and which physician to see. Dietitians can ask patients who have been helped by nutrition therapy to write insurers about the nutrition-related economic and quality-of-life benefits they have received.

that offers a benefit to the hospital, not just to the nutrition department, like good media exposure for the hospital or improved community relations, is more likely to be accepted.

Dietetics professionals develop and market products and services in the acute and long-term care settings using a variety of approaches. Some of these strategies are highlighted next.

THE ACUTE-CARE SETTING

Nutrition Screening Programs

Nutrition screening is the process of reviewing selected patient data in search of characteristics associated with either impaired nutrition status or the likelihood of developing impaired status. In large institutions, screening is often completed by diet technicians within 24 to 36 hours of admission, while in smaller facilities, it may be completed by the dietitians. In some cases, the results of screening are used to assign staff to provide nutrition care. For example, a diet technician may complete the nutrition assessment and initiate the care plan for patients with a low nutritional acuity, while the dietitian assumes responsibility for patients with more severe nutrition problems.

Although nutrition screening is usually completed at or near the time of admission, all routine assessment and care processes completed during hospitalization should be reviewed to determine the feasibility of incorporating nutrition-screening protocols. Nutrition screening can be promoted to hospital staff as a quick, accurate method of early identification of patients' nutritional needs. When you identify problems early, you can start working on them sooner. It also means more time to plan for discharge and home, long-term, or other care arrangements. Also, the nutrition screening and referral system is a way to collaborate with other disciplines in the assessment process, as required by the Joint Commission on Accreditation of Healthcare Organizations (JCAHO).

In all practice areas, dietitians should train nurses, social workers, occupational therapists, speech pathologists, enterostomal therapists, geriatric nurse specialists, and discharge planners to be alert to indicators of nutrition problems. The screening alerts listed in the *Nutrition Interventions Manual for Professionals Caring for Older Americans,* published as part of the Nutrition Screening Initiative, can be used by these staff to identify nutrition problems specific to their areas of professional practice. When patients are at moderate to high risk, they should be referred to the dietitian.

For example, more and more enteral feeding tubes and central lines for nutrition support are being inserted in the outpatient setting. A nutrition screening protocol can be established with the manager or nurse in the outpatient clinic for all patients having nutrition support lines placed to receive automatic nutrition referrals to the dietitian. With computer networks, an electronic referral can be sent as an "explosion order" (an order sent to all involved parties for comprehensive patient care) to the nutrition services office at the same time the order for line placement is entered into the system.

In some institutions, nutrition screening is being shifted to the preadmission setting. In these facilities, patients who are scheduled for elective surgery are assessed, or worked up, in a preadmission center anywhere from a few days to a few weeks before they are admitted to the hospital. Nutrition screening can be completed by staff who are already working in the center or by a diet technician assigned for this purpose.

At the author's institution, the patients who go through the preadmission process are less acutely ill and have less impairment in nutrition status. To date, the Preadmission Assessment Center seems to provide a better setting for evaluating educational needs and providing nutrition counseling on postsurgery nutrition guidelines. It also provides a good opportunity to introduce patients to Nutrition Services procedures. Each patient coming through the Preadmission Assessment Center is given a brochure with this information. Also, patients can preselect their hospital menus, which increases their satisfaction with food service.

Clinical Paths and Collaborative Care. Clinical paths, also known as clinical practice guidelines or managed-care maps, are being developed and used by many hospitals. By definition, a clinical path is an organized plan of care specific to a particular procedure, such as hip replacement, or a clinical condition, like stroke or pneumonia. Paths specify the care to be provided for the selected patient category by day of hospital stay. Daily outcomes, as well as discharge outcomes, are also defined. Variances in the expected care processes and in the achievement of expected outcomes are documented. Patterns of variance and reasons for these are evaluated over a period of time. Based on the results of the evaluations, changes are made in the paths as needed to achieve desired outcomes.

The goal of paths is to assure quality of care by identifying protocols that streamline the process of care giving. The use of paths can be limited to the inpatient acute-care setting. But ideally, their use crosses many settings, from preadmission to postdischarge, resulting in "seamless care." At some institutions, simple versions of the paths are given to the patient and family so they can monitor the patient's progress.

Ideally, a multidisciplinary team works together to plan a path. The team is composed primarily of individuals who are directly involved in the provision of care to patients in the selected category. Clinical dietitians need to be involved. You can incorporate your own nutrition practice guidelines into the different sections of a clinical path, such as nutrition consults, discharge planning, and postdischarge follow-up.

It is important for dietetics professionals to define and measure the achievement of outcomes for the nutrition care provided in addition to the outcomes defined for the path as a whole. Resources used to achieve these outcomes can also be measured, providing dietitians with institution-specific data on cost per nutrition outcome. This information is valuable in selling nutrition services to third-party payers.

Nutrition-Support Teams. The use of nutrition-support teams can be a cost-effective way to monitor the selection of patients for nutrition support, adherence to established guidelines for product selection, and patients' responses to therapy. The visibility and recognition of a nutrition-support team highlights the importance of nutrition therapy in achieving positive clinical outcomes and cost savings.

In many institutions, nutrition-support teams are well established; but in others, they are not. At the latter institutions, given the current health-care climate, it can be a challenge to convince administrators to allocate staff to nutrition-support teams when other valuable positions are being eliminated.

At the author's institution, a large non-university teaching hospital with primarily private-practice physicians, there is no nutrition-support team per se.

However, multidisciplinary collaboration on nutrition support is still the goal. It was decided that the dietitian on each unit would be responsible for the nutrition care of all nutrition-support patients on that unit, which takes the place of a "nutrition-support" dietitian.

When the Pharmacy Department implemented a system of total parenteral nutrition (TPN), the pharmacists and dietitians initiated daily reviews of patients' lab values and the adequacy of TPN solutions in meeting nutrition requirements. These miniteams are charged with reviewing nursing records and collaborating as needed with the patients' primary nurses and other patient-care staff. Any recommendations for changes in TPN are communicated to the primary physician or resident responsible for the patient prior to the cutoff time for orders. Over time, patients on enteral nutrition (EN) will also be included in the daily reviews.

Discharge Planning. Hospitals are now required to have a process for assessing and planning for patients' discharge needs. This process is known as *discharge planning*. It includes activities undertaken to prepare the patient and family for discharge and for successful adaptation to the postdischarge setting.

Nutritional needs are an important component of discharge planning. While not all patients need the dietitian's involvement in individualized discharge planning, assistance can be provided to other staff to ensure that nutrition problems are not overlooked. Discharge planning rounds and unit care conferences allow the dietitian to hear reports on these patients and be alert for unrecognized nutrition problems.

Discharge-planning procedures vary from one institution to another. They may include the activities of a team or only one or two individuals. Discharge planning may be completed for all patients or for only selected groups, such as oncology or geriatric patients. Dietetics professionals will want to be informed about institutional procedures and will want to examine these procedures for opportunities to take a leadership role in this important aspect of patient care.

Cost Containment and Reimbursement for Nutrition Services

Any effort to market nutrition services in the acute-care setting must include a focus on cost control and on developing systems to increase revenue and decrease the cost of care. There are many ways to demonstrate this focus.

Obtaining reimbursement for nutrition services is a top priority. Getting approval to charge and implementing the process of charging are major undertakings that require dietitians to negotiate with administrators as well as with staff from the admissions, billing, and patient accounting departments. In some institutions, there are different staffs for inpatient and outpatient charges. (See the sidebar on managed care.)

The information obtained from retrospective charge audits is also a powerful sales tool to use when promoting nutrition care in a new setting. For example, physicians who are hesitant to make referrals to the dietitian may be willing to do so when presented with a list of insurance companies that provide policies covering nutrition care.

Dietitians can promote nutrition care and the coverage of nutrition services in the outpatient setting by communicating directly with third-party-payer case managers. Who better to describe the importance of nutrition care to positive clinical and financial outcomes than the registered dietitian!

An Interview with Cindy Brylinsky, MS, RD, CNSD
  Geisinger Medical Center,
  Danville, Pennsylvania

AUTHOR: How have you marketed nutrition services at your institution?

BRYLINSKY: Twice a year, the Nutrition Services Department hosts a dinner with the hospital's administrators at which we feature a specific case study. The food served corresponds to the diet featured in the case study. We've also had dinners featuring our nutrition-screening and nutrition-support programs. For these, we served menus that met the daily food guidelines.

We send all physicians on our staff a copy of a monthly newsletter, *Food for Thought*. The newsletter focuses on current issues and provides information on topics their patients may ask about. We let new physicians on staff know who we are by sending them a letter explaining our services, along with a copy of our formulary, our Nutrition Reference Booklet, and the latest *Food for Thought*.

Continued page 121

Documentation. The way in which dietitians document information in the medical records can be used to promote nutrition and the knowledge and skills of the dietitian. Concise, outcome-oriented notes are effective, while notes that lack specificity may send the wrong message.

Recently, in an attempt to improve the quality of documentation, dietetics professionals have implemented systems of documentation that present alternatives to the standard SOAP format. These newer systems concentrate attention on patients' nutrition problems and on the specific interventions that are implemented to achieve desired outcomes.

The initiation of the use of clinical paths has affected the way dietitians document their services. In hospitals using paths, dietitians initial the interventions and outcomes that are part of a path to indicate their completion and achievement.

Dietetic Technicians. The use of support staff in patients' nutrition care can be promoted as a means of demonstrating the provision of timely, high-quality care in a cost-effective way. As noted earlier, dietetic technicians can participate in nutrition screening and assessments of patients with nutrition problems of low to moderate severity. They can participate in patient education, reinforcing concepts presented by the dietitians. Dietetic technicians can attend patient-care conferences to report on patients under their care. They can document care provided in the medical record, and charges can be entered for services they provide.

OUTPATIENT NUTRITION CARE

It is well known that the inpatient setting, given its limited timelines and very ill patients, is not a good situation for offering involved nutrition consults and providing long-term follow-up, especially for problems like diabetes and weight loss. To allow inpatients sufficient time to learn new behaviors, the initial hospital nutrition consult should focus on survival skills and answers to the patients' biggest concerns. In-depth therapy and follow-up should be scheduled with the outpatient nutrition department, diabetes education class, or a local private-practice dietitian for group or individual care.

Clinical practice guidelines for nutrition care should be developed specific to the outpatient setting. Use the guidelines to promote nutrition care to both physicians and insurance case managers. After reviewing the specifics of care, physicians will have a better understanding of the rationale for repeated blood work and other measurements. Case managers will appreciate the focus on achieving defined therapeutic goals and the time limitation on services.

Registered dietitians have been working in hospital-affiliated outpatient clinics for some time. However, as the provision of health care continues to shift to the outpatient setting, even more opportunities are developing. The challenges are to identify these opportunities, shift staff to meet the new demands, and obtain reimbursement for the services provided.

Start by identifying situations in which nutrition status either is not being addressed or is being addressed in a suboptimal way. For example, a geriatric assessment team should include a registered dietitian who can follow high-risk patients at home. When a diagnosis of HIV positive is made, referrals for nutrition assessment should be automatic in the outpatient setting. To facilitate the inclusion of nutrition services into existing systems of care, the referral and counseling processes must be easy and consistent with existing procedures.

Continued from page 120

Soon we plan to initiate preadmission nutrition screening. We will continue actively marketing our services at the 24 clinics affiliated with our hospital. And we plan to review the records of a list of outlier patients obtained from our Medical Records Department to determine the impact that nutrition interventions could make on decreasing the length of stay and the cost of care for patients with similar diagnoses. This is the type of information administrators are looking for.

In hospitals with physicians in private practice, your department could contract with private-practice dietitians or assign staff dietitians to work on-site in the physicians' offices as a service provided by the outpatient nutrition clinic. Charge the dietitian's time to the physician on a retainer or per hour basis.

We initiated nutrition counseling services in a large group internal-medicine practice affiliated with our hospital. Having the dietitians on-site has added value to the physicians' practice and improved the quality of patient care. The physicians write referrals slips for nutrition counseling during their patients' office visits. Patients take the referral slips to the receptionist's desk to schedule their appointments.

The following strategies have been successful in increasing the number of referrals in this setting:

- Dietitians meet informally with the physicians' nurses to explain the referral and counseling processes and to answer questions.

- Dietitians attend the physicians' management meetings to promote the counseling program and to discuss additional areas for nutrition services.

- Drop-in appointments are taken when the appointment times are open. This works well for patients who live out of town and fills the gaps in the dietitians' schedules.

HOME HEALTH NUTRITION CARE

There is a definite need for dietetics professionals to extend their services into the home-care market to ensure the provision of high-quality care. However, the limited reimbursement for registered dietitians' services in the home setting has seriously restricted our ability to provide home care. In spite of this economic reality, more companies are hiring dietitians to provide home care, especially home nutrition-support monitoring.

For dietetics professionals who want to expand nutrition services into their hospital-affiliated home-care agencies, a knowledge of the market and an understanding of reimbursement in home care are essential. Networking with peers who work in home care is necessary to obtain this information.

At the author's institution, there are two home-care agencies, one for Medicare patients and one for patients with private insurance. Neither agency has had a dietitian on staff, although each has been asked several times to consider this service in various clinical activities.

The initial request was made to the home-care managers several years ago. This proposal was rejected due to the lack of reimbursement. However, an invitation for the clinical nutrition manager to join the advisory board was issued and accepted.

As more home-care agencies in the community began to hire dietitians, the decision was made to approach the two hospital agencies again. In preparation, a survey of home-care agencies was completed to determine the role of dietitians. Both agencies with hospital affiliations and those without hospital affiliations were surveyed for the following information:

- Number of dietitian hours worked
- Types of nutrition care provided

- Procedures for charging for nutrition services
- Reimbursement received

Another proposal was presented. This time we offered the services of a paid staff dietitian on a trial basis. This proposal was accepted by the agency providing services to Medicare patients. As intended, they perceived this as a no-lose situation. From the Nutrition Services perspective, a trial would allow the dietitian to get to know the home-care staff, establish systems for involvement with patients, and prove the worth of nutrition care provided by a registered dietitian.

The registered dietitian defined procedures for referrals and developed nutrition-assessment forms. It was decided that nutrition consults for patients recently discharged from the hospital would be handled in the same manner as consults for other services, such as nursing care, physical therapy, and speech therapy. The patient's home-care nurse, who serves as a case manager, assesses the patient and determines if the dietitian's services are actually needed. The nurse makes any referrals and communicates the type of care needed. The dietitian conducted an inservice on nutrition screening and care for the home-care nurses and began attending monthly case-conference meetings.

Soon the dietitian received referrals for patient consultations. The home-care manager created an account for nutrition and wrote an agreement between Nutrition Services and the home-care agency. The procedures and forms for this agency will be adapted slightly and implemented in the agency providing services to patients with private insurance. Recently, the clinical nutrition manager has been appointed to the position of chair of the home health advisory board. Persistence pays off!

MARKETING NUTRITION SERVICES IN LONG-TERM CARE FACILITIES

Many of the opportunities and challenges that exist in acute care also exist in long-term care. And many of the marketing strategies are the same as well. There are different types of long-term care settings, including nursing homes, skilled-nursing facilities, independent-living facilities, and group homes, to name a few. The types of residents and their nutritional needs vary, as do the regulations and standards under which the facilities operate. All of these factors affect the way in which nutrition services are marketed.

Long-term care facilities have become increasingly sophisticated in the types of care provided to residents. Many facilities have established specialty-care units, such as those for patients with head trauma, with spinal cord injuries, and on ventilators. Other facilities have disease-specific units, such as those for patients with AIDS and Alzheimer's disease. The creation of these units produces a demand for the expertise a dietitian can provide. In addition, the use of nutrition support has expanded greatly, with both enteral and parenteral nutrition support being commonplace.

Dietitians in long-term care frequently work in more than one facility. This diversity in work environments gives them a broad perspective and allows them to position themselves as experts at problem identification and solution. Dietitians in this setting also must know how to develop systems for ordering food, equipment, and supplies, and implementing effective inventory controls to ensure adherence to budget and cost-control guidelines.

Long-term care facilities are installing computer systems in much the same way that acute-care settings are. A dietitian's expertise in computer applications in nutrition care and food-service management can be valuable during the selection and implementation of systems and in the ongoing evaluation of data.

The enactment of the Omnibus Budget Reconciliation Act (OBRA) legislation has had a great impact on the provision of care in nursing homes and skilled nursing facilities. Under OBRA, there is an increased emphasis on resident assessment, quality of care, quality of life, and resident rights.

OBRA regulations have presented dietitians and dietetic technicians with increased opportunities to participate in patient care as members of multidisciplinary care teams. While parts of the resident assessment are completed by nurses or food-service supervisors, dietitians oversee the nutrition care provided to all residents, including those at no apparent risk and those with less severe nutrition problems. Dietitians complete the nutrition assessments, care plans, and ongoing monitoring of high-risk residents.

Dietetics professionals have initiated many strategies to increase resident satisfaction with their food. Offering residents choices seems to be essential, and menu selection is one area where choices are available. Salad and dessert carts are another way to give residents menu options. Theme meals are fun and increase residents' interest in eating. Restaurant service is a nice change of pace for special occasions, such as birthdays. Some facilities offer the option of eating out while still dining in. Different types of "restaurant menus" are offered once a month for residents who are interested. At some facilities, residents can invite their families to dinner in much the same way they did when living on their own.

The many activities and programs related to residents' food and nutrition care can be actively promoted in resident newsletters, calendars of events, and bulletin board displays.

SUMMARY

The marketing strategies of successful acute- and long-term care dietitians serve as models for us in our own institutions. However, every situation is unique. It is up to each of us to assess our own environment, consider the options, make plans, and take action – with the realization that we won't always have a map to follow and we won't always know if we're going in the right direction. In looking back, though, we will see that maintaining the status quo would have left us behind.

Case Study: MARKETING STRATEGIES FOR CLINICAL NUTRITION SERVICES

At Yale-New Haven Hospital (YNHH), Michele Fairchild, MA, RD, and clinical management staff, Deborah Ford, MS, RD, and Barbara Bush, RD, market their services in a variety of ways:

- They initiated the Yale-New Haven Hospital Nutritional Classification and Assessment Program, which evaluates seven patient risk factors and classifies patients into one of seven treatment categories. Use of this program enhances the image of the dietitians at YNHH by improving the consistency in their professional practice. It also simplifies procedures for the dietitians and enables them to place better priorities on their workload.

- An article in a 1991 issue of the *Bulletin*, the YNHH newsletter, described the incidence of malnutrition in YNHH patients and the dietitians' role in fighting it.

- Dietitians at YNHH become involved in their community. For an example, they participated in the development and initiation of the Caring Cuisine Program, which provides home-delivered meals for persons with AIDS. Since its initiation in 1988, the program has served over 3,000 meals annually to AIDS patients in the New Haven area. In 1990, Caring Cuisine was awarded the 283rd "Point of Light" by President George Bush in recognition of its contribution to solving social issues.

- Dietetic technicians, acting as department representatives throughout the hospital, implemented a career apparel program. A dress code was adopted, and a line of career apparel featuring tailored business suits was chosen. Results of this program include enhanced public relations, improved technician credibility, and increased praise from hospital administration and patients. In addition, the program received an honorable mention in the 1989 National Association of Uniform Manufacturers and Distributors' Image of the Year Contest.

- YNHH implemented an incentive and recognition program for its dietetic technicians. The program is based on a point system for attendance, punctuality, on-the-job training, creativity, and quality of work. A monthly award is given to the dietetic technician with the most points.

- The Department of Food and Nutrition created a patient-advocacy program with a dietetic technician as its patient advocate. The duties of the patient advocate include visiting patients, randomly and in response to patient complaints, reviewing complaints, and initiating solutions to any problems. The visits improve patient relations, and the resulting records provide valuable information to department managers.

- Dietetic technicians assisted in the development of a brochure to market careers in food and nutrition, and the production of an informational video for our department on positive patient interactions.

- The dietitians and dietetic technicians promote their accomplishments with peers through their many publications in professional journals. Not only have they provided direction for other dietetic professionals, but they have established themselves as leaders in the field.

Chapter 17

Wellness and Disease Prevention

Jean Storlie, MS, RD, President, JS Associates, Inc., Ithaca, New York

Wellness is a proactive concept that focuses on healthy habits and disease-prevention practices. Throughout the last decade, the role of wellness in the practice of dietetics has expanded considerably. It is difficult to quantify the actual proportion of the dietetic profession involved in the practice of wellness because nutrition is a component of wellness and wellness is an integral theme in the delivery of nutrition care.

The ways in which dietetics professionals practice in wellness settings reflect the evolving nature of the wellness movement. They work in private practice, corporate, university/college, clinical/hospital, government, and community settings. They market programs that are targeted to a wide range of audiences: employee groups, hospital and clinic patients, restaurant and grocery store patrons, community groups, and many others. In some instances, dietitians provide the nutrition expertise for an interdisciplinary team. In other cases, dietetics professionals have broadened their skills and expertise into other disciplines, such as stress management, sports nutrition, and exercise instruction, so nutrition is one of many strategies they use to promote health and well-being.

THE EVOLUTION OF NUTRITION IN WELLNESS

Wellness, a philosophical departure from traditional medicine, was embraced by a growing number in the health professions and the public during the 1970s and 1980s. At the same time, a swelling body of evidence linked disease to lifestyle-related factors: fitness, nutrition, stress, and smoking habits. Wellness programs sprang up in corporate and some community settings. The forerunners in corporate wellness focused primarily on fitness programs in the 1970s and broadened to include other dimensions during the 1980s. Not only did the breadth and depth of wellness programming expand throughout the 1980s, but wellness programs were also delivered in more diverse settings. Hospitals, HMOs, government and community agencies, and fitness centers began to sponsor wellness programs. By 1985, it was estimated that 84 percent of the nation's hospitals offered health-promotion programs to at least one of their target audiences (1). During this time, the term *health promotion* was introduced and began to be used interchangeably with the term *wellness*. The concept of *disease prevention,* referring to a process by which the occurrence and severity of diseases are reduced by influencing key risk factors, was also attached to wellness. These more clinically oriented terms may reflect the greater involvement of the medical and scientific communities in the wellness movement as a solid body of research emerged to substantiate the relationship between lifestyle and disease.

Anita Owen, RD, during her term as President of The American Dietetic Association, initiated a collaborative effort between the Society for Nutrition Education and the U.S. Department of Health and Human Services to promote the role of nutrition in worksite wellness programs. This collaboration resulted in the publication *Worksite Nutrition: A Decision-Maker's Guide* (2), which was widely disseminated and used as a tool for planning nutrition programs at the worksite. The second edition of this popular publication was published in 1993 (3).

The percentage of worksites offering nutrition-education programs increased from 17 percent in 1985 to 31 percent in 1992; similarly, the percentage of worksites offering weight-control programs expanded from 15 percent to 24 percent (4, 5). Cafeteria and other food-service programs sprang up at worksites throughout the country. Of the 43 percent of companies that have a cafeteria, snack bar, or food-service operation, 31 percent provide nutrition labels on the foods (5). Nutrition programming at the worksite mimics other emerging trends in worksite wellness: an emphasis on changing the corporate culture; use of communication technologies to deliver programs in more cost-effective ways; strategies to reach retirees, family members, and other special populations; and integration of wellness into organizational-development strategies, occupational safety, and medical self-care.

Several dietetic practice groups of The American Dietetic Association are adapting to reflect changes in the marketplace. The new name Sports, Cardiovascular & Wellness Nutrition Practice Group (SCAN) reflects the fact that a large number of the group's members also work in the wellness arena. The Consulting Nutritionist Practice Group actively promotes that it includes the entrepreneurial dietitians and the new emerging nutrition therapist interest area, which both work very heavily with prevention and wellness. One of the most significant findings of SCAN's Ad Hoc Committee on Wellness is that of the 301 SCAN dietitians surveyed, the majority indicated they need to develop marketing skills to enhance their wellness practice.

SUCCESSFUL MARKETING STRATEGIES IN WELLNESS SETTINGS

The marketing strategies dietetics professionals use in wellness depend on the practice setting, the target audience, and the background and focus of the dietitian who is promoting services. Although worksite wellness and private practice are probably the most developed wellness opportunities for dietitians, they are not the only settings in which nutrition practitioners have established practices. Other settings include hospital-based health promotion, sports nutrition services, and consumer-oriented nutrition programs.

To develop a broader perspective on how dietitians market wellness services, I contacted 25 dietitians who had practiced wellness for more than five years (July 1993). Seventeen dietitians responded to a brief questionnaire, and I conducted follow-up interviews with some of them. Most of these dietitians practice in more than one setting, using a base (such as a university, physician's office/clinic, hospital-based program, or private practice) from which they branch into other settings (such as freelance writing, workshops, speaking, and consulting to business, food manufacturers, or sports teams). They serve employee groups, students, community groups, healthy individuals, athletes, and consumer groups.

As a relatively new niche within the dietetics profession, practicing wellness tends to be an outgrowth of other professional activities. Some of the dietitians who responded to the survey are profiled in sidebars throughout this chapter. Each experienced a career turning point from which wellness or disease-prevention opportunities emerged. Sparked by an unexpected break, a personal decision, or a responsibility associated with a current job, these dietitians broke away from

Lisa Dorfman, MS, RD, LMHC

Lisa started her career as a dietitian and licensed psychotherapist, working with extremely ill people who suffered from eating disorders, mental illness, and chemical dependencies. She was thrust into the media limelight when Karen Carpenter died. Media exposure created new opportunities to work with well populations, and she eventually established a private practice that serves community and government organizations, corporations, physicians, and private patients. As an avid runner, Lisa is well connected in her local running community and the Consulting Nutritionist practice group. Her athletic accomplishments make her message more believable.

traditional dietetic roles and forged successful wellness practices. They have relied on a variety of marketing strategies to build and maintain their reputations as wellness or disease-prevention experts.

When the respondents were asked to identify their most successful marketing strategy, they ranked referrals highest, followed by public speaking and publishing (see Figure 17-1). Networking through membership and active involvement in various organizations were cited as critical strategies for building a referral base. Some dietitians used constant media exposure in local markets as the cornerstone of their marketing programs. Conducting promotional events, exhibiting, listing in the *Yellow Pages* and directories, cold calling, and direct mail techniques, which were cited as less-effective marketing techniques, are known to work for some products or services.

Figure 17-1. Most Successful Marketing Strategies*

1. Referrals from third parties

2. Public speaking

3. Publishing

4. Organization membership and involvement

5. Media exposure

6. Direct mail

*Based on a survey of seventeen wellness dietitians.

Since each dietitian's practice is unique, it is difficult to draw broad conclusions from these results. The common theme throughout the survey respondents' stories is a commitment to and a passion for both living and professing a wellness/fitness lifestyle. This makes them role models for their clients, who aspire to increased levels of wellness. They exude a caring and sharing attitude, and they demonstrate upbeat, enthusiastic personalities. When encountering low moments in their personal and professional quests for wellness, they said that perseverance, a tough skin, a sense of humor, and spiritual beliefs were essential. Several dietitians said they learned important lessons from their low moments that led to greater levels of success and personal satisfaction.

MARKETING WORKSITE NUTRITION PROGRAMS

Marketing worksite wellness services involves two levels of selling. First, the company's management must buy into the program enough to sponsor it. Management's support is critical for obtaining necessary resources and establishing policies that permit employees to participate in the program (such as time away from the job to attend classes). Once management approval is secured, the employee population must be sold on the program. Marketing and promotional strategies need to be carefully crafted for each corporate setting to maximize participation rates, which are critical to both short- and long-term success. If a majority of employees do not participate, the impact of the program will be diluted, and programs that fail to make an impact on quantifiable objectives tend to have short lives. Regardless of whether an external consultant or an employee is selling a worksite nutrition program, these two tiers of selling are critical. Both new and existing programs need constant attention to marketing at both levels to remain successful.

When Selling to Management

Careful preparation is crucial to marketing your wellness program to management. Taking the following steps will enhance your chances of success:

1. Learn as much as possible about how wellness is currently structured within your target company before making a sales call.

2. Target the highest management level you can reach. In small and medium-size companies, start with the CEO. This level of management may be harder to reach in larger companies, unless the CEO is a wellness advocate.

3. If upper level managers are inaccessible, start with the human resources, training and development, or medical departments.

4. Go into a sales call armed with facts.

   - Managers want to know the costs, benefits, and expected outcomes of worksite nutrition programs and of all health-promotion programs in general.

   - Before a sales meeting, research the company to learn about the demographics of the employee population. Identify the number of sites and other factors that can affect the design and delivery of a worksite nutrition program.

   - Tailor a proposal that speaks to the needs and existing structure of the company. Include statistics that document the cost-effectiveness of the program.

   - Demonstrate your track record as a program provider.

When Meeting with Middle Managers

When you meet with middle managers, provide documents that clearly and concisely build an argument for why a worksite nutrition program can make a positive difference in their company. Since they will face the challenge of selling your program upward, you need to convince them to sponsor the program idea, then arm them with the tools they need to sell it to their superiors. Identify who will be involved in making the final decision to purchase nutrition services. Focusing a great deal of time and energy on someone who only influences a decision can be a futile effort. Try to become acquainted with both the influencers and the final decision maker. Work cooperatively with everyone involved, addressing the concerns that each party raises. Be careful not to become entangled in internal controversies and rivalries.

Sales Calls with Upper-Level Managers

Plan to spend no more than a half-hour with a busy executive. You may be given only ten to fifteen minutes, so be well prepared. A polished proposal that succinctly outlines the program concept, critical logistical considerations, costs, and expected outcomes is essential when presenting to upper management. Keep to the point and allow plenty of time for interaction. Top managers typically have take-charge personalities – they may want to lead the discussion.

Identify objectives for each sales call. For example, if the first sales call is an exploratory discussion with a middle manager, a realistic objective might be to gain enough information so you can draft a proposal. Close each meeting with a clear understanding of what the next steps are (for example, you will submit a proposal for preliminary review and the manager will schedule a follow-up meeting to introduce you to the decision maker or other influencers). After each sales meeting, plan a follow-up strategy.

Martin Yadrick, MS, MBA, RD

Because of his interest in health and fitness, Marty was a dietitian for the Cardiac Rehabilitation program at Research Medical Center in Kansas City and nutrition consultant to HealthPlus Fitness & Wellness Center in Overland Park, Kansas. Presently, he is a Training Consultant with Computrition, Inc., in California. Marty has the distinction of being the first male Chair of SCAN, the Sports, Cardiovascular & Wellness Nutritionists Practice Group, the President of the Kansas City Dietetic Association, and Ambassador for The American Dietetic Association.

Karen Reznik Dolins, MS, RD, had an experience selling worksite nutrition services to Merrill Lynch that illustrates the importance of persistence and follow-up. She contacted the company in 1988, soon after the National Cholesterol Education Program guidelines were issued, and they hired her to conduct a seminar on the subject for their medical staff. Although they expressed an interest in contracting her services to deliver a program to their 10,000 local employees, they did not act on it. For three years, she kept in touch with them periodically. Finally in December 1991, her timing was perfect. They had just budgeted funds for wellness, the medical director remembered her favorably, and she was able to sell them on her ideas. Karen says that this experience taught her that perseverance is everything. "Never forget a contact," urges Karen, "and never let them forget you."

Internal Promotions to Employees

Securing management support will get your foot in the door; getting employees to participate will keep it there. Even the best program can go unnoticed if managers and workers do not know what is offered and how to take advantage of it. When marketing a worksite nutrition program to employees, it is important to identify target segments within the employee population, such as women, minorities, blue-collar workers, or retirees. If a needs analysis was conducted, use the results to learn about the employees' needs and interests.

Company-wide marketing strategies alone may not be effective in achieving high participation rates. Focused communications that reach the targeted groups and speak to their needs will maximize participation. For example, presentations at department meetings provide an opportunity to reach employees in their work groups.

One target audience that requires special attention in launching a worksite wellness program is management. Meet with managers and supervisors to identify any concerns they have about how the program might affect their work unit. They may resent and resist the program because they perceive it as a disruption. Alleviating these concerns at the onset and tailoring the program to the needs of each employee work group will prevent serious problems later. Sell the program from the top down.

An employee wellness committee fosters grass-roots support, which is useful in marketing a program. Members provide valuable insights into the needs and interests of their co-workers, and they can help distinguish between effective and ineffective communication strategies. Members can play a role in the actual implementation of program promotions by volunteering to distribute materials, speaking on behalf of the program, and assisting in planning and conducting promotional events.

Joan Horbiak, MPH, RD, sets up a nutrition task force with every corporate client to guide her in tailoring her program to the company's needs. She believes that her most effective marketing technique is being an excellent speaker. Therefore, each year, she attends a formal training program in New York to enhance her speaking skills, and she gets herself in front of a group as part of her sales process. Joan provides two free presentations: the first to sell management (a targeted sales tactic), the second to generate employee participation (a value-added service intended to improve her ultimate outcomes).

Figure 17-2 presents strategies for internally promoting a worksite wellness program to both management and employees (6).

Figure 17-2. Promotional Techniques for Management and Employees

TO MANAGEMENT	TO EMPLOYEES
Presentations at management meetings	Written communications
Meetings with supervisors	Letters from CEO
Management health retreats	Fliers
Status reports on program development	Posters
Reports on program results	Memos
	Brochures
	Check stuffers
	Special events
	Kick-off event
	Health/nutrition fair
	Open house
	Introductory session
	Keynote speaker
	Presentations to employees
	Employee referral system

Adapted from Guidelines for Employee Health Promotion (p. 31) by Association for Fitness in Business, Champaign, IL: Human Kinetics Publishers. Copyright 1992 by Association for Fitness in Business. Reprinted by permission.

MARKETING HOSPITAL-BASED HEALTH-PROMOTION PROGRAMS

While hospitals have tremendous resources for building health-promotion programs, traditional hospital systems also have a number of economic, legal, political, and philosophical barriers that inhibit the success of wellness programs (7). Due to ever-tightening fiscal conditions, complex organizational structures, and an orientation to crisis medical intervention, hospitals sometimes have difficulty positioning wellness effectively within their organizations. And if a program is not positioned effectively internally, it has little chance for success externally. For this reason, leaders in hospital health promotion have recognized the importance of strategic planning in marketing hospital health-promotion programs. Strategic planning efforts hinge on the answers to three critical questions: Who are we? Where are we going? How will we get there?

Important questions to answer in strategic planning for hospital health promotion include: How does the hospital strategically position health promotion within

Donna Israel, PhD, RD, LD

After spending thirteen years as a counselor in social work and having five children, Donna returned to school to become a dietitian and earn a PhD in nutrition. At her first hospital job, Donna assumed the role of the Hospital Wellness Director, working with an interdisciplinary team. After one year in that role, she left to start her own company. The Fitness Formula is currently a thriving business in Richardson, Texas, that provides individual and group nutrition consultations, as well as nutrition consulting at a drug rehabilitation center and health-promotion programs to large companies and federal employees throughout the United States. Donna is active in the Consulting Nutritionist practice group and healthpromotion organizations like the Association for Worksite Health Promotion.

the organization? What is going on in the market? What is the program all about as a business unit?

Many community hospitals position health promotion as a community-outreach service. It is viewed as an attractive way to build goodwill, enhance the community's loyalty to the hospital, and strengthen relations with large employers. In light of this mission for health promotion, direct profits may not be as important as the more intangible benefits, such as public relations. Other hospitals have profit motives for health promotion, which affects how the program is marketed and operated.

Figure 17-3. Target Markets and Related Services for Hospital-Based Health-Promotion Programs

TARGET MARKETS	WELLNESS-RELATED SERVICES
Corporations	Health education Health risk appraisal Screening Occupational health Fitness Nutrition and weight control Smoking cessation Stress management
General public	Health education Fitness Nutrition/weight control Smoking cessation Stress management
Hospital employees	Health education Fitness Nutrition/weight control Smoking cessation Stress management
Women	Health education Nutrition/weight control OB/GYN Screening Fitness Prenatal Birthing Osteoporosis

Adapted from Health promotion young, but growing: the Optimal Health/Price Waterhouse health-promotion survey. Optimal Health, July/Aug. 1987: 22-24. Permission granted by Jeffrey M. Bensky, The Benfield Group, St. Louis.

Interpreting market conditions involves a thorough understanding of existing, as well as potential, competition. Knowing what factors will influence a given segment of the market to buy wellness services can be the most important determinant of longterm success. After identifying market segments, it is essential to gather information that will reveal their purchasing motives through focus groups, interviews, or surveys.

As Figure 17-3 depicts, hospital health-promotion programs may target a number of markets, and offer a wide range of services. Matching internal capabilities to the needs and interests of the buying groups is the cornerstone of creating an effective marketing plan. The ability to design specific promotion and sales strategies that communicate the benefits and features of a program in a manner that motivates purchasing behavior is what distinguishes successful from unsuccessful hospital health-promotion programs.

At the Baptist Center for Health Promotion in Nashville, the program director and the nutrition coordinator recognized an untapped market niche in selling nutrition counseling services to well populations (8). This represented a departure from the way nutrition counseling was traditionally offered through the hospital (that is, only through a physician's referral or a hospital stay). They believed that nutrition counseling could be marketed as a stand-alone product line, capable of producing revenue, enhancing the institution's image, and actively cross-selling other hospital services. Identifying that many well populations desired nutrition information and personal guidance, they packaged counseling services in the areas of weight control, heart health, sports nutrition, and food allergies.

The critical success factor in marketing these services was not the type of services, credentials of the provider, or sales strategy (although all three factors played influential roles), but rather the delivery mechanism that was put in place. Realizing that to reach well audiences, they had to cater to hectic schedules, personal appointments were offered during evenings and weekends, as well as during the day. Clear directions for parking and locating the counseling center (which can be quite confusing in large hospital complexes) were provided. Because image and service are very important when serving well populations, and because nutrition counseling is an optional service people purchase, care was given to the ambience and setting for counseling. A receptionist greeted clients. The facility featured an attractive waiting room and pleasant, private counseling rooms. By making the dietitians accessible between appointments and accepting credit cards as a form of payment, they further catered to clients' needs.

The primary promotional strategies were a listing in a quarterly health-education catalogue and word-of-mouth referrals from satisfied customers. In addition, they used free media appearances, minimal newspaper advertising, physician referrals, and participation in hospital-sponsored publicity events to enhance their visibility. All these strategies resulted in preventive nutrition-counseling services becoming a profitable and viable business venture for the hospital.

MARKETING IN PRIVATE PRACTICE

Over the years, thousands of dietitians in private practice have been successful in selling private counseling sessions to well populations. The most successful marketing strategies in private practice are:

- Word-of-mouth referrals
- Marketing to physicians, nurses, and clinic managers
- Appearing in local media
- Writing newspaper and magazine articles
- Joining local professional or health and fitness groups
- Speaking at community, sports, professional, and school meetings
- Attending and speaking at health fairs and fun runs

For over twelve years, Evette Hackman, PhD, RD, consulted private clients, most of whom sought her services for support of their wellness goals, rather than for help in coping with an illness. She found that constant media exposure in her local market was the most effective marketing strategy for her. In fact, she said that if a month went by when she was not in the media, her patient load dropped. To keep herself in the media, Evette wrote a bimonthly column in the daily newspaper, developed relationships with local media contacts, and served as nutrition editor for *Shape* magazine. She sent out press releases regularly, and, as a result, she was frequently invited to appear as a guest expert on local television and radio shows.

Theresa Wright, MS, RD, CDE, relies on referrals from a broad network of health professionals: psychologists, mental health counselors, and diabetes care providers. She also finds that word-of-mouth referral from satisfied clients helps to expand her client base. Theresa makes sure that each client leaves her office feeling like the most important person she counseled that day. She stresses the importance of showing that she cares about her clients through little touches, like birthday cards, Christmas cards, and a phone number where clients can reach her during evenings and weekends.

MARKETING SPORTS NUTRITION SERVICES

Dietitians have increasingly become involved in providing sports nutrition services to a wide range of athletic populations: high school, college, professional, Olympic, masters, and recreational athletes. Nutrition services are delivered

Georgia Kostas, MPH, RD, LD

Exposed to preventive medicine and heart-healthy programs in undergraduate and graduate school, Georgia was committed to finding a full-time job in prevention. In 1979, she wrote a proposal to Dr. Kenneth Cooper, who hired her to design and implement a nutrition program for the Cooper Clinic. Still with the Cooper Clinic, Georgia manages a comprehensive nutrition program that provides individual counseling on preventive nutrition, community-outreach weight-control classes, and worksite nutrition services. She has recently started consulting with the Mavericks professional basketball team and also with restaurants to help them develop healthier menu items.

through individual counseling sessions, group education, training programs for coaches and sports medicine professionals, and nutrition columns for newsletters and popular magazines.

When a dietition works with an athletic team (from high school to professional), the athletic trainer or coach typically plays a key role. Therefore, when marketing nutrition services to athletic teams, it is important to build relationships with coaches and athletic trainers. Speaking at conferences for these professionals and writing in their trade publications will help build visibility. A mailing to local coaches and trainers followed by a personal sales call can be an effective way to explore the level of interest in your area and generate qualified leads. Once a contact is established, keep in touch. If a coach shows no interest the first time, call again a few months before the next year's season begins. It can take a long time to break in.

Dietitians provide individual counseling services for athletes through their private practices, sports team contracts, sports medicine clinics, and physicians' offices. When marketing to athletes in a private-practice setting, it is important to maintain a high level of visibility among consumers, particularly those active in sports and fitness. Exposure in media that are targeted to athletic populations and focus on athletic events will augment broad-based media coverage. When marketing services as part of a sports medicine clinic or physicians' practice, you must first set up a relationship with the clinic or practice, then build relationships with the professionals on staff, as well as the patients, to establish a referral network.

MARKETING CONSUMER-ORIENTED PROGRAMS

Consumer-oriented nutrition programs have considerable potential for success in today's marketplace. Supermarkets, restaurants, and employee cafeterias are ideal locations to influence eating behavior. The introduction of the Nutrition Labeling and Education Act (NLEA) brings about many opportunities to teach consumers how the new food label can help them lead to healthier food choices. Programs that feature the new food label can be offered at supermarkets, as well as other locations (see Chapters 18).

Pending legislation may force restaurants to comply with stricter requirements when using descriptive terms, like *light* and *heart healthy*, on their menus. According to Diane Welland, a dietitian and former manager of nutrition services for the National Restaurant Association, this could expand the potential for dietitians to consult with restaurants in developing menu items and properly labeling them (9). Since restaurant owners do not know how to find a dietitian who can help them comply with the new regulations, it is up to dietitians to market their skills to restaurateurs. Welland suggests that it is best to start with local, single-owner operations. Before making a sales call, she recommends becoming well acquainted with the restaurant – its patrons, menus, and (if possible) kitchen capabilities. When scheduling a sales call, try to reach the local manager or owner between lunch and dinner service. Sell your services in terms of tangible benefits (such as drawing in new customers, improving satisfaction among existing customers, increasing food sales, and avoiding regulatory risk). Present specific ideas about what you can offer. For example, you could propose to analyze the existing menu items and provide advice on the appropriate use of descriptive terms, or consult with the chef to develop a line of health-oriented menu items.

Jean Storlie, MS, RD

I became involved with the Chicago White Sox in 1987, when the athletic trainer called me in response to a referral from a colleague. He was contacting me on behalf of the Executive Vice President, who wanted to start a cafeteria nutrition program for the employees (not the team). In providing wellness services for the employees, I brought in another dietitian, Mary Mullen, who assisted in designing the kitchen for the new stadium the club was building. Mary and I kept planting seeds about the possibility of working with the team, stressing the link between nutrition and performance, and we cultivated our relationship with the athletic trainer, who controlled access to the players. In 1991, we succeeded in expanding our services to include the team. Now the team receives a pregame snack, a full meal after each game, and a bimonthly newsletter. The two of us develop all menus, and Mary works with the kitchen staff to introduce and reinforce healthy food-preparation techniques. We attribute our success with this account to building good relations with the athletic trainer, kitchen staff, and management.

TRENDS THAT AFFECT NUTRITION AND WELLNESS

To quote Naisbitt, "Trends, like horses, are more easily ridden in the direction they are already moving." (10) Keeping abreast of trends that affect the future of the wellness movement is critical when marketing wellness services and programs. Wellness grew out of larger trends and continues to be influenced by forces that shape health care, the economy, corporate America, and society. Within a climate of change, there are both opportunities and threats to consider. As the costs of health insurance and acute care steadily rise, it appears that the need for corporate wellness and health promotion programs will continue.

A trend that can be viewed both positively and negatively by dietetics professionals is the emergence of nontraditional therapies. Those who view nontraditional therapies as a threat see other professionals (such as chiropractors) and unqualified providers encroaching on the turf of dietitians. Others realize that wellness is multifaceted and that to practice wellness, it is important to embrace the whole person and keep an open mind about new strategies. Practitioners who work in wellness should read what their clients read and stay abreast of emerging philosophies as well as new consumer rip-offs.

Wellness opportunities can be found among groups with special needs, such as women, children, the elderly, and people with disabilities. The Nutrition Labeling and Education Act (NLEA) creates the need for new roles and services, including teaching consumers to use the new food label to make healthier choices and helping food companies develop healthier products.

Dietitians marketing wellness services should monitor these and other trends, looking for creative ways to capitalize on the opportunities and, more importantly, turn threats into new avenues for success.

KEY LINKAGES FOR PROMOTING THE NUTRITION ASPECTS OF WELLNESS

Since wellness is an interdisciplinary field, building and maintaining relationships with professionals outside the dietetics profession expands a dietitian's base of resources and expertise and enhances the potential for referrals. Connection to a larger network also stimulates new learning and makes it easier to stay at the cutting edge.

As part of their Strategic Thinking Initiative, the leadership of ADA recognized the importance of key linkages in the implementation of strategic actions. They identified two key linkages important in positioning the profession at the forefront of the wellness and disease-prevention movement: the federal government, and the media and communications industry. The rationale for focusing on the federal government as the top priority is that health-care reform was identified as the most significant issue facing the profession because such reform will determine access to health-care services. The media were identified as the second priority because of their tremendous influence in shaping public perceptions of food choices and ways to ensure wellness.

The dietitians involved in wellness whom I contacted identified many other linkages important to sustaining and broadening their wellness practices. As illustrated in Figure 17-4, they recognized a wide range of alliances that can be important to marketing wellness: federal and state governments, local communities, professional organizations, business and industry, health-care organizations, food purveyors, and media. Developing specific contacts within each of these areas will increase the potential for dietitians to expand their wellness opportunities.

Figure 17-4. Key Linkages for Promoting the Nutrition Aspects of Wellness

KEY LINKAGE	SPECIFIC CONTACTS
Federal and state governments	Politicians Governmental officials Government agencies
Local communities	Fitness centers YMCAs HMOs Hospitals City recreation departments Universities and colleges Beauty salons Elementary and high schools Day-care centers

Professional organizations	Exercise-related professional organizations:
	    American College of Sports Medicine
	    National Athletic Trainers Association
	    National Strength Conditioning Association
	Wellness-related organizations:
	    Association for Worksite Health Promotion
	    National Wellness Institute
	    Wellness Councils of America (WELCOA)
	Spa industry

Business and industry	CEOs Human resource professionals Training and development professionals Occupational physicians Occupational nurses Occupational-safety managers Food-service managers
Health-care organizations	Hospitals Managed-care organizations Physicians' practices Health researchers and policy makers
Food purveyors	Restaurants Supermarkets Food industries
Media	National, regional, and local print and electronic media

Theresa Wright, MS, RD, CDE

After working in hospital intensivecare centers and burn units for nine years, Theresa took a parttime job in a fitness center, where she built a reputation in weight management. She helped several clients to lose and maintain losses of more than 100 pounds, and her success earned her a loyal following. Using her contacts with established mental health therapists for referrals, she set up a private practice that serves people who suffer from compulsive eating problems. As a certified diabetes educator, she also counsels people with diabetes and is seeing that part of her practice grow.

CONCLUSION

A wide range of marketing strategies can be successfully employed to promote a wellness practice. The success of a given strategy will depend on the setting in which the practice is based, the services offered, and the target audience. The following hints will enhance your attempts to market your wellness practice:

- Realize that referrals are critical. Credentials, establishing a solid reputation, and building relationships will foster both client and professional referrals.

- Use strategic alliances (or partnerships) as springboards to other opportunities.

- Seek media exposure in front of your target groups.

- Get training, if necessary. Professional sales skills are critical.

- Sell to the decision makers.

- Know your niche.

References

1. Northwestern University's Center for Health Services and Policy Research, American Hospital Association's Center for Health Promotion. Health promotion programs flourishing: survey. *Hospitals.* August 16, 1985:128-135.

2. The American Dietetic Association, Society for Nutrition Education, Office of Disease Prevention and Health Promotion (PHSHHS). *Worksite Nutrition: A Decision-Maker's Guide.* Chicago, IL: The American Dietetic Association; 1986.

3. The American Dietetic Association, U.S. Public Health Service. *Worksite Nutrition: A Guide to Planning, Implementation, and Evaluation.* 2nd ed. Chicago, IL: The American Dietetic Association, 1993.

4. Office for Disease Prevention and Health Promotion, U.S. Public Health Service (HHS). *National Survey of Worksite Health Promotion Activities: Summary Report.* Washington, DC: U.S. Government Printing Office; 1987.

5. Office for Disease Prevention and Health Promotion, U.S. Public Health Service (HHS). *National Survey of Worksite Health Promotion Activities: Summary Report.* Washington, DC: U.S. Government Printing Office; 1993.

6. Association for Fitness in Business. *Guidelines for Employee Health Promotion Programs.* Champaign, IL: Human Kinetics Publishers; 1992.

7. Storlie J, Daly-Gawenda D. Hospital innovation and entrepreneurship. In: Sol N, Wilson PK, eds. *Hospital Health Promotion.* Champaign, IL: Human Kinetics Publishers; 1989:229-262.

8. Kelley L, Scheer J. Nutrition counseling in a hospital-based wellness program: keys to success. *SCAN's Pulse.* 1991; 10(3):811.

9. Welland D. RDs and restaurants: recipes for success. *J Am Diet Assoc.* 1993; 93(10):1005.

10. Naisbitt, J. *Megatrends: The New Directions Transforming Our Lives.* New York, NY: Warner Books; 1982.

Chapter 18

Marketing Strategies in Food Service

Cathy Powers, MS, RD, Director of Nutrition, Culinary Institute of America, Hyde Park, New York

In the not-too-distant past, the terms *nutrition* and *healthy food* were synonymous with bland, boring, and unappetizing food. Dietitians were the "enjoyment police." You ate either a good meal, or a healthy meal, but never one and the same.

Today, eating well has taken on new meaning. Healthy food can and should taste good and look as appealing as traditional fare. There are many opportunities for chefs and dietitians to work together toward the common goal of preparing good-tasting, nicely presented, well-balanced meals. In other words, people can have their cake and eat it too. Additionally, surveys show that the consumers want good healthy fare and are willing to pay for it. The opportunities for dietetics professionals have exploded in the area of commercial food service.

The popular press and the newly reformed like to give the impression that marrying culinary skills with healthy cooking is innovative and new. Yes, there is some innovation, but it is hardly a new concept. Dietitians did know about food at one time; we understood where it came from, what to do with it, how to advise our clients about it, and even how to enjoy it. Over time, however, we became removed from food because it was too simple and not serious enough. However, you cannot talk about nutrition and healthy eating practices without talking about how to prepare food. The two concepts are connected and dependent upon each other.

If the dietetics professional represents one side of the healthful eating coin, the flip side, and the ally or partner, is the culinary professional. In the past, chefs and cooks may have dismissed efforts by well-intentioned but culinarily naive dietitians as "too many cooks spoiling the broth." But this is no longer the case. Culinary professionals know that if they are to succeed, they must respond to demands from the popular press, trade journals, their own professional organization, their peers, and, most important of all, their guests for healthful, nutritionally correct meals. For some managers, owners, and chefs, the quest for a greater emphasis on healthy cooking may take a truly personal slant; many who have had personal health problems are especially keen to implement changes on their menus. Operations can turn completely around because the general manager has had a heart attack.

The opportunities to market your services within the commercial food-service segment are bountiful. Many operators, managers, and chefs are anxious to implement some sort of healthful eating and dining program but lack the time and expertise to know where to begin.

Americans continue to spend a significant portion of their food dollars on meals eaten outside the home. Dining out has become a way of life for many and is no longer just a special occasion. These patrons have become more conscious of what they eat away from home. Business travelers traditionally suffer health problems that can be laid at the door of a lifestyle that includes high-fat restaurant meals. They have become more vocal about their needs, and restaurants have become more responsive to their rising clamor for healthier meals. Those same restaurants, trying to respond to their guests, have gotten lost in a sea of conflicting reports, misinformation, and consumer confusion.

A great many cooks and chefs are ready to work together to form new partnerships with health and nutrition professionals, but are we? Our opportunity to impact on school-lunch, health-care, and commercial food-service markets is *now*, and we cannot let it pass us by.

WHAT YOU HAVE TO OFFER THE FOOD-SERVICE INDUSTRY

Your services could run the gamut from a simple menu evaluation to a complete recipe-development project. When consulting in this area, remember your role and tailor your services to the expertise of the people with whom you are working. When working with highly trained culinary professionals, capitalize on their expertise and offer guidance on ingredient substitution, menu balance, and portion control. Enhance their creativity, do not stifle it. When dealing with someone with less training, step forward with more input on correct cooking methods, recipe development, and ingredient selection.

Recipe Analysis (Nutrient Analysis)

Whether you are assisting in the development of an operation's recipes or are evaluating the menu, providing nutritional analysis of recipes is a valuable and often lucrative service. It is often easier for a chef to relate to a recipe analysis and use it to make modifications than to conceptualize a healthy recipe.

The process of recipe development and evaluation will take several steps: develop the recipe, analyze the recipe, make modifications, reanalyze the recipe, and so forth. Recipe analysis calls for a specialized database, so you may need to spend some time customizing the database you use. Items such as stocks, dried cherries, sundried tomatoes, specialty meats, and fishes may not be found in traditional databases.

Recipe-analysis also calls for an understanding of cooking and how ingredients will react. For example, when marinating items, how much of the marinade will be absorbed, or how much alcohol is burned off from heating or flaming a product?

Recipe analysis services are used by many segments of the industry and can be quite lucrative. Fees can range from $5.00 to over $35.00 per recipe.

Creating Standards of Operation

Before starting the actual recipe evaluation and development, it is important to set standardized nutritional criteria, as shown in Figure 18-1. There are no set rules or absolute values. The nutritional criteria will vary depending on the style of operation. For example, a spa might have a lower caloric limit, and a sports-training facility might have a higher caloric limit. It is important for both the patrons and the food-service operators to have specific values to relate to.

One potentially difficult area in implementing a healthy cuisine or menu into an operation is setting standards of practice, or agreement and evaluation procedures. We all know that what is done on paper (such as a printed recipe) and what is

Figure 18-1. Example of Nutritional Cooking Criteria: Suggested Menu Parameters (enlarged in Appendix)

Weight Maintenance					
		1800 to 2500 calories			
		60 to 75 grams fat			
		70 to 100 grams protein			
		250 to 350 grams carbohydrate			
		less than 3000 mg sodium			
		less than 300 mg cholesterol			
	Breakfast	400 to 600 calories			
	Lunch	500 to 700 calories			
	Dinner	700 to 1000 calories			
	Snacks	max. 200 calories per day			

Weight Maintenance	DINNER				
Course	Calories	Fat	Protein	Sodium	Cholesterol
Appetizer	<150	<5 gm	<10 gm	<300 mg	<50 mg
or Soup	<100	<2 gm		<300 mg	
Salad	<100	<5 gm		<150 mg	
Entree:					
Main item with sauce	<225	<10 gm	<30 gm	<500 mg	<100 mg
Starch	100	<2 gm		<150 mg	
Vegetable	<50	<2 gm		<100 mg	
Dessert	<200	<4 gm		<100 mg	
Bread	<100	<2 gm		<200 mg	
Beverage	80 to 100	trace	trace		
Total	less than 1000	less than 30 gm	approx. 50 gm	less than 1500 mg	less than 150 mg

done in practice may not be the same. It is important to protect your credibility by setting evaluation standards.

After setting evaluation standards, set enforcement and monitoring procedures. A good idea is to have "mystery customers" (for quality control) assisting in the monitoring of a program. These costs must be built into the contract.

Recipe Evaluation, Revision, and Development

Evaluating Existing Recipes. Many items that are prepared and served in restaurants can be identified as healthy and would meet the defined nutritional criteria without any major changes. Examples of such items may be clear soups, poached fish, pasta with marinara sauce, and fruit desserts.

When evaluating recipes, look for the following:

- Recipes that use lower-fat main ingredients, such as lean meats, fish, poultry, or grains and legumes.

- Recipes that have light sauces, such as fruit and vegetable coulis, natural reductions, and alternatives to roux, such as arrowroot or cornstarch as thickening agents.

- Recipes that use lower-fat cooking methods: poaching, simmering, broiling, grilling, roasting, hot smoking, stir-frying, or dry sautéing.

Modifying Existing Recipes. Many traditional or classical recipes can be adjusted or modified to meet the defined nutritional guidelines. One word of caution: when modifying recipes, be careful not to compromise taste or appearance. Customers will not accept a dish that is not as satisfying as the traditional counterpart. The kiss of death is "this isn't too bad – for a healthy alternative."

When adjusting recipes to meet nutritional guidelines, look to the following:

- Modifying portion sizes, particularly with the main item.
- Substituting ingredients that are lower in fat and/or higher in flavor.
- Using alternative techniques, such as smoke roasting, dry sautéing, and poaching.

Creating New Recipes. Using the chef's skills and your knowledge of the nutrients in ingredients, you can create and develop new and exciting recipes specifically intended to meet the nutritional guidelines. New recipes can be marketed from the start as healthy alternatives and will not invite comparisons to traditional items.

When creating a new recipe, keep the following points in mind:

- Use the freshest ingredients available.
- Use lean meats, fish, and poultry.
- Keep sauces light and flavorful.
- Use low-fat cooking techniques.
- Use low-fat products when possible.

Ingredient Selection

Consulting services could include advice and guidance on product selection and development of purchasing specifications. Showing the commercial market the wide range of healthy alternatives to standard products will help professional cooks and chefs understand how a dietitian with in-depth knowledge of foods can assist in the development of a healthful menu.

An interesting approach to this service might be to develop comparison or selection grids that compare different items within a product line. Comparison criteria might include taste, color, texture, usability, fat content, calories, sodium, overall palatability, as shown in Figure 18-2. Items that lend themselves to comparisons are regular and reduced-fat cheese, alcoholic and nonalcoholic beverages, commercially prepared soups and bases, and various grades of meats or cuts (prime versus choice beef, or free-range versus factory-raised poultry).

Figure 18-2. Food Product Evaluation

For product acceptability, use a scale of 1 to 5:

5 *excellent*
4 *good*
3 *average*
2 *fair*
1 *poor or unacceptable*

Date__________

Evaluator__________

Nutrition Profile				Product Acceptability				
Food Item	Calories	Fat (gm)	Sodium (mg)	Taste	Texture	Usability	Overall Palatability	TOTAL

Also arrange tastings to broaden the kitchen staff's flavor repertoire and update menu selections. Interesting and useful items to taste include flavored or infused vinegars and oils, sun-dried tomatoes, sun-dried fruits (cherries, blueberries, strawberries, or cranberries), chilis, tropical fruits, less familiar grains (quinoa, spelt, amaranth), and legumes.

Tastings may be expanded to include others in the organization. Consider including as many of the following individuals as appropriate: the chef, the sous-chefs, the maitre d' or dining room manager, lead servers or waiters, and cafeteria supervisors.

Staff Training

Many healthy dining programs fall through the cracks because of inadequate staff training and support. The kitchen and service staff must buy into a program's philosophy wholeheartedly to keep momentum high.

Training for the back-of-the-house staff needs to include the following points:

- Basic nutrition information that will explain why changes are being made (Staff members need to understand the why's of the change to relate to the how's.)
- Portion control and ingredient-measuring techniques
- Proper cooking techniques and the need for conscientious application each time a dish is prepared
- Translating customers' special requests into specific menu items (such as broiling fish instead of sautéing, frying, or cooking à la meunière)

Training for the front-of-the-house staff needs to emphasize basic nutrition information so they communicate more accurately with the guests, as well as some information about cooking techniques and ingredients. Only then can the waitstaff help guests meet their individual needs and help the kitchen staff provide carefully prepared and nutritious food. Emphasis needs to be placed on communicating how the restaurant accommodates guests by changing a cooking style, replacing a high-fat sauce with a lower-fat one, preparing a smaller portion size, and so forth.

Simply having a dietitian as part of an operation provides credibility and reliability for a promotion targeted at healthful dining. Such a person becomes a source of information in many key areas, such as marketing, generating local support, and acting as a resource.

Menu Development

A natural extension of recipe development and menu revision is working with the manager or operator to determine how the new information will be communicated to guests and potential customers.

There are several schools of thought concerning how best to identify healthy items on menus. The classical approach relies on symbols or icons to designate items on a menu as healthier alternatives. Symbols assist guests in making selections without a lot of server assistance and eliminate guesswork. They are also clear and concise. Nonetheless, the jury is out regarding the overall benefit of symbols. As the FDA continues its movement toward tighter control over what constitutes a health claim, the use of symbols on menus in restaurants may have many ramifications. Interestingly, when one restaurateur removed the "healthy" symbols and claims from his menu, he found that healthy items increased in sales because they were stigma-free.

Another approach is to design a separate menu or section of the menu that is specifically for healthier items. All courses from soups to desserts, and maybe even beverages, are segregated. The obvious benefit for the guest is that healthier alternatives are easier to find. The great disadvantage of having a separate menu is that the guest must specifically request it to see the healthier alternatives. It is possible that more people might order these items if they were right on the main menu.

Another approach is *not* to highlight the healthy alternatives. This approach is based on the reasoning that special labeling sends a negative message about the rest of the menu and leads guests to wonder, "If these items are 'healthy,' does that mean the rest of the menu is 'unhealthy'?" This reinforces the old "good food/bad food" approach to eating. Often when people are trying to make healthy changes in their diets, they do not want to call special attention to themselves by making selections from a segregated menu category that ends up sounding like yet another series of diet plates. A more positive approach is to let the items speak for themselves and rely on a combination of the guests' knowledge and personal interest in healthful selections and the servers' education about and ability to promote the items appropriately.

TAKING THE SERVICE TO THE CUSTOMER

Independent Restaurants

Let's look at the specific needs of the commercial food-service industry that cry out for the assistance of a dietetics professional who knows food. One area with great potential is independent restaurants. Such restaurants are usually small and often have limited resources. They cannot afford to hire a full-time dietitian, but are willing to hire a consultant.

The easiest way to begin consulting with such restaurants is to assist them with menu modifications and recipe evaluation. The best place to begin is at a restaurant that you frequent. Arrange a meeting with the manager and/or chef to discuss your personal desire for lower-fat meals or healthier alternatives and turn it into an opportunity to assist. If you know the operation, their menu, their customer base, and their basic operating philosophy, you will have a distinct advantage.

A second networking opportunity can be tapped into by joining a local chapter of either the American Culinary Federation (ACF) or the American Institute of Wine and Food (AIWF). Develop a formal presentation for the organization. Most groups welcome interesting and informative speakers who help members meet the needs of their current customer base and attract new clients. Nutritional concerns are viable marketing and profit-generating tools.

Once you have identified potential food-service clients, put together individual proposals to meet each operation's needs. Present all the consulting services you can offer, such as reviewing menus, staff training, and assistance with marketing to specific groups, including senior-citizen centers, weight-loss programs, and other likely candidates. You are offering a service that the commercial food-service market wants.

Recognize that consumers and restaurants want to affiliate with someone with credentials in healthy dining. Consumers want to trust that a restaurant is meeting certain standards and that it is carefully monitored.

Restaurant-Marketing Ideas

As a first step, identify your client restaurant as a leader in healthy dining. Do this by creating a program that both consumers and the food-service industry recognize as in touch with sound nutrition principles.

Consider, for example, aligning the operation with a hospital outpatient clinic, wellness center, weight-loss center, or health organization. Arrange for the chef to provide cooking demonstrations or classes. Bring groups into the restaurant to experience healthful dining at a new level. Market the restaurant through cooking competitions, food tastings, and media interviews to promote healthy dining.

Restaurant Chains, Hotels, and Resorts

Another segment of the commercial food-service industry to work with is restaurant groups or chains. Within this segment, you can develop a wide range of opportunities beyond those discussed previously. From signature dishes to special brochures to cooking demonstrations for customers, the dietetics professional and restaurant chain can develop a unique relationship and extensive list of services.

Hotels and resorts need your services in more than their restaurants. Getaway weekends with themes are becoming more popular, and cooking as a theme is as popular as ever. Combine your expertise with the chef's skills and innovation to put together a series of getaway weekends that include cooking demonstrations, nutrition seminars, exercise workshops, and other lifestyle enhancers. If a venture of this sort is developed for a hotel chain, it could be marketed across the country.

One interesting idea that several hotels are marketing is healthier bedtime treats. Rather than sending their guests to bed with a high-calorie, high-fat snack, they send a healthy alternative: fresh fruit, fresh-squeezed juice, or a specially created house item.

Don't forget to tie into the hotel exercise center, a natural potential for seminars, private consulting, and product promotion. Make recommendations for additional profit opportunities for the hotel or resort. Natural extensions in the fitness center include creating a juice bar, offering-body fat testing, and developing a menu for the restaurant that is "sponsored" by the fitness center.

Many hotels host conferences that could use special nutrition seminars for programs such as spouse activities or lifestyle-enhancement seminars. A series of seminars that could interest a range of guests might include "Healthful Entertaining," "How to Survive Business Lunches," "Staying Fit on the Road," and "Eating to Increase Your Productivity."

Resorts, including cruise ships, spas, island resorts, ski resorts, and dude ranches, also present some unique marketing opportunities. Menu-consulting and recipe-development opportunities can be found in any of these entertainment arenas, but to realize the fullest potential, you need to look beyond the standard fare. Complete service packages are often more enticing to such organizations, which may not know they need or could benefit from your services.

Services can range from menu consultation to seminars, cooking demonstrations, fitness-center evaluations, nutrition consultations for guests, wine tastings, and employee wellness programs. Keep in mind that people will often pay more for services when they are on vacation or on business than they would at home.

Apart from this new avenue, there are many ways that dietitians can incorporate aspects of the culinary field into traditional avenues of practice to enhance their marketing potential.

Health-Care Food Service

The food served in health care has long had a reputation for being unappealing and bland. First, let me say that in many cases, I do not think this is just. Given the limitations of meal production in many facilities, miracles are often created. However, food service was once an area of great pride, some of which has been lost along the way. As hospitals and other health-care operations are trying to differentiate themselves from the competition, patients often look to auxiliary services. The food served is certainly an area for differentiation, and good food is always appreciated.

Many food-service operators want to hire a professional chef, but cannot afford to. In fact, when the situation is analyzed, they cannot afford *not* to hire a professional chef. The increase in patient and employee satisfaction, the increased revenue from the cafeteria and catering, and the savings from limiting mistakes can often pay for a professional's salary. This is a case of doing the right thing right.

There are many marketing opportunities within health care that can bring the culinary and nutrition worlds together. Once you have made a hospital's food healthy and delicious, invite the board, medical staff, and auxiliary for lunch. Show off the new fare at catered functions, and invite the local media to taste the food and interview satisfied patients. Invite guest chefs from local restaurants or hotels to appear at fund-raisers, promotional activities for the hospital food service, or educational activities for the outpatient center. Give cooking demonstrations to send a sound nutrition message and draw new clients.

It is almost impossible to discuss diet modifications or nutritional concerns without discussing food and its preparation. When dealing with patients or clients, it is essential that you also discuss how theory is translated into practice. The public wants to know what ingredients they can substitute, how they can change traditional recipes, what cooking methods are recommended, which yogurt is best to use, how many grams of fat are in specific products, and the like. It is clear that people are dealing with food – not theory – and that we need to relate to them on that level.

School Food Service and Other Large-Quantity Feeding Operations

Students and institutional residents of all ages appreciate the strides food-service directors are making to serve food that is more nutritious and appealing. Many food establishments are adding salad bars, baked potato bars, soup and salad lines, vegetarian and stir-fry entrees, homemade whole-grain breads, low-fat entrees and dairy products, lite salad dressings, and grilled and petite meat portions.

The new food options can be promoted in newsletters to parents or residents, on bulletin boards and posters, on table tents in the cafeteria, and in presentations to classes or group meetings. Again, it helps first to instruct the cooking and serving staff, residents, and teachers on the nutrition benefits and reasons for change before introducing the change.

Dietetics professionals can teach good food habits directly to students or through class curricula from preschool through graduate school. Nutrition presentations, cooking demonstrations, food and wine tastings, catered parties, and holiday or theme meals are all popular with retirement residents.

Teaching in Culinary Schools

The American Culinary Federation requires thirty hours of nutrition studies for their chef-certification program. There are several ways of obtaining the requisite training, but they are often unsuitable. Dietitians in various localities have developed nutrition-education programs for chefs and have worked with local ACF organizations for sponsorship and promotion. It is from such programs that many other opportunities have followed.

Most community culinary programs offer some level of nutrition education to their students, or if they don't offer it yet, they are looking to add it. In the past, such programs have been taught by the culinary faculty or well-intentioned management instructors. Openings certainly exist for exciting nutrition-education curriculums within culinary programs.

PROFESSIONAL DEVELOPMENT FOR DIETITIANS

Traditional education requirements do not necessarily prepare a dietetics professional for working within the culinary field, and we often need to supplement or enhance our food knowledge. But beyond all required skills and knowledge, we must first have a passion for food and enjoy working with it. On this, we must build our understanding of basic culinary terminology, cooking techniques, functions and uses of ingredients, current food trends, ingredient combinations, and flavorings and seasonings, and develop your sense of taste.

There are many ways to enhance your culinary knowledge, and some are actually fun. The first way is to experience food as much as possible. Eat out and enjoy. You learn about food by touching and tasting it. The second way is to read about food. Each year, more food magazines enter the market; some are directed toward consumers and some toward professionals, but all can be valuable resources. There is a wealth of food books and cookbooks that make enjoyable reading. The third way is to cook, both at home and with professionals.

There are many opportunities to collaborate with other professionals and professional organizations to highlight nutrition and healthy cooking. At the 1992 annual meeting of the American Culinary Federation, the First ACF National Championship, entitled "Healthful Cooking – Balancing the Art," was held. This competition paired chefs and dietitians in a competition to highlight healthy cooking. This event, organized by Victor Gielisse, CMC, and Nancy Skodack, MS, RD, LD, created much excitement and set the trend for future collaborative efforts. Beyond being an enjoyable time and a personal challenge, such an event can be turned into a fund-raiser, community adventure, and media event to highlight a product promotion or business.

Other organizations, such as the American Institute of Wine and Food, are actively working on incorporating taste and health. Several years ago the AIWF initiated a program entitled "Resetting the American Table," which brought together culinary professionals and nutritionists to discuss strategies that will promote our common goal of improving the taste and healthfulness of the food we consume. This initiative opened many doors for dietitians to form partnerships and establish collaborative projects.

On a more formal level, many local community culinary programs have short courses that enable you to continue your education. The Culinary Institute of America, in Hyde Park, New York, has developed a specific 30-hour course just for dietitians that is designed to provide a broad introduction into the culinary world. The American Institute of Wine and Food has developed a short course for dietitians that is team taught by a chef and a dietitian that was premiered at the 1993 American Dietetic Association Annual Meeting and Exhibition.

In conclusion, the plate is clean, the pot is empty, the opportunities for dietitians in food service are wide open, and the time is now.

Recommended Culinary Resources and Reading

Books

Culinary Institute of America. *The New Professional Chef.* 5th ed. New York, NY: Van Nostrand Reinhold; 1991.

Culinary Institute of America. *The Professional Chef's Techniques of Healthy Cooking.* New York, NY: Van Nostrand Reinhold; 1993.

Prosper M. *Larousse Gastronomique.* American ed. Lang JH, ed. New York, NY: Crown Publishers, Inc.; 1988.

Escoffier A. *The Complete Guide to the Art of Modern Cooking.* A, trans. New York, NY: Van Nostrand Reinhold; 1990.

Brillat-Savarin JA. *The Physiology of Taste.* Dreyon A, trans. New York, NY: Penguin Books; 1970.

McVane AJ. *The Encyclopedia of Fish Cookery.* New York, NY: Holt, Rinehart and Winston; 1977.

Tannahill R. *Food in History.* New York, NY: Crown Publishers, Inc.; 1988.

Root W, De Rochemont R. *Eating in America.* New York, NY: William Morrow; 1976.

Coyle PL. *The World Encyclopedia of Food.* New York, NY: Facts on File; 1982.

McGee H. *Curious Cook.* New York, NY: Charles Scribner's Sons; 1990.

McGee H. *On Food and Cooking: The Science and Lore of the Kitchen.* New York, NY: Charles Scribner's Sons, 1984.

Johnson H. *Hugh Johnson's Modern Encyclopedia of Wine.* 2nd ed. New York, NY: Simon and Schuster; 1987.

Zraly K. *Windows on the World Complete Wine Course.* New York, NY: Sterling Publishing Co.; 1985.

Project LEAN. *Chef's Handbook. Low-Fat Quantity Food Preparation.* Chicago, IL: The American Dietetic Association Foundation; 1993.

Journals

Art Culinaire, P.O. Box 238, Madison, NJ 07940

Gourmet, 560 Lexington Avenue, New York, NY 10022

Food & Wine, 1120 Avenue of the Americas, New York, NY 10036

Culinary Trends, 6285 East Spring Street #107, Long Beach, CA 90808

Chocolatier, 45 West 34th Street, New York, NY 10001

Food Arts, 387 Park Avenue South, New York, NY 10016

The Wine Spectator, M. Shanken Communications, Inc., 387 Park Avenue South, New York, NY 10006

Professional Associations

American Culinary Federation, *National Culinary Review*, P.O. Box 3466, St. Augustine, FL 32084

International Association of Culinary Professionals, 304 West Liberty, Suite 201, Louisville, KY 40202, 502-581-9786, FAX: 502-581-3602

The Friends of Wine, Les Amis du Vin, 2302 Perkins Place, Silver Springs, MD 20910

The American Institute of Wine & Food, 1500 Bryant Street, San Francisco, CA 94103, 1-800-274-AIWF, 415-255-3000

Case Study: **ADDING CULINARY SERVICES TO A PRIVATE PRACTICE**

Alanna Benham Dittoe, RD, Principal, Dittoe and Associates, Menlo Park, California

The 1990s will present the opportunity for dietitians to debut nutrition services directly to the consumer. With consumers' elevated interest in nutrition, our company decided to deliver products directly to our customers throughout the culinary world. What is closer to our consumers than great-tasting food? From a business point of view, it is more subtle marketing, and the direct contact with the public results in a more powerful increase in new business and revenues.

Our initial idea was spurred by the expansion of an elaborate grocery store called Draeger's in Menlo Park, California. It was started in 1923 by the Frank Draeger family in San Francisco and is considered unique in the United States. It offers every possible gourmet item, from specialty produce, meat, fish, and poultry to imported caviar and cheeses. In addition, it has a wine and hors d'oeuvre bar, a coffee bar, culinary equipment and gift sections, and a cooking school. The culinary director hires famous chefs from all over the United States as well as Europe to teach cooking classes and culinary workshops.

We met with the culinary director and proposed a series of seasonal light cooking classes. We opted to joint-venture the project to gain the opportunity to participate in the marketing campaign and help determine program content. To ensure program quality from our end, we invited Patricia Hart, a registered dietitian and chef who teaches at the Culinary Academy in San Francisco, to participate. Her wealth of knowledge, passion for food, and creative technique were essential to creating a cutting-edge concept. By working together, we produced a service superior to anything either of us could have done alone, one with long-term potential.

We offer five classes per season, each with a different food interest: Salads and Salad Dressings, Pasta and Pizza, Entrees, Desserts, and Appetizers. We also provide full menus with themes such as Lite Italian, Lite Asian, and Lite Holiday. The classes run two to three hours each. The fee is $35 per class, with a 30-person maximum. A discount is given for purchasing a season series. We vary the times and days of classes to reach more potential clients. The classes are marketed through an elaborate brochure, newspaper advertisements, and word-of-mouth.

Four to five individuals assist in these classes. I orchestrate all the introductions, the presentation of nutrition information, the food product tasting, and some equipment and cookbook presentations. Chef Hart handles the food and recipe demonstrations with her Chef's Assistant. A helper serves all recipe samples and food products. The Culinary Director may float in and out and offer words of wisdom. The guests are greeted by the Food and Wine Steward, who serves them the beverage of their choice and gives them the class notebook of nutrition publications and recipes. I introduce the class members to each other. Our attempt is to create a warm atmosphere conducive to "learn today, apply tonight, and return seasonally with a friend." Theatrical glass surrounds the cooking school, creating a focused entertainment center within the store.

We offer nutrition information and guidelines for fat and calories, while allowing room to ad lib for attendees' input and questions. Guests learn how the recipe portions fit into their usual meal plans. We provide workbooks, called *Hidden Fat*, to assist them with planning.

The culinary skills are presented by Chef Hart. She provides food demonstrations and incorporates techniques such as smoking, herb infusion, reduction, flavor balancing, and marinating. Students also learn sanitation, easy methods for cutting items to reduce calories, how to make items from scratch, and food-presentation tips.

We include samplings of all recipes and a number of food tastings throughout the class. Students experience textures, taste comparisons, and new flavor combinations. The highlights have been balsamic vinegars, frozen yogurts, sorbets, fresh herbs, nonfat sauces, and assorted roasted peppers.

We present equipment, new light cookbooks, newsletters, and cookbooks written by dietitians, and offer a 10 percent discount if the items are purchased on the day of the class. We also promote the grocery store tours that Karen Ross, another dietitian, provides.

We provide and encourage verbal as well as written evaluations. The overall response has been fabulous. We expect that our best marketing tool will be word of mouth. The classes provide great exposure for our firm and give us the opportunity to inform attendees about our other individual, group, and corporate nutrition consultation services.

Future ideas? Soon we will provide the same culinary concept at a more elaborate level at Fetzer Winery in the Alexander Valley of Northern California. We will also be providing classes entitled Lite Menus from Draeger's Deli, Cooking for Teens, Cooking Lite for Singles, and How to Prepare a Healthy Lunch Box. In addition, we want to highlight guest speakers, especially registered dietitian cookbook authors (please call if you are interested).

Whether we cook it, taste it, dip it, top it, or soak it, we have something light to offer everyone in these classes, whether the person is a gourmet cook, weekend cook, new cook, or only-want-to-entertain-for-an-evening cook. It is a win-win situation, and certainly a success for everyone involved.

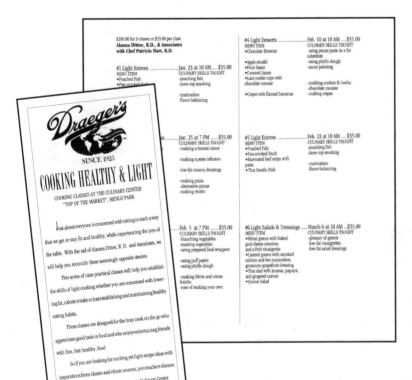

Culinary/Nutrition Class Brochure

Sharon O'Melia Howard, MS, RD, CEO, Nutrition For Living,
Kennett Square, Pennsylvania

In 1988, before low-fat eating was trendy in our area, I was working with a successful restaurateur who was trying to lose weight and control her hypoglycemia. She was the owner of the Firehouse restaurant, a lively eatery with a bar, where many repeat customers come for business lunches. One day after having successfully lost weight, she said to me, "I can't eat anything I serve in my restaurant! You must come and talk to my chef and tell him what to make for me."

Not long afterward, I met with my client, her first chef, Joe, and second chef, Pat. We decided that some customers might also want interesting low-fat meals, so I designed one 400-calorie low-fat lunch platter. Pat, the college-trained chef, was assigned to work with me. He had no trouble understanding the need for portion control and low-fat cooking methods to ensure each meal's validity.

The new Nutritious and Delicious lunch platter was marketed with a special menu insert. We naively thought we would run the same platter for a month to see what happened. Within four days, the customers were asking for other Nutritious and Delicious™ platters — both for lunch and for dinner.

Chef Pat and I scrambled to create twenty 400-calorie lunches and twenty 600-calorie dinners. Again, we mistakenly thought that only weight-conscious women would be interested, but we were delighted to find that the men also greatly appreciated our watching their waistlines. Chef Pat was amazed that he constantly sold out of the meals, and the sales reached 20 percent of gross at lunch and 12 percent at dinner.

My client, the restaurateur, used Nutritious and Delicious™ in her advertising, displaying my name and phone number on the advertisements, as well as on the menu. This brought many new private clients to my office. She also sent out a press release, which resulted in stories with photos in three newspapers.

That year the Firehouse hosted the annual county Restaurant Association Meeting. We served

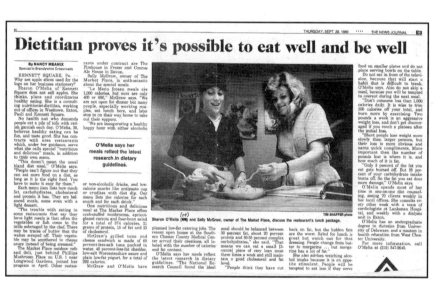

News Article to Promote Healthy Restaurant Items

a special Nutritious and Delicious™ meal, and I was featured as the guest speaker. The interest of the other restaurants was peaked, and I extended the concept to include a gourmet deli, a beef and beer establishment, a salad bar luncheonette, a pizza shop, and an upscale dining restaurant. My income increased, the publicity and exposure were priceless, and my private practice grew. Six years later, the Firehouse restaurant continues to offer my meals.

In time, the product's life cycle aged, competition became stiff, and my idea lost its uniqueness. Local hospital nutrition departments started to offer healthy heart menu items, and food brokers offered their dietitians' services for free. Good ideas don't last long. Looking back, I know I could have capitalized on this project on a grander scale and pursued larger accounts while the idea was new. What is it they say about hindsight?

Chapter 19

Consumer Education

Molly Gee, MEd, RD, Methodist Hospital, and TV Nutrition Reporter, Houston, Texas

The mission, vision, and philosophy of The American Dietetic Association focus on best serving the profession through serving the public by promoting optimal nutrition and health. The public awareness of the relationship of diet to health positions dietetics professionals in an advocacy role in food and nutrition consumer education. The well consumer, rather than simply the patient, now becomes the customer for our information.

The Strategic Thinking Initiative (STI) identified public and consumer education as the fourth key market that dietitians and diet technicians should pursue. This market is huge (over 250 million Americans) and diverse (requiring many ethnic, age, health, and gender considerations). The competition for the consumer's attention and dollar is stiff. The consumer is more knowledgeable and sophisticated about nutrition. What was good enough to sell ten years ago is old news now.

Dietitians have established a reputation for their professionalism, hard work, and dedication to improving the health of the public. This is not enough. Judith Dodd, a past president of ADA, defined the fifth P of the marketing mix as pizzazz. She stated, "It is an individual's perception of the worth of the product that may be the prime motivation in the decision to choose a product. The energy, creativity, style, or flair that a product or service represents in the mind of the potential consumer affects the perceived value. The 'sale' may go to the seller who has applied pizzazz successfully (1)."

ENVIRONMENTAL TRENDS IN THE CONSUMER MARKET

Change is a certainty. Today's environment is one of constant change. Many environmental trends will affect dietetic practice, especially as it relates to the consumer. It is important to respond aggressively to trends rather than merely react.

Traditional Families: A Disappearing Act

In years past, television series like *Father Knows Best* and *The Donna Reed Show* represented the traditional family, complete with the father as the breadwinner and the mother who stayed home to raise the children. Today, the many different forms of families provide additional challenges. Two-income families and single-parent families are becoming the norm rather than the exception. More adults are living alone instead of marrying or living with a roommate. Children are being left at home alone or with extended family members. Convenience and speed become major commodities as increased numbers of women enter the workforce. Cooking at home is fast becoming a novelty. The family dinner with all members present is fast becoming a rarity.

Wellness and Disease-Prevention Issues

Nutrition has become a priority for some Americans. Many federal reports have given nutrition a jump start. The relationship between diet and disease was documented in the 1988 Surgeon General's Report on Nutrition and Health. The

United States Department of Agriculture (USDA) and Health and Human Services (HHS) Dietary Guidelines and the Food Guide Pyramid are major social marketing campaigns designed to improve the eating habits of Americans. Unfortunately, science alone does not command action.

Legislation

The 1990 Nutrition Labeling and Education Act (NLEA) set a specific timeline for the Food and Drug Administration (FDA) to propose and finalize new labeling regulations. The new label, Nutrition Facts, was developed to help consumers make informed food choices. However, it will require additional information to be consumer friendly.

Constance Geiger, PhD, RD, established a private practice to fill this niche. Dr. Geiger has been involved in food-label design since 1981. Her technical background in food science, combined with studies in consumer behavior and economic and nutrition public policy, were keys to her success. Food companies need experts to translate the technicalities of the FDA rulings onto the panels of their products before the established deadlines. Dr. Geiger's strong belief that the food label is a primary way of communication to consumers has fueled her continuing efforts.

Health-care reform will result in greater emphasis on wellness and disease prevention. As a cost-containment strategy, consumers will be assuming more responsibility for their own health. Dietetics professionals have both the opportunity and the responsibility to position themselves to help set health policy (see Chapter 17).

Women

Another major consumer trend of this century is the growing power base for women in business and politics. While political clout is moving into Congress, governors' mansions, and city halls across the country, the glass ceiling is cracking slightly as women slowly move into leadership roles in corporations. According to the Small Business Administration, women are starting their own businesses at twice the rate of men, perhaps because of glass ceilings and walls, which restrict upward and lateral career movement. These changes have increased research monies for women's health issues. It is yet to be seen whether nutrition-related programs like child care, school breakfasts and lunches, and school-based nutrition education will become higher priorities.

The improvement in the opportunities for some women comes at a time when many others are not faring so well. The poor economic times have played havoc with family incomes and job security. Unemployment is known to increase the incidence of depression, suicides, and heart attacks (2). With the break-up of marriages, many women and children are thrust into poverty. Increasingly, women and children are victims of domestic violence. Feeding programs, community food pantries, and food-stamp and family-shelter programs can help these people in need.

Risk Avoidance

Today's consumers want to avoid risk in the foods they eat and in their environment. Some food-safety issues include bacterial contamination; the use of pesticides, food additives, and preservatives; and product tampering. Apples and Alar, grapes and cyanide, and hamburgers and E. coli are examples of highly publicized foodsafety worries. In addition, according to *Advertising Age*, consumers consider environmentally friendly issues in packaging to be important (3). Consumers will change their buying habits, especially of their children's food, to avoid potential problems.

Changing Communication Technology

Advances in communications will dictate how business will be conducted. *Speed* would be the appropriate one-word summary. Electronic mail is quickly replacing the fax machine. A growing phenomenon is the computer bulletin board system. Users merely go online for educational, business, or social interaction with other users of the system. Young people are especially responsive to this type of communication.

Magazines, direct mail companies, and other marketers use an interactive phone system to meet the needs of their customers and increase their revenues at the same time. A customized recorded message awaits customers based on their inquiries. Combine this with a fax machine, and readers can request and immediately receive a reprint of an article or other information.

Emerging Food Technology

Frequently, technology moves more quickly than consumer acceptance. Irradiated food and fat substitutes are two examples. Incidents like the apples and Alar scare sparked fear among consumers and moved them to resist advancing technology in favor of natural and organic produce. Professionals who work as consumer advocates are in a precarious situation as we begin to research and support new technology.

Biotechnology is the use of part or all of any living system for the production of different useful products; for example, the use of a hormone to increase milk production in cows. Common fruits, such as nectarines and tangelos, are the results of genetic engineering. Food irradiation ensures an increased shelf life for many highly perishable fruits, like strawberries. The combination of these technologies will revolutionize all aspects of the food industry. However, in the final analysis, the will of the consumer and the market will prevail.

CHALLENGES OF WORKING WITH CONSUMERS

Presently, there is no typical consumer. Identifying today's consumers can be a challenge. Age, ability, and race are just a few variables to consider.

The New Consumer Diversity

Today, 80 percent of Americans are white, up 6 percent from 1980. However, by the year 2000, whites will represent only 72 percent of the nation's total. Hispanics are the fastest growing group and are projected to reach 10 percent of the population by 1998. By 2050, one of every five Americans will be Hispanic. Currently, 12 percent of the population is African American, up 13 percent from 1980. By 1998, they will represent 9 percent of the population. Our ethnic population is projected to double to 48 percent by the year 2050 (4).

The Food Guide Pyramid does not take into account the cultural food preferences of our diverse population. Ann Miller, MS, RD, chair of the Nutrition Education for the Public practice group contends that one educational piece cannot be simply translated to meet the needs of every culture. Dietetics professionals must begin developing culturally sensitive education materials in preparation for the emerging population shift. The best way to begin is by working closely with community leaders and organizations of other cultures. (See the case study on creating an English-Spanish consulting nutrition business, at the end of this chapter.)

Consumers with Disabilities

Another type of diversity is added by the 43 million Americans with disabilities. People with physical challenges, especially with challenges to hearing and sight, need their messages appropriately interpreted for communication. Specially developed materials are not readily available. This is a growing segment of the population with unfulfilled needs for nutrition information.

Consumers with Limited Education and Low Literacy

When literacy is low, our messages about nutrition must be simple and visual. The USDA and HHS Dietary Guidelines and the Food Guide Pyramid provide the best examples of appropriate social marketing campaigns. Much of the responsibility lies with government agencies, hospitals, and other large businesses, but they need experts like us to assess the nutritional accuracy of the information and carry the message to the public.

Older Americans

The Nutrition Screening Initiative is a tool to identify at-risk older Americans. In 1988 the median net worth of households headed by someone over age 65 was $73,500, well above the US average of $35,800. These consumers have special needs as a consequence of their advancing years, chronic illnesses, and yet overall satisfactory health. Many also have the resources to afford nutrition care. Some estimate that 75 percent of the fluid capital in America is owned by persons over the age of 55.

Niche Marketing

To respond to the increasing diversity of our population, dietetics professionals must match their message to their target audience. This is called *niche marketing*. In niche marketing, we identify a small segment of the market and customize a message for that segment. In *Making Niche Marketing Work*, Linneman and Stanton state, "Today's customers look for products and services developed especially for them." (5) Such behavior creates many opportunities for dietetic professionals.

EMERGING MARKETS

Timing and speed become important factors when providing a service or product that is targeted to specific consumers. Entrepreneurial spirits are driven to be the first to take action on emerging trends. The growing number of small businesses is a trend itself. Dietetics professionals should use their expertise and credibility in food and nutrition to establish themelves in developing food-related businesses.

COMPETITION IN THE PUBLIC ARENA

Providing information is a business. Dietetics professionals do not have a monopoly on dispensing nutrition information. Much of the information on health is in the public domain. The media, other allied health providers, dentists, physicians, chiropractors, health-food retailers, health clubs, and the food industry are just some groups that supply nutrition information. Are they friends or foes? Ask the consumer who is faced with sorting out the facts.

Why would consumers listen to dietetics professionals? College degrees do not suffice. It is also necessary to stay up-to-date on the latest research. Conducting your own original research increases your credibility. The definition of research can be broadened to include local surveys or questionnaires in addition to well-controlled and designed clinical trials. Seek monies from a variety of public and private grants and foundations and publicize your results.

THE CHANGING TOOLS OF NUTRITION EDUCATION

There is tremendous competition in providing nutrition information. Many of the trends and emerging markets influence how dietetics professionals can successfully get their messages out. The reach and penetration vary with each tool and how it is targeted to the specific consumer. (See the case study at the end of this chapter.)

The Media

It's impossible to ignore the powerful influence of the media in our lives. With thousands of print and electronic media outlets reaching millions of Americans daily, there are endless opportunities waiting to be explored by dietetic professionals. Most consumers have access to television, radio, newspapers, and magazines. Working with the media provides immediate visibility and credibility for dietetics professionals. The media and the communications industry are key partners to get our messages to consumers.

Many dietetics professionals join the ranks of the media in addition to serving the media as valuable sources of information. Becoming a regular in the print or electronic media is the perfect way to reach consumers.

The author can provide personal testimony about the impact of having a regular television segment. In 1989, after a number of guest appearances on the local Houston ABC affiliate, I was asked to join the medical team of experts for the morning talk show. Then in 1992, I joined the morning news team to provide a weekly nutrition news segment. This 90-second segment reaches over half a million viewers weekly.

In 1982, the ADA Ambassador Program was launched as a public relations initiative to develop media spokespersons and nutrition advocates. The success of this national media effort is demonstrated by the fact that ADA receives about 700 clippings per month from newspapers and magazines with circulations of more than 50,000. A recent study reported that ADA or registered dietitians represent 20 percent of the sources cited in local and national print stories on food and nutrition.

Obviously, the media appreciate the benefits of using experts. However, there is no need to wait for the media to call. Be proactive and pitch your story to local dailies and radio and television stations. Use The National Nutrition Month Press

Kit to launch many successful placements. (See Chapter 13 for more information on working with the media.)

Also, do not overlook the reach of local cable stations. Joanne Lichten, PhD, RD, used the Houston Access Cable to publicize her book, *Dinin' Lean,* in Houston. The affordable studio fee for a 30-minute taped session has paid off handsomely. Her book sales remain brisk as a result of the reruns of her original segment.

Community Reach

An effective way to reach consumers is as a volunteer giving something back to the community. All local civic, religious, and professional organizations need help. It is a good strategy to broaden your network and contacts beyond medical and health professionals. In addition to committee work, speakers' bureaus and health fairs provide opportunities to showcase your services or products. If an organization is unable to provide an honorarium, negotiate for other benefits, such as use of a membership mailing list or an advertisement in a newsletter. You don't want to miss that one person in the audience or corporation who will provide your next big opportunity.

Publishing

Writing is an effective form of communication that can enhance visibility and credibility and reach a variety of consumers. Unlike radio and television, the written word can be carefully crafted and redrafted to clearly represent the author and the message. No one ever sees the first draft.

Writing talent is not a genetic trait. Learning to write effectively requires study through formalized courses, workshops or seminars, and constant practice. Start out with contributions to community or school newsletters. Seeing your article published with a byline will build your confidence and motivation to seek other outlets for publication. Joining the ranks of nutrition health journalists requires skill, creativity, and persistence, plus a well-crafted plan to get published. (For more information, see Chapter 33 on how to publish a book.)

Public Speaking

The thought of standing in front of an audience to give a speech is the number-one fear of most people. However, public speaking can be an effective tool to establish credibility, educate consumers, and market your services or products. To build confidence, speak on familiar topics to smaller audiences, such as school or civic organizations. Practice, practice, practice is the only way to control any fear you may feel. Toastmasters is an excellent organization to join for practice in extemporaneous and prepared speech making.

When preparing a speech, target a specific audience and plan to use visual aids to reinforce your message. A polished, professional talk can be expanded to a series of lectures, workshops, or seminars for other audiences, such as professional or corporate groups. Giving an effective speech is more than saying something to an audience, it's the ability to persuade the audience to take some action. (See Chapter 35 for hints on how to market yourself as a public speaker.)

ESTABLISH ALLIANCES

Building alliances with industry, corporations, coalitions, government agencies, and others creates opportunities to move your message, service, or product.

The Food Industry

Dietetics professionals and food companies enjoy a symbiotic relationship. Such a partnership offers a variety of potential opportunities, including endorsements and recommendations of products, creation of health messages, nutrient analysis of products, and development of educational materials.

In 1989, Guiltless Gourmet, Inc., was founded by Doug Foreman, who recognized that there was no low-fat tortilla chip to support consumers' interest in low-fat snacks. Mr. Foreman utilized dietetics professionals as public relations agents to add credibility to his new product and introduce it to consumers. In addition, Linda McDonald, MS, RD, was hired to develop nutrition education materials about low-fat snacking for the public. Today, Guiltless Gourmet Chips are among the top ten in chip sales. (In Chapter 34, Linda tells how she wrote a proposal and created her job.)

Other nutrition- or health-related food producers hire dietetic professionals with communication skills as spokespersons and consultants. Kraft General Foods, ConAgra (Healthy Choice), Quaker Oats, and Kellogg are just a few of the companies that include dietetics professionals in their marketing strategies.

Corporations

Fast foods and a nutrition message? McDonald's Corporation collaborated with The American Dietetic Association to support ADA's 1993 National Nutrition Month activities. This provided opportunities to reach millions of children with basic nutrition information.

Health-care reform has placed an emphasis on wellness and prevention. Corporations are beginning to recognize that good health is good business. Weight-control classes, brown-bag talks, heart-healthy classes, and prenatal nutrition are just a few possible offerings on the corporate front. Corporations are joining the ranks of learning centers for employees. You can market your services to these businesses to spearhead and carry out their programs.

Coalitions

In 1990, the American Institute of Wine and Food (AIWF) organized a historic coalition-building project called "Resetting the American Table: Creating a New Alliance of Taste and Health." Its purpose is to unite health professionals, culinary leaders, and the media to improve the taste and health of Americans simultaneously. The simplistic classification of foods as "good" or "bad" based on nutrient content has not been effective in bringing about change. Low-fat substitutions may look great on paper, but could produce an inferior product. Consumers will always use taste as the deciding criterion for food selection.

Dietetics professionals are already identified as nutrition experts. The nutrition and health communication expert and former ADA President Mary Abbott Hess, LDH, MS, RD, suggests that dietetics professionals go that next step to become food experts.

Government Agencies

The 5-A-Day program is the first national public-private nutrition program to approach Americans with the simple, positive message to eat five or more servings of fruits and vegetables every day. The program is jointly sponsored by the National Cancer Institute (NCI) in the U.S. Department of Health and Human Services and the Produce for Better Health Foundation (PBH), a not-for-profit consumer education foundation representing the fruit and vegetable industry. The original grant for the pilot study in California was spearheaded by dietitians.

Pharmaceuticals

The Nutrition Screening Initiative is a five-year, multifaceted effort promoting routine nutrition screening and better nutrition care for older Americans. This effort is a project of the dietitians in ADA, the American Academy of Family Physicians, and the National Council of Aging, Inc. The Initiative was made possible in part through a grant from Ross Laboratories, a division of Abbott Laboratories. A blue-ribbon advisory committee of more than 27 key organizations and dietetics and other professionals from the fields of medicine and aging also play an important role in guiding this effort.

Grocery Stores

Look for grocery stores and restaurants to be the new learning centers for nutrition. Point-of-purchase education is an industry concept that began with complimentary food samplings to introduce new product lines. Recipes and coupons are constants in the grocery aisles. The 5-A-Day Campaign for Better Health has a well-established place in many grocery produce sections.

Since 1988, Lori Valencic, MEd, RD, has been providing grocery shopping tours and contributing nutrition news for a major Texas grocery chain. In 1992, she wrote a cookbook for the supermarket. She attributes her years as a teacher, clinical dietitian, and food-service manager as stepping stones to her current focus on helping people as a food and nutrition communicator. (Chapter 36 contains specific information on how to market nutrition in grocery stores.)

Commercial Weight-Loss Programs

Many dietetic professionals are qualified in the management of obesity. In the past, commercial weight-loss programs were perceived as their competition. Now, most commercial programs rely on the expertise and credibility of dietetics professionals and respect their ability to translate the latest scientific research into practical consumer information. Weight Watchers, International, regularly uses professionals as guest lecturers. Because most weight-loss programs are franchises that are independently managed, they offer many opportunities for dietetics professionals to market grocery shopping tours and other services. In addition, these programs are recruiting dietetics professionals for management positions.

SUMMARY

Consumers want nutrition information that will help them improve their health and lifestyle. Such demand, combined with new technologies and environmental trends, will continue to provide exciting opportunities for dietetics professionals.

To succeed in marketing consumer education, remember to tailor your message to meet the diverse needs of the marketplace. Build partnerships with the media, food and health organizations, corporations, government agencies, and others. Improve your food knowledge and communication skills. Finally, never forget that people eat food, not nutrients.

References

1. Dodd J. President's Page: The Fifth P. *J Am Diet Assoc. 1992;92:616.*

2. Stress management and heart disease. *Harvard Heart Letter.* July 1993.

3. Rehak, R. Green marketing awash in Third Wave. *Advertising Age.* Nov. 1993;22.

4. *Statistical Abstract of the United States: 1991.* 11th ed. Washington, DC: US Bureau of the Census, 1991.

5. Linneman RE, Stanton JL. *Making Niche Marketing Work.* New York, NY: McGraw-Hill Book Co; 1991.

Case Study: **A BILINGUAL, CULTURALLY SENSITIVE NUTRITION CONSULTING BUSINESS**

Nancy Magaña, MS, RD, Nutrition Consultant, Yakima, Washington

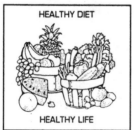

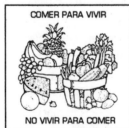

Bilingual Business Card Samples

Ten years ago, I began working as a public-health nutritionist in the Hispanic community. I quickly realized there was a void of culturally sensitive, culturally relevant nutrition education materials for this population. After years of adapting materials, creating my own, and networking with other frustrated public-health professionals, I realized that my ability to speak and write Spanish could open doors to a vast market. Thus, I became an entrepreneur.

My bilingual consulting company provides a variety of services: Hispanic diet consultations, cultural-awareness presentations, evaluation or design of culturally sensitive and relevant education materials for Hispanics, and English-Spanish, Spanish-English translation. I also volunteer my services occasionally to the State of Washington Department of Health Spanish translation review board and to The American Dietetic Association.

Prior to developing my first commercial product or submitting my first contract for services, I carefully researched my potential enterprise. I conducted an exhaustive search of the professional literature in my area of interest to update my knowledge base and augment my reference library. Other research included a market analysis and a study of the target population, such as literacy level, preferred education methods, and so on. Then I explored options for financial support and the economic feasibility of starting a business. I calculated the start-up costs and costs to produce a given product and performed a break-even analysis. I also devised a marketing strategy, which included a cost-benefit analysis.

Most of my business opportunities come as a result of networking. To help people remember me, I designed a business card that stands out because one side is printed in English and the other in Spanish. It serves as a constant reminder of my bilingual, bicultural English-Spanish skills.

I have achieved the competitive edge in dietetics because I provide a unique service in my profession and offer products in the early stages of the product life cycle. I maintain communication with my established customer base. I continually watch the changing market and anticipate who potential competitors are, hypothesize about how they will enter the market, and determine what my response will be. Seeking new markets and developing new products are ongoing processes.

Case Study: PURSUING THE PUBLIC MARKET THROUGH VIDEOS

Dayle Hayes, MS, RD, Nutrition Consultant, Deaconess Medical Center, Billings, Montana

In 1987, I began consulting to the Public Relations and Cardiac Rehabilitation Dedpartments of Deaconess Medical Center (DMC), a 272-bed secondary-care facility in Billings, Montana. Our service area, larger in square miles than 24 states, isn't just rural — it represents frontier America of the 1990s. Patients travel great distances for care at DMC, and during their short crisis-oriented hospital stays, they have minimal opportunities to learn new patterns of heart-healthy shopping, cooking, and eating.

The video series, *PRO-HEART KITCHEN: The Food-Heart Connection*, was born out of the needs expressed by cardiac patients and their families. Having developed an appreciation for the power of video in my training as a State Media Representative, I suggested that we tape nutrition information for patients in rural areas who have limited access to dietetics professionals and educational materials in their own communities.

Initial taping was done in the occupational therapy kitchen of the hospital using in-house equipment and personnel. Realizing that the video format was perfect fro the material but deserved more professional attention, Deaconess committed the resources to tape eight videos in the summer of 1988 and two more in 1989. Eight of the videos were taped in my home kitchen, and the other two were filmed in local restaurants.

As a video program, *PRO-HEART KITCHEN* is unique. First, the series covers virtually every aspect of selecting and cooking heart-healthy food. Secondly, the information on the tapes is reinforced both through the recipe and information cards that accompany every tape and through presentations in the hospital and community, in radio spots, in a monthly newspaper column, on grocery store tours, and on restaurant menu markers.

DMC shoes the *PRO-HEART KITCHEN* tapes on its in-house TV channel, lends free tapes to residents in our service area, and sells them as a package (including a facilitator's manual) to other health-care facilities. It sells three of the tapes separately through a catalogue of health education materials.

PRO-HEART KITCHEN programs are enormously popular. Tapes are checked out 2,000 to 3,000 times per year, and dozens of complete sets have been sold. The hospital recouped its initial investment many times over, and I received thousands of dollars as my percentage of the sales.

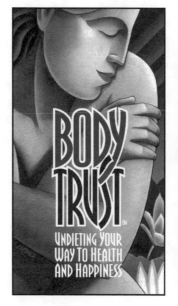
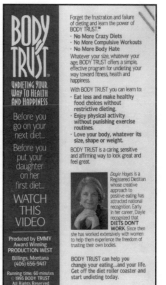

Cover of *Body Trust* Video

TOOT YOUR OWN HORN

For me, the success of the *PRO-HEART KITCHEN* project and its marketing has been far more than financial. The recognition I received for creating the program advanced my career in every possible way. Getting that recognition was as simple as applying for it. In 1991, the ADA National Center of Nutrition and Dietetics (NCND) announced the first Anita Owen Award of Recognition for Innovative Nutrition Education Programs for the Public. With the help of several departments at DMC, I evaluated the effectiveness of our program and applied for the award.

PRO-HEART KITCHEN was honored with the first Anita Owen Award in 1991, then with a Governor's Health Promotion Award from the Montana Department of Health and Environment Science in 1992, and an Outstanding Community Health Promotion Award from the Centers for Disease Control and Prevention in 1993. These awards, all based on applications we submitted, garnered excellent publicity and marketing opportunities for Deaconess — and for me personally.

THE SKY IS THE LIMIT

Based on the popularity of *PRO-HEART KITCHEN*, I realized many professional goals. I've been credited with making low-fat eating a household word in Billings, and I've been nationally recognized for creative approaches to positive eating. My connection with the NCND allowed me to be a part of first the ADA Consumer Education Champion Team, and now, the NCND Strategic Advisory Team, and to network with the movers and shakers of the dietetic profession. I am frequently asked to speak at local and national meetings.

The expertise I gained from working with the *PRO-HEART KITCHEN* project is invaluable. In 1992, I produced a video for the Montana Child Care Food Program called *Beans, Peas, and Broccoli Trees: Implementing the Dietary Guidelines in Child Care Programs*. It has been distributed to child-care providers across the country.

All of these projects provided the springboard for a wonderful opportunity in 1993. I formed a partnership with the video company that made *PRO-HEART KITCHEN* and produced the first video about the nondiet approach to weight issues for women. A limited partner completely underwrote the production costs based upon the success and sales of *PRO-HEART KITCHEN*. We introduced *BODY TRUST: Undieting Your Way to Health and Happiness* at the 1993 ADA Annual Meeting and Exhibition in Anaheim and received fantastic response from both health professionals and the public. So far, our national marketing campaign, including media coverage, magazine advertising, and direct mail, have met our sales goals and expectations.

For me, the rewards have been many: personal confidence, professional recognition, financial gain, and the chance to speak out on issues near and dear to me. Sure, I've struck out on occasion, but like Babe Ruth, it is the home runs everyone remembers!

How to Write a Marketing Plan

Marketing and Business

Plans Are the Tools Used

to Research,

Organize, and

Check the Feasibility

of Your Ideas.

They Communicate

Your Intentions

in an Orderly,

Business-like Fashion.

How to Write a Marketing Plan

Chapter 20

Writing Business and Marketing Plans

Kaye Jessup, MS, PH, RD, Ross Laboratories, Dallas, Texas

All dietetics professionals are businesspeople in business for themselves. We are all in sales because sales are what business is based on. Think about all we do to make our jobs happen. In clinical practice, we work with physicians on recommendations for nutritional care or teach patients to change their eating habits to manage a medical problem. In food service, we plan foods that patients and cafeteria customers select, and advise and write justifications to administration about the needs of our department. Research dietitians often provide information to companies or foundations for grant money to continue their work.

There is no mystery in sales. Selling means knowing and understanding the needs of the customer and then meeting those needs. We sell all the time, we just do not call it by that term.

Marketing defines your product (for our discussion, the term *product* includes both services and products). It defines the group or groups of individuals most likely to use product, and educates them on the product's features and benefits. Marketing is all of these things combined with how you package and communicate your information and sell and promote your product.

Dietetics professionals must learn these marketing skills to survive the growing competition and all of the changes in the health-care industry. Learning to write business and marketing plans is necessary to communicate our skills, knowledge, and effectiveness to others. The following pages will guide you through writing a business and marketing plan. The best way to get started and complete your plans is to ask questions of people who have the information and experience you need. People generally like to share their knowledge with others, so ask, ask, ask!

The components of a business and marketing plan and some tips on assembling them are outlined below.

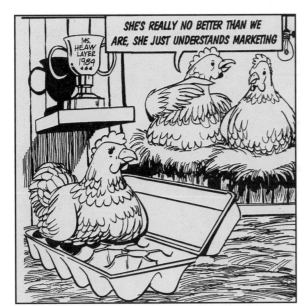

When Practice Is Equal, Marketing Can Make the Difference.

From Roger F. Smith, Entrepreneur's Marketing Guide, © 1984, p. 27. Reprinted by permission of Prentice-Hall, Englewood Cliffs, NJ.

I. *Business Idea Statement.* Write a clear statement of the business idea or goal that you want to research and develop. Answer the following questions:

    A. What business do you want to be in?

    B. What needs do you wish to serve?

    C. What clients do you wish to serve? (client profile demographics)

    D. How will you go about offering your product or service?

II. *Determining Your Target Market Through Market Research.* Market research of the environment must be done to determine the feasibility of the business idea and whether the time and conditions are right for your business idea to be a success. Market research has been defined as "the systematic, objective and exhaustive search for and study of the facts relevant to any idea or problem in marketing." The typical procedure for a marketing research investigation is outlined in Figure 20-1.

Figure 20-1. Procedure for Marketing Research Investigation

1. Define the objectives for the project or define the problem.
2. Conduct a situational analysis.
3. Conduct an informal investigation.
4. Determine if further investigation is necessary.
   If no, skip Step #5; if yes, plan and conduct a formal investigation of items listed under Step #5.
5. Conduct a formal investigation.
   a. Select the sources of information.
   b. Select the methods for gathering data.
   c. Prepare data-gathering forms.
   d. Pretest the questionnaire or other forms.
   e. Plan the sample.
   f. Collect the data.
6. Analyze and interpret the data.
7. Prepare a written report for management.

A. *Step 1* in the market research investigation is to define the objectives for the project or define the problem. Use the business idea statement that you develop during this first step in your market investigation.

B. *Step 2* is to conduct a situational analysis. This involves learning about the internal and external environments of the company or organization through library research and interviews of company officials. The goal is to learn about the company's organizational structure, products, or services, market, competition, and industry in general.

Ask questions about the organization's strengths and weaknesses in each area. If you are starting your own business, you may have an advisory committee that you can consult about the organizational structure you want to establish, the market for your business idea, the competition, and the industry.

C. Once you develop a general impression about the business, proceed to *Step 3*. An informal investigation consists of talking with people outside the organization, such as competitors or colleagues, physicians, customers, job-search firms, and, possibly, advertising agencies to get their opinions and ideas about the feasibility of the business idea.

D. In *Step 4*, if you are satisfied that you have sufficient information, you can start analyzing and interpreting the data. If you would still like further facts, you can plan and conduct a formal investigation.

E. *Step 5* is the conducting of a formal investigation of the market. Two types of data can be gathered to help analyze the business idea:

Primary data are original data gathered specifically for your project. For example, standing in a store and observing people's buying habits is a way of collecting primary data. Focus groups are another way of gathering primary data. If you are a beginner, primary data collection is not recommended, unless you are going to investigate something relatively simple, like the number of cars that pass by a location at certain times of day. Primary data-gathering tools must be carefully designed to obtain answers that have meaning to your study.

Secondary data are data that already exist. You must decide what type of information you want and then locate it. Reference librarians can be of great help in locating certain information. Examples of secondary data are total referrals and number of referrals by ICD9 code or by DRG, average number of admits by physician, number of admits from each zip code in the marketing area, average length of stay, demographic information, and client-profile information. Such data can help you establish the position of your product in the marketplace (who will buy it) and determine if there are other similar audiences that should be included in your marketing strategies.

The profile of your customer can often be drawn from secondary data. Such information will lay the foundation for your marketing strategies. Customer-profile information includes such demographic information as sex, age range, education level, marital status, and number of children. Depending on your business idea, you may need other information, such as height and weight, clothes size, shoe size, and buying habits. Incredible amounts and types of market research information are available. You just need to define what information you want and then ask knowledgeable people where to find it.

Secondary information is readily available in libraries, local Chambers of Commerce, and state, federal, and local governmental agencies. A growing source of information is computer database services, such as Find S.V.P. and Dialogue Lockheed. These are often available in libraries. A fee may be associated with some of the information searches. A detailed profile of your target patient or client is an important component of your business and marketing plan.

F. In *Step 6*, to analyze and interpret your data, you need to organize it into a manageable format. One approach is to use the format of the SWOT analysis. SWOT stands for Strengths, Weaknesses, Opportunities, and Threats. A SWOT analysis lists all aspects of a business idea, such as location, competition, and demographics. Then, for each aspect, all pertinent research data are placed in the appropriate SWOT category, as shown in Figure 20-2.

Figure 20-2. SWOT Analysis for Locating Nutrition Consultation Private Practice

STRENGTHS	WEAKNESSES
1. In professional office building next to hospital	1. Office next to food court smells of pizza
2. Adequate space in office, well laid out	2. Rent is $1.50/sq ft more than planned
3. Access to building is user-friendly	

OPPORTUNITIES	THREATS
1. Medical director of nutrition-support team has office on same floor	1. Hospital Nutrition Services Department is starting outpatient consultation service
2. Hospital installed a new service referral program and will include nutrition consultation service	

It may take more time to SWOT each component of your business idea, but when you prepare your final analysis, your SWOT charts will be very useful in assisting you to make decisions based on an organized set of information.

G. *Step 7* is to prepare a written report of the information that will be formatted into your actual business and marketing plan. Market research can be done on many levels and, if incorrectly conducted, can lead to misleading conclusions. Therefore, if you need primary data beyond the very simplest level, consider hiring a market research company. They will most likely save you money in the long run.

It is crucial to know who will be reading and approving your plan. You want to write your plan to show the dimensions of the business, but you also want to write it in the language of the ultimate decision makers. Find out what their "hot buttons" are and how they like information written and presented. If they are CPAs, include detailed financial information. If you are asking for venture capital money from a bank, find out what kind of ventures they have funded in the past. Try to avoid taking your business and marketing plan to someone you will have to educate about your idea.

III. *The Marketing Mix.* The marketing mix is important to keep in the forefront as you investigate business ideas and operate your business. The four P's of marketing – product, place, price, and promotion – are dynamic elements whose synergy yields sales, referrals, and business. Carefully evaluate their roles in the development of your business idea.

A. Product. Whether you are talking to a banker or a client, always describe your product in terms of the benefits it delivers, rather than just listing its features. If the benefits are things that people want, they can translate into sales. In defining your product's features and benefits, you must also be able to define its U.S.P., or unique selling proposition. Define in writing what differentiates your business idea from the competition.

Another important phase of product evaluation is to plot the phase of the product on the product life cycle, or P.L.C. There are four phases of the product life cycle: introduction, growth, maturity, and decline. A company's marketing success often depends on its ability to understand and manage the life cycle of its product. The P.L.C. is important to understand because the phase your product is in can indicate what marketing strategies to use.

B. Place. In evaluating place, or distribution, consider the following:

1. Is the place of product availability or service delivery accessible to clients? Do you take the service to them, or do they come to you? If they come to you, carefully list all types of clients who will come to the premises and evaluate its accessibility. Does the location offer wheelchair access, bus transportation, and parking?

2. Is the space attractive, but not overdone? Clients need a clean, comfortable space, but should not be led to wonder if their money goes to furnish and decorate an elaborate office.

3. Are you considering changes in the location or decoration? If so, carefully examine all of the above points and your budget. Will the expenditure enhance the environment in proportion to the expense?

C. Price. Establishing price is an ongoing challenge because it is crucial to the success or failure of any business. In establishing prices within an organization, consult the administration about your role. For example, assume that you work for a not-for-profit hospital and that its mission includes charity care to the needy. Would you be expected to provide charity care, and if so, at what level? Does the administration expect you to be a cost center (a nonrevenue producer), to break even, or make a profit? Sometimes, programs or services are purposely priced lower and used as a strategy to attract patients to feed into other, profit-making services.

Pricing certainly can be and has been calculated by hand. A fast, efficient way to evaluate pricing strategies is to use an electronic spreadsheet, such as Lotus 1-2-3; load in the costs, the profit margin, and the prices; and run scenarios by changing costs, profit margins, and prices to see the effects of different variables. If you are unable to run an electronic spreadsheet yourself, perhaps a colleague, friend, or neighbor could assist you. If that fails, ask an accountant to recommend someone, consult the *Yellow Pages*, or ask at the public library for possible references.

The what-if system of an electronic spreadsheet is excellent for evaluating many variables in a variety of combinations, which will give you the best picture of the overall financial impact of prices. Remember that price is the perceived value as a direct correlation between the price a buyer is willing to pay and the value of the product.

To set prices you need the following information:

1. Competitive Pricing. Find out and record competitors' pricing. When researching pricing, ask enough questions to confirm that you are comparing like products. Businesses often position their services or programs by packaging several components, such as a nutrition consult and an exercise session, which can make direct comparisons difficult.

2. Costs of Operating Your Business. Know your costs! The main categories of costs and expenses are personnel, operations, and marketing. A more complete discussion of costs appears later, in the section entitled "Financial Information."

3. Pricing Strategy. Discuss pricing strategy with the administration, or if you have your own business, define your pricing strategy. In general, there are three pricing strategies.

a. Charging more than your competitors is called *premium pricing*. This strategy will be successful for hospitals or organizations that enjoy an image advantage over the competition or when normal competitive factors are not effective in controlling prices.

b. To charge the same or about the same as your competitors is known as *market pricing*. In health care, this strategy is the most common form of pricing because of insurance reimbursement and the fact that no one service provider has a significant competitive advantage.

c. To charge less than your competitors is called *bargain pricing*. This is not recommended if you want to stay in business. Do not confuse bargain pricing with *introductory prices*, which are temporary and designed to launch a new product.

D. Promotion. Promotion is essential to the continued success of a business. For this example, there are two major types of promotion: paid advertising and public relations. *Paid advertising* is the placing of prepared messages or ads where they will be seen by the target market you have determined to be the most likely to utilize your product. The objective of paid advertising is to inform consumers and referral persons about your product and to motivate them to come in or refer someone to your product. *Public relations* includes participating in health fairs, placing stories with reporters, doing radio and TV interviews, and holding open houses, seminars, and continuing education programs.

Choosing the most appropriate mix of promotional activities is important because such activities cost money. Remember that to make money, one must spend money wisely. In selecting promotional activities, consider the following:

1. What are your target markets and who are your customers? Use the client profiles you have established from primary and secondary research. Examples of target markets for a medically supervised weight-management program are physicians, nurses, the profiled consumer, professional organizations, HMOs, PPOs, insurance carriers, and corporations.

Figure 20-3. Audiences and Effective Media

AUDIENCE	EFFECTIVE MEDIA
Consumers	Citywide and suburban newspapers Billboards, *Yellow Pages* Direct mail Local and regional magazines Radio and television Health fairs
Physicians	Medical Grand Rounds Hospital medical staff meetings Open houses One-on-one presentations Direct mail
Hospital staff	Open house Informational programs Events Posters, paycheck stuffers, and hospital newsletters
Businesses	Special presentations Direct mail

2. The next step is to identify where your target markets seek information. Ask questions like: Which magazines do they read? Which radio station do they listen to and at what times? At what times do they watch TV? Which newspaper do they read, and which sections do they read first? There are so many questions you can ask to identify the best places and times to attract the attention of your target customers. In dealing with the media, ask similar questions as you investigate pricing, placement of ads, and the like. They have much information regarding their readers and viewers. Examples of audiences and effective media are shown in Figure 20-3.

3. The mix and level of promotional activities change based on the product's phase in the product life cycle. An example is shown in Figure 20-4.

Figure 20-4. Promotional Activities Appropriate for Introduction Phase of Product Life Cycle

Direct Response Marketing
- Print advertising — Heavy
- Radio/TV — Heavy (if affordable)
- Direct mail — Introductory information to target markets
- Public relations — Press releases, contact media for news story coverage

Physician Referrals
Physician referrals build slowly. It may take eight to eighteen months to see results from these strategies.
- Telephone — One call per week to physicians' offices to educate physicians and staff about the program
- Print — Articles in hospital newsletters and advertisements in local medical association publications
- Grand Rounds — Presentation by medical director to medical staff
- Medical section meetings — Meet with each section about the program

Word of Mouth
Spread the word in the hospital community first.
- Print — Articles in employee newsletters
- Informational programs — Department presentations

E. Marketing Planner. Once you have selected the promotional activities that you are going to use, it is time to plan them. A marketing planner like the one shown in Figure 20-5 can be used to list the promotional activities and advertising that you are going to do and mark the months when they will occur. A marketing planner is particularly helpful when planning a product promotion that has any seasonality or cycle. Marking things on the planner makes it much easier to plan your time and resources carefully. For example, you may

Figure 20-5. Marketing Planner

Marketing Planner												
	DEC	JAN	FEB	MAR	APR	MAY	JUN	JUL	AUG	SEP	OCT	NOV

want to plan special low-fat cooking classes during February for Heart Month or offer a series of nutrition classes for teenagers in the summer.

When marketing to a business, it is necessary to know when their fiscal year begins and ends so you can present your product in time to have any related costs included in the next year's budget.

Another useful form is a marketing activity schedule, shown in Figure 20-6. It is a daily calendar on which you mark when activities will happen. Finally, a business development planning form (Figure 20-7) will help you plan your strategies and tactics.

IV. *Statements of Action and Achievement*. The business world and the health-care world use different terminology to define the "what are we going to do" and "how are we going to get there" components of a business plan. The business world uses the terms *mission statement*, *objective*, *goals*, *strategies*, and *tactics*. The health-care world uses the terms *mission statement*, *goals*, and *objectives*. Whatever you call the action component of your plan is fine, as long as you use the preferred terminology of the ultimate decision maker.

A. Definitions: Business World

1. Mission statement: A summary of what business you are in, whom you will serve, and how you will go about fulfilling clients' needs

2. Objective: A statement synonymous with a mission statement; an open-ended statement with no time limits or quantitative targets

3. Goal: A statement that expresses the objective with numbers and a time frame

4. Strategies and Tactics: Specific activities that name resources, costs, time frames, and projected results that will accomplish goals

B. Definitions: Health-Care World

1. Goal: A sweeping, open-ended statement of what you want your business to achieve

2. Objectives: Specific, measurable activities that name resources, time frames, and projected results

3. Mission statement: For example, the OUTLOOK Program is a cost-effective, comprehensive approach to weight management. It serves the medical profession as well as the community at large, including individuals, institutions, and corporations. See attached example for strategies and tactics.

V. *Key Operating Indicators (KOIs)*. Ongoing evaluation strategies must be determined for your product and monitored at regular intervals, whether daily, weekly, or monthly. This management function is necessary to identify and correct problem areas and operational weaknesses. Be proactive! Key operating indicators are important to discuss during the interview phase of marketing research. Suggested areas in which to establish key operating indicators are marketing, product quality, operations, and finance. Key operating statistics are often expressed as ratios. Figure 20-8 shows some KOIs for a medically supervised weight-management program.

Once the key operating indicators are determined for your product, develop or adapt forms to facilitate systematic documentation.

Figure 20-6. Marketing Activity Schedule

JANUARY	SUNDAY	MONDAY	TUESDAY	WEDNESDAY	THURSDAY	FRIDAY	SATURDAY
		N-Release	1 T	2 T	3 T	4 T	5 T
	6 P	7 T	8 T	9 T	10 T	11 T	12 H Women's health fair
	13	14 Orientation	15	16	17	18	19
	20	21	22	23	24	25	26
	27	28 N Release on holiday weight gain	29	30 D	31		

FEBRUARY	SUNDAY	MONDAY	TUESDAY	WEDNESDAY	THURSDAY	FRIDAY	SATURDAY
						1	2
	3	4 R	5 R	6 R	7 R	8 R	9 R H Heart health fair
	10 P	11 R	12 R	13 R N Release on cardiac risks of obesity	14 R	15 R	16 R
	17	18 P PE Grand rounds presenation	19 Orientation	20	21	22	23
	24	25	26	27	28		

MARCH	SUNDAY	MONDAY	TUESDAY	WEDNESDAY	THURSDAY	FRIDAY	SATURDAY
						1	2
	3	4 Orientation	5	6	7	8	9
	10	11	12	13 N Release on exercise programs	14	15	16
	17 P	18	19	20 P	21	22	23
	24 P	25 Orientation	26	27 P	28	29	30
	31						

Key: N - News Release H - Hospital PR Event **P - Print Advertising** **R - Radio Advertising** **T - Television Advertising** D - Direct Mail PE - Physician Education Event
Reprinted with permission. Copyright Abbott Laboratories.

Figure 20-7. Business Development Planning Form

Business Development Planning Form

RECOMMENDATION/GOAL: *To increase physician referrals of patients to 20% of total enrollment* Page _____ of ____

OBJECTIVES	STRATEGIES AND TACTICS	PERSON RESPONSIBLE	RESOURCES REQUIRED	START DATE	DUE DATE	EVALUATION/ COMMENTS/POA*
1. Present a Grand Rounds on the Outlook Program		Medical Director	slides, make appointment with Dr. Price, 35 mm slide projector		Apr. 23	
2. Make 3 sales calls to physicians and their staffs educating them about the Outlook Weight Management Program each week.		Manager	Outlook physician office packet			
3. Take a healthy luncheon into a medical group practice office once a quarter to discuss the Outlook Weight Management Program with the physicians and staff.		Manager	Lunch: maximum of $50.00 each flip chart, packets.		Quarterly Dec. 3 Feb. 22 June 8 Sept. 10	

* POA: Plan Of Action

VI. *Customer Service.* Marketing campaigns are designed to bring your target market to your door. You and your staff, if you have one, take it from there. The service customers receive will determine to a large extent whether or not they correctly utilize your product and whether or not they will return if follow-up is needed. Always be courteous to clients, consider their feelings first, and make everything associated with your product as easy for them as possible. A few examples are to provide easy-to-understand payment-information sheets, have a suggestion box, offer customers a beverage (like coffee or tea) when they arrive, and supply a list of all of the products

Figure 20-8. Sample KOIs for Medically Supervised Weight-Management Program

Marketing
- *Inquiry – Conversion Rate*: Of the number of people who call for information, how many actually come in for an orientation? This figure would indicate the program's effectiveness in translating a telephone inquiry into a face-to-face orientation visit.
- *Sign-Up Rate*: Of the number of people who attended an orientation, how many actually signed up for the program? This figure would suggest how effectively the program closes the sale.

Quality
- *Attendance Rate*: Of the total number of people enrolled, how many actually attended the class? This is one indicator of the quality of the program and the effectiveness of the instructor.
- *Drop Out Rate*: The number of patients who leave the program before completion divided by the number of patients who start the program is a measure of how effectively the program keeps patients active in the program.
- *Labor Cost per Group*: This is the labor cost for both full- and part-time employees divided by the total number of class meetings during the period, expressed as a dollar amount. As the program grows, labor cost per group is expected to decrease.
- *Finance*: Return on net revenue: Profit divided by net revenue for the period is a relative measure that allows management to determine if the program is operating above or below the expected range of profitability.

Figure 20-9. Break-Even Analysis (enlarged in Appendix)

The purpose of a break-even analysis is to determine the amount of revenue (sales) necessary to pay all expenses incurred by the business. In preparing this analysis, you must determine the cost of goods sold and all other expenses that are associated with the business. This is normally done as follows:

1. Variable expenses tend to change directly with the amount of revenue, and include such items as the cost of goods sold, hourly labor, copier/office supplies, credit card fees, and cash over/short. These are normally expressed as a percentage of revenue (a video that sells for $60.00 and costs you $30.00 will have a cost of sales of 50%; $30.00/$60.00 = .50 = 50%). These cost relationships remain essentially constant regardless of the revenue volume. If you have multiple products and/or services, it is important to determine a cost for each:

Product/Service	Cost %
Nutrition consultation	0.0%*
Cookbooks	25.0%
Videos	50.0%
Educational materials	15.0%

*The cost of this product is the registered dietitian, which is fixed and not included in the variable cost of sales.

2. Fixed expenses tend to not change directly with the amount of revenue, and include such items as the management salary, utilities, rent, and insurance. These expenses tend to change due to nonrevenue relationships (i.e., electricity is a greater expense in the summer months in Texas).

3. Segregate expenses into variable (expressed as a percent of revenue) and fixed (expressed in annual dollars) as shown in Figure 20-12.

4. Select a revenue volume for each type of goods or service that you will provide. In the early planning stage, it is often easier to think of what percent of total revenue each product will represent. If you use a total revenue number of $100, then the percent of the product and its dollar amount are the same:

Product/Service	Revenue %	Revenue $
Nutrition consultation	41.0%	$41.00
Cookbooks	20.0%	20.00
Videos	19.0%	19.00
Educational materials	20.0%	20.00
	100.0%	$100.00

Don't worry if your actual revenue volume is higher. The percentages will remain valid regardless of the revenue.

5. Calculate total expenses with the following emphasis:

Variable: Percent of expense and profit
Fixed: Total dollars

Prepared by Eric P. Jessup

Figure 20-10. Pro Forma Income Statement (enlarged in Appendix)

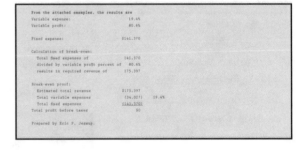

From the attached examples, the results are
Variable expense: 19.4%
Variable profit: 80.6%

Fixed expense: $141,370

Calculation of break-even:
Total fixed expenses of 141,370
divided by variable profit percent of 80.6%
results in required revenue of 175,397

Break-even proof:
Estimated total revenue $175,397
Total variable expenses (34,027) 19.4%
Total fixed expenses (141,370)
Total profit before taxes $0

Prepared by Eric P. Jessup.

you offer. Train your staff to be customer-service-oriented and to deliver quality services in an efficient, friendly manner.

VII. *Financial Information.* Decision makers scrutinize financial information more than any other part of a business and marketing plan. Businesses must make money, or at least break even, to continue operating. Decision makers may require that your business and marketing plan contain the following types of financial information. (They are presented in the order in which they are usually developed.)

A. A break-even analysis indicates the amount of revenue (sales) required to pay all expenses incurred by your product. Break even is discussed in Figure 20-9.

B. A pro forma income statement presents projected revenue, expenses, and income for several scenarios. Normally, it will present the most likely scenario, a scenario at 10 percent less revenue, and a scenario at 10 percent more revenue. (See Figure 20-10.)

C. A budget (financial plan) presents the target revenue and costs in a monthly and whole-year format. This document may also have supporting subschedules for revenue, personnel, marketing, and operations that show specific items in detail. A budget for the most likely pro forma scenario is shown in Figure 20-11.

Figure 20-11. Budget (enlarged in Appendix)

	Jan	Feb	Mar	Apr	May	Jun	Jul	Aug	Sep	Oct	Nov	Dec	Total
Revenues													
Nutrition consultation	6,370	5,753	6,370	6,164	6,370	6,164	6,370	6,370	6,164	6,370	6,164	6,371	75,000
Cookbooks	2,123	1,918	2,123	2,055	2,123	2,055	2,123	2,123	2,055	2,123	2,055	2,124	25,000
Videos	4,247	3,836	4,247	4,110	4,247	4,110	4,247	4,247	4,110	4,247	4,110	4,242	50,000
Educational materials	6,370	5,753	6,370	6,164	6,370	6,164	6,370	6,370	6,164	6,370	6,164	6,371	75,000
Total revenue	19,110	17,260	19,110	18,493	19,110	18,493	19,110	19,110	18,493	19,110	18,493	19,108	225,000
Cost of sales													
Cookbooks	(531)	(479)	(531)	(514)	(531)	(514)	(531)	(531)	(514)	(531)	(514)	(529)	(6,250)
Videos	(2,123)	(1,918)	(2,123)	(2,055)	(2,123)	(2,055)	(2,123)	(2,123)	(2,055)	(2,123)	(2,055)	(2,124)	(25,000)
Educational materials	(955)	(863)	(955)	(925)	(955)	(925)	(955)	(955)	(925)	(955)	(925)	(957)	(11,250)
Total cost of sales	(3,609)	(3,260)	(3,609)	(3,494)	(3,609)	(3,494)	(3,609)	(3,609)	(3,494)	(3,609)	(3,494)	(3,610)	(42,500)
Labor													
Registered dietitian	(4,167)	(4,167)	(4,166)	(4,167)	(4,167)	(4,166)	(4,167)	(4,167)	(4,166)	(4,167)	(4,167)	(4,166)	(50,000)
Secretary	(1,667)	(1,667)	(1,666)	(1,667)	(1,667)	(1,666)	(1,667)	(1,667)	(1,666)	(1,667)	(1,667)	(1,666)	(20,000)
Taxes and benefits	(1,750)	(1,750)	(1,750)	(1,750)	(1,750)	(1,750)	(1,750)	(1,750)	(1,750)	(1,750)	(1,750)	(1,750)	(21,000)
Total labor	(7,584)	(7,584)	(7,582)	(7,584)	(7,584)	(7,582)	(7,584)	(7,584)	(7,582)	(7,584)	(7,584)	(7,582)	(91,000)
Controllable expenses													
Educational supplies	(191)	(173)	(191)	(185)	(191)	(185)	(191)	(191)	(185)	(191)	(185)	(191)	(2,250)
Office supplies	(200)	(200)	(200)	(200)	(200)	(200)	(200)	(200)	(200)	(200)	(200)	(200)	(2,400)
Copier supplies	(153)	(138)	(153)	(148)	(153)	(148)	(153)	(153)	(148)	(153)	(148)	(152)	(1,800)
Books and subscriptions	0	0	(250)	(1,000)	0	0	(600)	0	0	0	0	(150)	(2,000)
Cash over/short	(19)	(17)	(19)	(18)	(19)	(18)	(19)	(19)	(18)	(19)	(18)	(22)	(225)
Travel	(75)	(75)	(75)	(75)	(1,000)	(75)	(75)	(1,750)	(75)	(75)	(75)	(75)	(3,500)
Professional fees	0	(1,000)	0	0	0	(500)	0	0	0	0	(500)	0	(2,000)
Telephone	(306)	(276)	(306)	(296)	(306)	(296)	(306)	(306)	(296)	(306)	(296)	(304)	(3,600)
Utilities	(204)	(184)	(204)	(197)	(204)	(197)	(204)	(204)	(197)	(204)	(197)	(204)	(2,400)
Repair and maintenance	(102)	(92)	(102)	(99)	(102)	(99)	(102)	(102)	(99)	(102)	(99)	(100)	(1,200)
Equipment rental	(200)	(200)	(200)	(200)	(200)	(200)	(200)	(200)	(200)	(200)	(200)	(200)	(2,400)
Total controllable expenses	(1,450)	(2,355)	(1,700)	(2,418)	(2,375)	(1,918)	(2,050)	(3,125)	(1,418)	(1,450)	(1,918)	(1,598)	(23,775)
Controllable profit	6,467	4,061	6,219	4,997	5,542	5,499	5,867	4,792	5,999	6,467	5,497	6,318	67,725
Administrative and general													
Advertising	(400)	(400)	(600)	(800)	(1,000)	(1,000)	(1,000)	(400)	(600)	(600)	(800)	(400)	(8,000)
Accounting service	(150)	(750)	(150)	(150)	(150)	(150)	(150)	(150)	(150)	(150)	(150)	(150)	(2,400)
Total administrative and general	(550)	(1,150)	(750)	(950)	(1,150)	(1,150)	(1,150)	(550)	(750)	(750)	(950)	(550)	(10,400)
Occupancy expenses													
Rent expense	(1,000)	(1,000)	(1,000)	(1,000)	(1,000)	(1,000)	(1,000)	(1,000)	(1,000)	(1,000)	(1,000)	(1,000)	(12,000)
Common area	(50)	(50)	(50)	(50)	(50)	(50)	(50)	(50)	(50)	(50)	(50)	(50)	(600)
Insurance	(108)	(108)	(108)	(108)	(108)	(108)	(108)	(108)	(108)	(108)	(108)	(112)	(1,300)
Depreciation	(548)	(547)	(548)	(547)	(548)	(547)	(548)	(547)	(548)	(547)	(548)	(547)	(6,570)
Total occupancy expenses	(1,706)	(1,705)	(1,706)	(1,705)	(1,706)	(1,705)	(1,706)	(1,705)	(1,706)	(1,705)	(1,706)	(1,709)	(20,470)
Profit before taxes	4,211	1,206	3,763	2,342	2,686	2,644	3,011	2,537	3,543	4,012	2,841	4,059	36,850
Add depreciation	548	547	548	547	548	547	548	547	548	547	548	547	6,570
Cash flow before taxes	4,759	1,753	4,311	2,889	3,234	3,191	3,559	3,084	4,091	4,559	3,389	4,606	43,420

Prepared by Eric P. Jessup.

VIII. *Budgets.* Budgets are guidelines for monitoring the current year's revenues and expenses. They also serve as the foundation for future budget planning. Budgets are prepared for the fiscal year (FY). A fiscal year always consists of twelve months, but it may start with any month. A fiscal year may run from January 1 to December 31, from July 1 to June 30, or from October 1 to September 30. It does not matter which twelve months you select, but you must be consistent. If you are part of a larger organization, the fiscal year will already be established. In developing a budget, the usual steps are as follows:

A. List all sources of revenue (income).

B. List all expenses, including such small items as name tags and paper clips.

C. Group expenses into categories such as "Controllable Expenses," "Administrative and General," and "Occupancy Expenses" (see Figure 20-12). If you work in a larger organization, you will use an established budget format. If you are starting your own business, use a budget format suggested by your CPA or bookkeeper.

D. Group like expenses into categories known as *subaccounts*. Examples of subaccounts are office supplies, travel, and telephone (see Figure 20-12). Since tracking of expenses by subaccount is so very important, select enough subaccounts to make such monitoring possible. Avoid having a subaccount named

Figure 20-12. Expense Analysis (enlarged in Appendix)

```
Revenues
   Nutrition consultation                                41
   Cookbooks                                             20
   Videos                                                19
   Educational materials                                 20
   Total revenue                                        $100

Variable Expenses
   Cost of sales
      Cookbooks                      25.0%             (5.00)
      Videos                         50.0%             (9.50)
      Educational materials          15.0%             (3.00)
   Controllable expenses
      Educational supplies            1.0%             (1.00)
      Copier supplies                 0.8%             (0.80)
      Cash over/short                 0.1%             (0.10)
   Total variable expenses           19.4%            (19.40)

   Total variable profit             80.6%             80.60

Fixed Expenses
   Labor
      Registered dietitian                           (50,000)
      Secretary                                      (20,000)
      Taxes and benefits                             (21,000)
   Controllable expenses
      Office supplies                                 (2,400)
      Books and subscriptions                         (2,000)
      Travel                                          (3,500)
      Professional fees                               (2,000)
      Telephone                                       (3,600)
      Utilities                                       (2,400)
      Repairs and maintenance                         (1,200)
      Equipment rental                                (2,400)
   Administrative and general
      Advertising                                     (8,000)
      Accounting service                              (2,400)
   Occupancy expenses
      Rent expense                                   (12,000)
      Common area                                       (600)
      Insurance                                       (1,300)
      Depreciation                                    (6,570)
   Total fixed expenses                             (141,370)

Prepared by Eric P. Jessup.
```

"Miscellaneous" as it will become a catch-all account. Sub-accounts may also be called *line items*.

E. When an expense is incurred, you or a staff member should write the correct subaccount number on the invoice. This is called *coding the invoices*. Invoices should be coded by you or a staff member in your office before sending it to the Accounting Department or to the bookkeeper.

When these invoices are entered into an accounting system, a "detailed trial balance" report will be generated and sent to you. Check this sheet every month for discrepancies. If you question an entry, research the question to make sure that the expense is for your business or department. If it is an error, write the Accounting Department a memorandum and ask it to reverse the charge.

F. Prepare a chart of accounts. This is an alphabetical listing of everything your business purchases with the correct subaccount number beside the name of the item. Each time you add a new item to be purchased, assign it the correct subaccount number and add it to the Chart of Accounts listing.

G. You will need to provide projected numbers for revenues, personnel, and operations. Marketing may be a major part of your total budget dollars, so it is important to prepare the marketing budget numbers carefully and include them in the operations section of the budget.

1. Revenue budgets: Determine how many products you will provide each month and multiply the volume times the price of the product. An electronic spreadsheet is a fast and accurate way to make these calculations.

2. Personnel budgets: People who work full-time work 2080 hours per year or 40 hours per week. This status is known as one full-time-equivalent, or FTE. In most cases, someone who works less than 40 hours per week is a part-time employee. Full-time employees often receive benefits, such as paid vacation time, sick time, and health insurance. Part-time employees often receive vacation and sick time, but not health insurance. For each employee you expect to need, multiply the number of work hours times the hourly wage rate and calculate a total for each of the months for the budget period. Also calculate the cost of each employee's benefits. If you work in a large organization, ask the Personnel Department how much to allow for benefits. If you own your own business, ask your CPA for such data.

3. Marketing Budget: Determine all expenses you will have related to promoting and advertising your product. If you offer a discount on the product, the dollar amount of the discount is an expense in the marketing budget. It is not subtracted from the Revenues. For example, assume that students who take your cooking class receive a $10 discount on the cookbook you wrote. If 65 people take the class, the amount of the discount for the cookbook is $650, which you would show in the marketing budget as a line item called "Discounts."

H. A budget is a guidepost for monitoring expenses in the current year plus serving as a basis for planning for future years. In any one month, if the subaccount is over spent or under spent by 10 percent, write a memorandum to the file as to why the overage or shortage occurred.

I. Reading financial reports is a major management function. Some budgets and monthly financial reports often show expenses in parentheses ( ) or with a minus sign in the subaccount section of the budget. On the profit lines, if the numbers have parentheses around them or a minus sign in front of the number, that means you are losing money, or are "in the red." At that time, the situation needs to be researched and corrective action taken.

Example of losing money:

- Profit Before Tax: ($1,250) (loss)

    versus

- Profit Before Tax: $1,250 (profit)

Do learn how to read the financial reports that are provided to you. Know where all of the numbers come from. If you have different numbers, do find out why and make necessary corrections.

J. *Fixed cost* and *variable cost* are terms you will encounter and will need to be able to discuss with the accounting people. Fixed costs tend not to change directly in response to changes in revenue, and include such items as rent, marketing, and full-time salaried employees. Variable costs tend to change directly with the amount of revenue earned, and include items such as cost of goods sold, copier supplies, office supplies, and cash over or short. One major point to remember is that different businesses define fixed and variable costs to match their specific needs.

Bibliography

Cohen WA, Reddick ME. *Successful Marketing for Small Business*. AMACOM; 1981.

Key Operating Statistics for the New Direction Weight Control Program. Columbus, OH: Ross Laboratories; 1991.

Ross Marketing Associates. *SWOT Analysis*. Columbus, OH: Ross Laboratories.

Smith RF. *Entrepreneur's Marketing Guide*. New York: Reston Publishing Co; 1984.

Staton WJ. *Fundamentals of Marketing*. New York: McGraw-Hill Book Co; 1978.

System Manager's Manual, New Direction Outlook Weight Control Program. Columbus, OH: Ross Laboratories; 1992.

Quick How-to Reference

Quick How-to Reference

When You Need Help

On Some of the

Basic Skills of Marketing,

Turn to This Section.

Chapter 21

How to Set Prices and Fees

Elizabeth Hamilton, RD, Executive Director, Be Trim Canada, Winnipeg, Canada

O f all the marketing decisions that must be made, the one that likely causes dietetics professionals and other members of the helping professions the most anguish is the setting of prices and fees. How much should you charge?

KNOWING YOUR WORTH

Perceived Value

People buy more than products and services. They buy what they perceive the products and services will do for them. In other words, they buy benefits. A weight-loss program does not make them exercise and eat less food, it makes them happier and more attractive. Your challenge is to package your service or product at a price that does not exceed the customer's perceived value of it. Arriving at this figure is a process of trial and error or negotiation.

A low fee is sometimes perceived as indicating lesser quality. A fee that is too high stifles sales. Your reputation, name recognition, years of experience, and expertise all factor into the fee you can charge. Your fee can be higher when your work requires more skill and expertise, which fewer people possess. Your fee can be higher, or you can ask for a fee and a royalty, when your product or service is going to be used to generate profit for your client – for example, when you write a script for a video series, write a weight-loss program for a fitness center, or write a cookbook for a food company.

If your product or service does not have any perceived or actual advantage over those of the competition except for price, a simple price cut by a strong competitor might put you out of business. In other words, you might reconsider going into a business venture if your products or services aren't different or better than those of the competition and if price is your only advantage.

Competitive Analysis

A competitive analysis is simply an in-depth look at who your competitors are, what they are selling, and what they are charging. You then use this information to create or adjust your services or products so they are different and better – that is, you competitively position them to have advantages in the marketplace against your competitors. Price is just one factor to use; others could be easy-open packaging, home delivery, child care during classes, accepting payment by credit card, phone orders, and overnight delivery.

Value Added

Another strategy that is popular in business today is value added – the addition of something more in the way of service or accompanying product to give customers more value for their money. For example, you could offer a free computer diet assessment for new clients or give a lean and healthy holiday cookbook with each catered event through the holidays.

PRICING STRATEGIES

The prices and fees you set need to match your target market's ability to pay and perception of value. For example, a person with limited funds may be willing to pay for an outpatient consultation for a medically related diet, but be unwilling to pay for healthy catering at parties or for a personal nutritionist. The image you wish to create, your competitive positioning, and your client's ability to pay will help you decide how much to spend on the quality of your materials, meeting space, packaging, promotion tools, and other overhead.

The six common pricing strategies for services or products are:

1. *Skimming*: charging a very high price to reach a small, elite, and profitable market

2. *Trading down*: adding a lower-priced, less-prestigious service to an existing elite service – a technique used to expand to a less elite or affluent market segment

3. *Trading up*: introducing an expensive service or product to increase the status of other generally low-priced services and to attract new buyers

4. *Cost plus*: starting with what it costs to offer the service or product and adding a markup based on a standard policy (commonly used on books and clothing)

5. *Demand-oriented*: setting a price according to an estimate of what the market is willing to pay (All the strategies use a little of this method.)

6. *Underbidding*: setting a price with a low profit to be more attractive than competitors (This is a very common method among dietitians; but it often means that you could work very hard just to break even. Also, consider your image: do you want to position yourself as the least expensive or one of the best? In tight economic times, underbidding can be an appropriate option. WalMart has certainly succeeded with this philosophy.)

Setting Product Prices

In the manufacture of goods, estimates vary, but most experts suggest that manufacturing costs should not exceed one-sixth to one-eighth of the suggested retail price. If you think your product will sell best at $40 retail, but you have to sell it through distributors or brokers to reach retailers, you may have to give 10 percent of the price to the distributor and 40 percent to the retailer to sell it. That means you have $20 left to pay for the product, its packaging, insurance, transportation, marketing (advertising and public relations), salaries, postage, phone, and your salary and profit. By knowing your probable expenses and how much consumers are willing to pay (determined through focus groups or competitive analysis), you have a better idea of what price you must manufacture the product for to make it worth your time to sell.

ESTABLISHING PROFESSIONAL FEES

Quoting Fees

Do not rush into quoting fees. Do your homework first. Ask questions about the job and carefully evaluate what the client wants you to do. Consider any additional costs, such as travel expenses (additional time away from home, added day care), or tight deadlines (you might need to pass on other job opportunities, use the phone and overnight mail more, hire additional help, and pay overtime for secretarial work).

When you have a job opportunity that is new to you, talk to businesspeople in your area, call employment services that place dietitians and technicians, and call practitioners in other parts of the country. Take the time to find out what the going rates are for the kind of work you plan to do. Be sure to compare like services and economic conditions.

If a business calls and wants to know your fees, don't answer immediately unless you know exactly what you want. Say instead, "I need to know more about the job and then I need to work the numbers to see what it will take. Do you have a ballpark amount that you want to offer?" You play a game. You don't want to commit to a low amount when they may be willing to pay you more – and they don't want to offer too much in case you may be willing to work for less.

The Cost of Doing Business

A salaried person may not give much thought to the cost of doing business. When you have to cover all your business expenses as a consultant, private practitioner, or entrepreneur, however, rent, telephone bills, and health insurance premiums take on new meaning.

You must determine your cost of doing business. To more accurately establish your fees, you need to consider both direct and indirect costs. *Direct costs* are costs incurred while working with a specific client, such as educational materials, billable research time, travel, special messenger service, faxes, and long distance phone charges. Such costs are usually passed along to the client or patient. *Indirect costs* are your overhead to run and maintain your business venture, for example, rent, telephone, secretarial service, computer, furniture, supplies, photocopying, postage, advertising and marketing, legal and accounting services, licenses, insurance, continuing education, professional dues, social security, and taxes.

One way to estimate a range for consultant fees is to determine the hourly pay range of salaried dietetics professionals in your area. It is against the law to discuss fees in a manner that might suggest price fixing. However, calls to Human Resources Departments of several hospitals and clinics or to consultants will probably provide you with usable figures.

To determine where you might place yourself within the range you have found, consider how much experience you have, what the work entails, and what unique expertise you can bring to the table. Then multiply the hourly pay of a similar full-time employee by 2.5 to 3 times to determine your hourly rate as a self-employed professional who must also cover all the business overhead (1).

Example: Assume the salaried worker's pay is $20 per hour. Your rate would be $20 x 2.5 or 3 = $50 to $60 per hour.

You may use $50 to $60 per hour as your *first* rough estimate. Keep those figures in mind as you proceed.

Billable Hours

How much time are you willing to work? As an entrepreneur, you may enthusiastically commit to a 60-hour week. However, those will not be 60 billable hours.

Professionals consider that they are doing well if they can bill 50 to 75 percent of their working hours (1). The remainder is spent on paperwork, administration, preparation, travel, and marketing. That brings your 60-hour week down to 30 to 40 billable hours or less (zero on projects like writing a book for royalty only). How soon will you burn out at that pace? How many weeks per year are you going to work? Remember, there's no paid vacation.

Is It Worth It?

You have considered your number of billable hours and your overhead, but now there is something else to consider – your profit. What is going to be left over for you? The low bid that landed you the contract may find you working for less than you had anticipated. Businesspeople hope to make a 20 percent profit. Use your own figures to check the validity of the original hourly rate you made by extending the formula as follows (1):

1. Billable hours per week x number of working weeks per year = billable hours per year

2. Annual overhead ÷ billable hours per year = hourly costs

3. Hourly costs + hourly pay + 20% profit = hourly rate

You may want to adjust the resulting figures. It may or may not be possible to raise your hourly rate without pricing yourself out of the market. If that is the case, you need to look at how you might lower your costs or increase your number of billable hours.

FEE STRUCTURES

There are six common ways of charging for products or services. Depending on the nature of your business, you may choose to use any number of them.

- *Flat rate*. The same fee is charged for the same service to any client. People use flat rates when selling the same service again and again because they have a good idea of the time and expense involved. Such rates are easy to use for speaking engagements, routine clinical consults, and group classes.

- *Per-hour rate*. If the number of required hours of work is variable or unknown in advance, it is logical to charge only for the hours worked. Such rates are used for subcontracting, long therapy sessions, and consulting projects. To set clients' minds at ease, it is helpful to estimate an approximate time frame or maximum number of hours.

- *Per-head rate*. With this rate, the amount of money you make depends on the number of individuals who participate in an event. This rate is often used for workshops, courses, and speeches to groups when attendees pay at the door. It does involve some risk, but if attendance is good, you can do very well.

- *Project rate*. This rate covers your direct and indirect costs, provides a profit, and leaves some room for unexpected delays or miscalculations in developing something (educational materials, a kitchen plan, a marketing tool, and the like) for a client. Clients like this rate because they know what the final cost will be and because you will usually be expected to absorb any cost overruns (unless the clients created them). To protect yourself from nonpayment, have your agreement in writing and ask for one-third to one-half of the total fee up front.

- *Retainer fee.* This fee is charged, usually monthly, for your availability. Dietitians receive retainers for being on-call consultants to food companies and public relations firms. You could charge a clinic a retainer to see patients every Tuesday. No matter how many patients you see, you are paid the same amount, so the clinic takes the risk for inconsistent patient loads, not you. If the patient load is more than you can handle in one day, renegotiate the retainer to include another partial or full day. A retainer should be tied to an amount of time (like ten hours per month), with any time over that amount billable at an hourly or daily rate. If a commercial client wants to state that you are a staff member or consultant, ask for a retainer fee and draw up a letter of agreement on your rights (including the right to review all materials and ads associated with your name) and liability limitations. Talk to your advisers before signing anything.

- *Contingency fee, commission, or royalty.* Such fees are paid only as money is generated. The product or book must sell, or the recruiter must place a prospect. The risk is high because a lot of time and overhead may be invested without any promise of income. If someone asks that you work on commission, make sure the reward is worth it, either financially or professionally.

ANNUAL EVALUATION OF FEES

It is necessary to evaluate your fees at least annually. When reviewing annual statements with your accountant might be an appropriate time. Determine whether your fees covered your expenses and gave you the profit you had predicted. If not, decide if you can increase your fees without charging more than the market will bear and if you can cut your costs. Other possibilities might be to add a new service or trade up into a new target market.

SUMMARY

Remember when setting fees that, unless you are subsidized, they must be high enough to cover your expenses and generate a profit. At the same time, your fees must give customers value that is equal to or higher than expected and not be higher than they are willing to pay.

Reference

1. Kelly K. *How to Set Your Fees and Get Them.* New York, NY: Visibility Enterprises; 1989.

Bibliography

Helm KK. *The Entrepreneurial Nutritionist.* Lake Dallas, TX: Helm Seminars; 1991.

*Felicia Busch, MPH, RD, Owner, Felicia Busch & Associates,
St. Paul, Minnesota*

The biggest mistake I made when starting my private consulting practice in 1986 was charging fees that were too low. While $35 an hour may have been double the hourly rate I earned at the county health department, it was not a reasonable value for the services I provided when I subtracted my overhead, fringe benefits, marketing, and other expenses. Dietetics is a profession. Charging fees well below the market price of similar professional services is not only a poor business practice, but also detrimental to the advancement of our profession.

I quickly learned that if I offer services that exceed my clients' expectations and surpass my competition, fees are not an issue. Not only do higher fees mean a more successful practice for me personally, but they also garner more respect for the high-quality services I provide to clients. It is not easy to negotiate a competitive fee, especially when there are still individuals giving away their services for $10 to $15 an hour. But it can be done successfully if you lay the right groundwork, as the following example will show.

Several years ago, a colleague of mine suggested that I contact a major department store chain based locally in Minneapolis. The management wanted to add a new line of light items to their Marketplace restaurant's menu. Their dietitian menu consultant was moving out of town, and they needed help developing the new idea. I learned they paid $15 an hour for the dietitian's services.

I wanted this account because it would open a whole new area of practice for my business. On the other hand, I knew I must earn a competitive rate. As I interviewed people, I learned a great deal about how the store worked with their previous consultant and what was completed on the new project. It became clear that to meet their deadline would require almost full-time work.

I decided to ask for $75 an hour, or five times more than they currently paid for the position. As I prepared to negotiate the fees for my services, I developed three selling points to explain why they needed me and how cost-effective my rates would be in the long run. First, I use a state-of-the-art computer analysis program customized for each client, while the previous consultant hand-calculated the nutritional values of recipes. I showed numbers that proved it was cheaper for me to analyze recipes at $75 an hour by computer. Second, I offered to provide assistance in recipe development to speed up the approval process and help meet the looming deadline. Third, my credentials, professional contacts, and name recognition in the local media lent added value to the services I provided.

My price and terms were accepted because I brought a professional offer to the table and backed it up with strong selling points. The store was no longer hiring a registered dietitian to calculate calories for menu items. They hired a professional nutrition consulting firm to develop healthful food concepts for all their restaurants and other food-service operations. They were buying creativity, a professional image, and state-of-the-art nutrition services.

Since my initial agreement with the store, they have purchased two other department store chains. Felicia Busch & Associates now provides comprehensive nutrition and menu consulting services for all three chains. Our current contract calls for a monthly retainer instead of hourly rates. Our services are seen as so critical that the department store chain executives view us in the same light as their legal counsel, and we are paid a fee each month to work on their behalf. In addition, I charge hourly for special projects outside the scope of our agreement.

ANOTHER ALTERNATIVE FOR BILLING AN ACCOUNT – BARTER

It's important to stick to your fee schedule. Of course, there are always instances in which a client simply may not be able to afford your rates. For example, a private university wanted assistance with the nutrition component of their health-promotion program, but had budgeted only $1,000. That was not enough money at my hourly rate to provide the kinds of services they needed. However, I determined this would be a good client for my business, and I felt there might be more opportunities for work in the future. We reached a bartering compromise. I still billed them at my normal rate, but to cover part of the payment, the university provided secretarial assistance, photocopying, and graphic arts services for my other projects. The value of my services was not diminished because I received full value. They now pay my regular rates and budget for them in advance.

TITHE YOUR TIME

Finally, there are times when it is better to offer a service for free than to accept a token payment. When groups call for presentations, I quote them my standard fee of $150. If they have budgeted only $25, they have an inappropriate idea of the value of a registered dietitian. As part of my business plan, I set aside a percentage of my time for volunteer work. If a group that calls for a presentation fits into the scope of my volunteer time, I may agree to do the presentation pro bono. They are still sent a bill for $150, but it indicates that the time has been donated and that no payment is expected. This ensures that the perceived value of the presentation is significantly more than if I had agreed to do it for $25.

USING UNDERCUTTING AS YOUR PRICING STRATEGY

A few years ago, the executive who negotiates my contracts told me a story. After concluding our session, which included a price increase, he pulled me aside and said, ""I just had another dietitian call me a few days ago and offer to take over your work with us. She said that whatever we were paying you, she would charge much less. I told her thanks anyway, but that we were more than satisfied with your efforts."

If the perceived value of your services meets or exceeds your clients' expectations, you will be in demand and price will not be the most important issue. The value of your service must be reflected in your fees. If you price your services too low, you demean your own value and that of other dietitians. I sometimes tell my clients that I may be the most expensive dietitian in town, but I work very hard to give them more than they pay for. My clients are satisfied with the value they receive, and I love my work and feel rewarded for what I accomplish.

Case Study: **ROSES NOT THORNS: CHANGING YOUR FEE SCHEDULE**

Theresa Wright, MS, RD, Owner, Renaissance Nutrition Center, Inc., Germantown, Pennsylvania

Setting your fee schedule in private practice is a thorny issue. Your fees influence other areas of your practice, how many hours you will work, how much you will earn, and how your practice grows. Your attitude as you discuss fees with your clients will affect how they feel about paying you, and will ultimately affect your practice. The purpose of this case study is to discuss how I change my fees. Maybe my experience can help you!

The first time I raised fees was really difficult for me. I thought long and hard about the effect of the increase on individual clients. I worried so much about it that a friend finally asked me to consider the effect on *me* of not raising fees when I really needed the money! I had to consider myself as well as my clients.

I checked my proposed fees against the fair market value of my services and the reasonable and customary fees in my area. (You can find this out by talking to your patients, listening at meetings, and reading published fee surveys.) What did other nutritionists charge, and what did other related programs cost? Would my fees be competitive with others' fees for similar services? I asked friends and associates how much they would be willing to pay for a service.

I have to balance my needs with what is appropriate for my practice. Many of my referrals come from psychologists and other therapists. I find that a fee two-thirds to three-fourths of what the referring therapist charges is generally acceptable to the client for shorter-term adjunct therapy. Because insurance companies will reimburse clients for therapist fees, but not for nutrition services, this amount seems affordable to the client who gets no reimbursement. I make my fees appropriate for my target population.

OTHER OPTIONS TO CONSIDER

Since I'm making fee changes, it's a good time to consider if I want to add or change other policies on fees. What about cancellation notices? Must clients pay at the time of the consultation or will they be billed? Being clear with clients about this and all fee-related matters is essential to avoid misunderstandings, resentments, and lost referrals.

Should I use a sliding scale? Clients frequently request sliding-scale sessions. They tell me about their financial difficulties and their need for my services. In the beginning of my practice, I wanted to meet everyone's needs, so I offered sliding scales. As a dietitian alone in private practice, I had no real way of assessing income and ability to pay. However, I often discovered that the sliding-scale clients could afford vacation trips and other amenities of life that I could never afford. Now, if people cannot afford my standard sessions, I offer them shorter sessions, less frequent sessions, or a group class. For clients I know well and have been seeing for a long time, I make other allowances, such as exempting them from a rate increase or allowing them to mail a check after the session. I now see my time as my most precious resource, and I guard it more carefully than ever before.

PLANNING FOR FEE CHANGES

As you plan fee changes, consider the following:

1. How long has it been since your last fee increase? It is best to maintain the same rate for one to two years. If you need to raise fees in less than a year, you probably did not plan properly. Moreover, frequent raises can make you seem unstable. However, if you delay a rate increase too long, the amount you have to increase to bring yourself up to the right level may be a shock for your clients. Better to make small increases every one or two years than significant increases spaced further apart.

2. Consider the general economy. In the middle of an economic recession or war may not be a good time to raise fees. If you wait a few months until conditions improve, will the reception be better?

3. It takes two to three months for a fee increase to be felt in your income. What are your plans for the next year? How much money will you need? Can you cut costs?

4. Make some practical decisions. Are you willing to have a long-term, favorite client continue to pay your old fee? Will all clients pay your new fee structure, or only new clients? You could decide that after a certain date, all new clients will pay the new fees while old clients stay at the same fee. If old clients stop coming for a time, you may want them to return at the new fee. Tell them this at the time the fee structure changes.

5. Write down your decisions. Talk about them with trusted advisers, such as your accountant, lawyer, or other professionals, and listen to their counsel. As you implement the fee structure you have chosen, give your clients adequate *written* notice. Four to eight weeks is adequate time for most people in your practice to see your notice and discuss it with you. In your notice, indicate why the change is necessary, if you can (see sample letter). Be prepared for questions from clients like, "You mean me? I don't think I can afford this!" Have some answers ready, like "There hasn't been a rate increase for two years, and my rent, taxes, and utilities all have increased. I'm sorry if this is a problem for you." Use your counseling skills to hear and validate your clients' feelings with comments like "I understand, it is difficult," and "It's really tough to make ends meet these days."

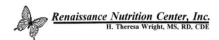

Renaissance Nutrition Center, Inc.
H. Theresa Wright, MS, RD, CDE

January 24, 1995

To all my clients.

While I am pleased to have maintained my hourly rate for nutrition counseling for the past several years, it has become clear that, due to rising costs, I cannot continue to do so. I have given this matter much thought and consideration, and find that I must raise my rates for nutrition counseling to $60.00 per session effective March 15, 1995.

My clients' welfare has always been of paramount importance to me, and I trust that the importance of our work together is apparent and valuable to you. If you have concerns, or if this fee creates undue hardship for you, please feel free to discuss the matter with me. Thank you for your understanding, commitment, and continued effort.

Sincerely,

H. Theresa Wright

H. Theresa Wright, MS, RD, CDE

231 West Germantown Pike, Plymouth Meeting, PA 19462 (215)825-4330 Fax (215)825-7131

Consider timing your rate increases to coincide with the introduction of other programs. New classes, courses, or support groups offer good opportunities to raise rates. If you want to change the time frame of client sessions, you may also coordinate that with a rate change. For example, if you offer a one-hour initial visit followed by 20-minute follow-up visits, you may want to change to 1¼-hour initial assessments followed by 30-minute follow-ups. (Be careful not to adjust your time so that you continue to charge at your old rate!) You can present the change so that clients will feel they are getting more for their dollar, and the rate increase will become part of "a package of expanded services to better meet your needs."

Remember, this is a business decision. Do not allow your clients to personalize it. Focus on the value of your services; talk about how much you want to see the client reach his or her nutritional goals.

Setting and maintaining a fee structure is a very important part of private practice. Just as companies adjust the prices for their products to reflect their costs and the economic environment, you must adjust the price for your time. Clients must believe that they have come to a quality provider and will receive excellent services delivered in a creative and caring atmosphere. Such belief lets the financial aspect of those services recede to its appropriate level of importance.

How to Obtain Publicity for Your Special Events

Chapter 22

Sue Bach-Baird, MS, President, Meet the Challenge,
Littleton, Colorado, and Former Special Projects Manager,
Swedish Hospital Wellness Program, Denver, Colorado

Part of my of job description as Special Projects Manager for Swedish Hospital Wellness Program in Denver, Colorado, was to create community events that would help educate the public about our hospital services. Our philosophy held that if we took care of people when they were well, they would come to us when they were sick. In the 1970s and early 1980s, this was not standard thinking for any hospital. We were considered a forerunner in the field of wellness and preventive care.

One of the most successful events I helped create was the Go for Gold Foot Race. It was sponsored in part by the hospital, a local television station, a national athletic shoe and clothing company, the local professional basketball team, and a race event company. We couldn't be sure of how many runners would turn out for a race sponsored by a hospital, so we invited the Denver Nuggets basketball team to be involved, and they attracted the media. The athletic company, in turn, was attracted to the potential for exposure to the runners and through the media.

We wanted to create an event that would appeal to local corporations as well as the community. To attract local corporations and the public, we provided free running shorts and a free ticket to the opening-night professional basketball game, as well as free food, music, and entertainment. There were also special drawings for merchandise, special guest appearances by the professional basketball players, and the local "runner" weather forecaster stations (see Chapter 23).

We publicized our event through *press releases* – factual documents that usually run no more than a page to a page and a half. They can be used for general news about a special event or program. The release should include the five W's: who, what, when, where, and why. If you don't think you can write an adequate release, substitute a fact sheet that simply lists your major points. Both a press release and a fact sheet should include:

1. The announcement of the event: what it is, when it will take place, where, and who will be participating

2. Ticket prices and where to get tickets

3. Names of participants as they become available

4. Facts and figures on the event

Send your press release to the media that will best reach your target audience, whether local or national. (See Chapter 12 for a bibliography of current media sources.)

Press releases are the staple of the public relations business. In addition to informing the press, they can keep your colleagues up-to-date on your activities. Releases can be used for various purposes:

1. To announce a new appointment or the opening of a practice

2. To give details of a special event or program

3. To announce a new product or publication, or the release of an association's position paper

You can also try to get your release on the "wire." A news wire service is a valuable way to gain broad exposure. A release sent over the wire reaches media throughout the country and costs less than a mass mailing.

Press kits are used to interest the media in a story about your event (see Chapter 25). Press kits should be descriptive, attractive, and to the point. They should provide solid information and explain why the public should be interested in the event. The kit should include the following:

1. A press release or a pitch letter describing the event you want to publicize

2. Samples of promotional giveaways and copies of related articles, advertisements, and critical reviews

3. Résumés or short biographical sketches of noteworthy organizers and participants

Press briefings are one-on-one deskside interviews or more formal editorial board briefings that are used to provide the media with in-depth, background information about your event.

SPONSORSHIP

Event marketing and sponsorship have grown into a billion-dollar industry. Virtually every major special event or program held today requires at least some financial support from commercial sponsors.

Three types of sponsorship opportunities are available at each special event or program: financial, media, and in-kind. All are important and worth pursuing. Financial sponsorship includes grants, donations, and corporate contributions. Media sponsorship includes radio, television, magazine, and newspaper support. And in-kind sponsorship is the donation of services or products in lieu of cash. These are services or products that you would normally have to buy to conduct the event anyway.

It is often best to secure your media sponsorships first. When print and broadcast sponsors commit their support and agree to promote your major financial sponsors, it becomes easier to secure cash-giving sponsorships. Media sponsors may contribute radio, TV, or newspaper advertising to promote the event. Today, when my company does a national program, we target sponsorships with specific magazines. Both *Shape* and *Harper's Bazaar* magazines have provided ad space to help promote our sports programs.

Corporate sponsors are often in a position to help promote an event at little or no cost to themselves. Printing on grocery bags, adding bill stuffers, and tagging existing radio ads are a few examples.

In-kind sponsors save you money by donating items that would otherwise have to be purchased. For example, a print shop may agree to print your brochures, signs, posters, or fliers at no charge. We also use a bulk mail company to help defray some of our bulk mailing and sorting costs. We get the service for free, and they get exposure in our promotional materials.

What are some of the benefits to the sponsor? Meaningful business returns can come in many forms:

- *Publicity.* Sponsors often benefit from the publicity generated by a community-wide or national event.

- *Enhanced image or public awareness.* Association with a popular or respected event can enhance a company's public image and is a good way for a new company in the community to get exposure.

- *Improved customer relations.* Special events allow sponsors to make their existing and potential customers feel very appreciated. Sponsors can show their appreciation by offering free tickets or underwriting a free special event for the entire community.

- *Sale of products or services at the event.* Certain types of companies will find that a community-wide special event enables them to sell large quantities of a product or service in a short period of time.

- *Increased employee morale.* Sponsorship of an event can include an opportunity for a company to provide perks for employees.

- *Opportunity to be a good corporate citizen.* More and more companies are realizing the long-term benefits of giving to the community in which their employees reside, and they are taking the responsibility seriously.

- *Economic development.* A special event can contribute to the quality of life in a community and provide monetary benefits as well.

Securing corporate sponsors for a worthwhile event need not be a difficult task since potential sponsors usually recognize a good investment. When soliciting a corporate sponsor, allocate sufficient time and follow a systematic process, which should include these steps:

- *Define the sponsors' opportunities.* Describe the event in detail, including the date, day, time, location, past attendance figures, and target audience. State your goals and any experience from past events to substantiate your position.

- *Identify potential sponsors.* Potential sponsors are looking for exposure to their identified market. They are also looking for event exposure. Propose that brochures, ads, T-shirts, banners, signs, posters, fliers, and other printed materials include sponsors' logos. It is important that sponsors' names and logos be involved in the program or event, and that the nature of their business match the needs of the event.

- *Research potential sponsors.* Learn as much as you can from your potential sponsors. What is the company philosophy? Do they budget for sponsorships? What type of events have they sponsored in the past? Who buys and uses their product? What is their advertising strategy? What are their corporate goals for image enhancement, publicity, customer relations, employee relations, community relations, and economic development? Who makes sponsorship decisions? The event organizer who has taken the time to gather specific information about potential sponsors may have an advantage over others competing for a limited amount of sponsorship resources.

- *Develop the sponsorship proposal.* Develop a sponsorship package for each desired sponsor and write a formal sponsorship proposal. Each proposal should include a description of the event, information from past events, and a description of sponsorship levels that details what you are requesting of sponsors. Also include a list of benefits the sponsor will receive from the event, a market profile, the names of past sponsors, any promotional materials from past events or testimonials, and a clearly stated deadline for responses.

- *Follow up on the proposal.* Be sure to include a cover letter in your proposal specifying the date you will follow up. It is helpful to allow companies a week to ten days of discussion time after the proposal has been received.

- *Sign a formal agreement with the sponsor(s).* Once you have an agreement with the sponsor, put the terms in writing. This can be done informally by a letter of agreement or formally by a contract. Either format should be signed by both parties.

- *Send a follow-up highlight report.* After the event's conclusion, put together a highlight report for your sponsors. The report should include the results of the event, photographs and stories from the event, copies of promotional materials focusing on the sponsors, and any other pertinent information.

OTHER MARKETING TOOLS

Celebrities attract attention and bring in the media and the crowds. When we held the Go for Gold Race, we used several celebrities. Some were members of the local pro basketball team. We also invited top runners and race walkers as well as local media celebrities. The local news people taped and narrated the entire event. The event was filmed and shown on cable in its entirety, and clips were shown during the 5 P.M. and 10 P.M. newscasts on the local TV station.

Posters, signs, and banners are potentially effective promotional tools if they are used appropriately. It is an important part of your master plan to determine the use of signs, banners, and posters. Make sure that they are eye-catching, provide pertinent information, and call your reader to respond. With signs and posters, you may want to include a tear-off mail-in card. Banners draw attention to your special event or program. At a large outdoor event, such as a bike or foot race, banners can assist in directing and educating the crowd. State-of-the-art sign shops now use computerized equipment. Your message is put into the computer by keyboarding or scanning. The computer then sends the information to a plotter, which cuts the letters or symbols from a vinyl material. The vinyl is then transferred to a sign, banner, or poster. There are several levels of quality to choose from. This approach is not only cost-effective, but also time-saving.

Giveaways are always popular, whether they be T-shirts, shorts, notebooks, mugs, bumper stickers, gym bags, sweatbands, or posters. For our upcoming four-day walking wellness getaway, every participant will receive a free pair of name-brand walking shoes from our sponsor. We worked out an agreement with our sponsor to sell us the shoes wholesale, and we allocated a very small amount of our per-person budget to cover the cost. The sponsor gets the name-brand exposure in all our promotions plus its normal wholesale cost for the shoes, and we get a very attractive perk for our program that the participants value at full retail price.

There are various opportunities for *promotional tie-ins* with every program or special event, but they are not always obvious. It may call for the promoter to use some imagination. A health or sports event may want a tie-in with a talk radio station. Not only is the exposure free, but it can be ten times more effective than any advertisement because of its direct relationship with the media. This is why Sue Campbell's walking clubs have been so successful (see her case study in this chapter). Without the proper promotions, your event or program may never get off the ground. In summary, there are several key steps to gaining publicity for your program or event:

- Make a written plan for your event and set deadlines for completing tasks.
- Develop a budget and determine sponsorship contributions based on levels of exposure.
- Research and identify the appropriate sponsors for your event. Make sure to offer a win-win proposition to all sponsors.
- Work out a written agreement with each sponsor that includes a breakdown of who is responsible for each task.
- Involve the media as sponsors to generate credibility in the eyes of potential participants in the event. Promotional tie-ins generate inexpensive or free media coverage.
- Bring your event to the media. The press release is a great way to introduce your program or event to the media.

Bibliography

Cicora K. Sponsoring special events. *Parks & Recreation*. December 1991: 2630.

Cipalla R. When staging public events, the Smithsonian reaches for the moon. *Communications World*. October 1990: 2832.

Decker J. Seven steps to sponsorship. *Parks & Recreation*. December 1991: 4449.

Ernst & Young. *The Complete Guide to Special Event Management*. New York, NY: John Wiley & Sons; 1992.

Event sponsorship: a useful tool. *Business Atlanta*. August 1992: 2224. Interview with Ardy Arani, founder and partner of Championship Group Inc.

How to tap different media to publicize your business. *Profit Building Strategies for Business Owners*. November 1991: 1416.

Case Study: **HEALTHMARK: A HEALTH PROMOTION COMPANY**

Sue Bach-Baird, MS, President, Meet the Challenge, Littleton, Colorado

HealthMark of Denver, Colorado, is a preventive medicine and education clinic with programs and services designed to create and maintain a healthier public. HealthMark's objective is to provide education and support for people interested in improving their health and preventing certain diseases. It was founded by a physician in 1985 and has helped thousands of people through primary health care, lifestyle education, and ongoing support services.

Three programs were developed as part of HealthMark's community outreach to help its patients make lifestyle changes. The programs strive to improve food selections in local restaurants, in supermarkets, and through a food-endorsement program. These three programs are successful in part because of the large following that HealthMark has established with businesses and private industries.

To carry out these programs, HealthMark's staff developed its own criteria from nutrition research and heart disease and cancer prevention guidelines for what it feels is the most healthy way to eat (the recommended fat level is 20 percent of calories).

For HealthMark, these programs are great tools for promoting wellness education, along with being additional sources of revenue. Since HealthMark did not have money for advertising when it began, these programs helped it stay very visible in the community.

THE RESTAURANT PROGRAM

In the 1980s, some of the top restaurants in Denver were being asked by their clientele to offer healthy meals. In answer to this need, HealthMark started consulting with local establishments on a no-fee basis because the service was new and didn't have a track record for success. Recipes were reviewed by HealthMark's registered dietitians. HealthMark's logo was affixed to the menu on all the food items that met its healthy criteria.

Later HealthMark started charging a fee for this service, which made some restaurants keep the food items but discontinue using the HealthMark logo. Currently HealthMark has approximately eighty local restaurants participating in its program. Every time a new restaurant joins it means more free publicity for HealthMark.

After a few years, HealthMark began monitoring the program. In response to program evaluations, HealthMark initiated waitstaff training and computerized nutritional analysis of each HM menu item. The results of these analyses are attached to the contract for each restaurant.

THE SUPERMARKET PROGRAM

The supermarket program began as a community service and a no-fee project. Its purpose was to make patients more aware of the healthy choices available to them in the grocery store. Two major grocery chains in Denver support the project by providing HealthMark shelf labels for foods that fit the HealthMark criteria. The two supermarkets also carried HealthMark cookbooks and information about HealthMark in their newsletters. The stores also printed a list of all the HM items for distribution to their customers. HealthMark sold thousands of cookbooks and received ongoing promotions each week in local newspaper ads purchased by the food chains.

PRODUCT ENDORSEMENTS

HealthMark's newest endeavor is certifying products that meet its nutritional guidelines. HealthMark evaluates each food's formula and, in many cases, requires a laboratory analysis of the product. Currently, HealthMark sets fees based on the sales volume and distribution area of the product. Its clients include over twenty food companies, 75 percent from Colorado, including local coffee, dairy, and pure water products. This program has been so successful that HealthMark is considering expanding. They are watching the labeling changes, and regulatory and marketing trends.

HealthMark continues to build a network of support for its patients and establish itself as a credible source of health information for the community. It receives a large majority of new patient referrals from the publicity it receives from the three community-based programs.

For further information, contact Jill Howell, Executive Director, HealthMark, 5889 Greenwood Plaza Blvd., Suite 200, Englewood, CO 80110, (303)694-5060.

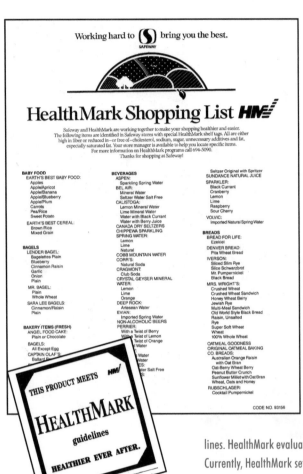

Healthmark Point-of-Sale Markers.
(Copyright HealthMark, reprinted with permission.)

Sue Bach-Baird, MS, President, Meet the Challenge, Littleton, Colorado

Dietetics professionals in wellness are always looking for ways to interest large groups of people in more healthy lifestyle choices. Professionals who work with clients who need to lose weight look for ways to make it fun and provide ongoing peer support. The following example can be used for its value in fulfilling both those objectives, or it can be used as a model of how to use publicity when you create public-oriented programs.

Walking for fitness has become the exercise of choice for over 70 million people. Once perceived as an exercise for the elderly, fitness walking has been adopted by professional athletes, runners, aerobic instructors, and the overweight population. It has also been used for cross training. Whether you are young or old, conditioned or not, walking is an easy, inexpensive way to get and stay fit.

Susan Campbell, the general sales manager for WLVU-FM in Port Richey, Florida, was out walking one day with her husband when she had the idea to start a walking club. She loved to walk and felt there would be opportunities for her to bring advertising revenue to her radio station through walking clubs.

In three years, Sue started three clubs representing over 3,000 members. These clubs generate $4,000 a month to the radio station for promotions of club events. Two more walking clubs will start soon in the local county. "Starting a walking club is an exciting adventure," says Sue. "It provides an opportunity for people to get together to share goals for fitness and health."

HOW TO START A CLUB

If you're thinking about organizing a club, find a name that communicates what you're all about. Create a logo or symbol that can be used on all your print materials for immediate recognition. Find out what special skills or services your members can contribute.

Structure your club so that it will continue to grow. Elect a director, secretary, historian, social director, and events and publicity chair. Among the probable costs your club will incur are membership applications, membership cards, logos, flyers, and newsletters. The club needs to decide what financial obligations they want to cover and what they will ask the participating sponsors to cover.

In trying to find sponsors, check with the marketing department of your local hospital. Be prepared to show them the benefits of their participation, such as the number of members you expect to solicit and areas where you'll distribute publicity. Ask them if they will provide free health screenings at major walks, including blood pressure, pulse rate, and so on.

Call your local medical society and ask for the names of physicians in several different fields, such as orthopedics, sports medicine, cardiology, and rheumatology. Doctors are great draws for seminars and may agree to be sponsors.

Another sponsor might be a local bank that has several branches. Request an appointment with the vice president or director of marketing. Prepare a written proposal requesting the bank to be the sign-up point for your club (see Chapter 34). Because you will be creating traffic for the bank, it will be difficult for them to turn you down.

Call your local newspapers and request a copy of their public service announcement (P.S.A.) form. Newspapers have a public service column available for nonprofit organizations, which you may be able to use to promote your walking club. Call your local radio stations and ask their public service directors for their format for P.S.A.'s.

Sue Campbell's tips for success are as follows:

- Always include all your sponsors in your promotions.

- Check your local shopping malls to see if they already have walking programs set up. When bad weather threatens, malls can save the day.

- Guest speakers can help motivate your club members. Registered dietitians, local athletes, celebrity walkers, and doctors all make good speakers.

- Having a theme walk, such as "Walk on the Wild Side," can help promote your club.

- Instead of charging members a fee, ask them to donate time, effort, refreshments, or in-kind items.

- Have a hospitality committee at each walk. Split walkers into groups so that the leaders of the pack and the first-time walkers do not feel left out.

Sue's formula for a successful walking club is *enthusiasm* among members. Her success with the right sponsors also put money in the radio station and was a wonderful public relations tool for the hospital and the bank.

For more information, call or write Sue Campbell, General Sales Manager, WLVU 106.3, 6214 Springer Drive, Port Richey, FL 34668, (813)845-1063, fax (813)846-1502.

How to Write a Press Release

Mona Boyd Browne, MS, RD, Owner, Nutrition Communication Services, New York, New York

A press release, also called a news release, is used to generate publicity and is the cornerstone of a successful public relations program. A press release is a newsy announcement from or about an organization that is written in journalistic style, follows a standard format, and is intended for publication or broadcast. Releases can be sent to print and broadcast media outlets, such as newspapers, magazines, and newsletters, and radio, television, and cable stations. Press releases are used by editors, writers, reporters, and other members of the media to tell worthwhile stories and report news. Many published news and feature stories originate from press releases. The most important part of a press release is information. A good release provides a newsworthy story or announcement, stated clearly and simply. Press releases that are poorly written, contain misspelled words or present sketchy or inaccurate information will likely end up in the trash. This quick how-to reference section shows you how to write a professional press release. It also contains several sample releases.

NEWSWORTHY TOPICS

Releases are used by dietetics professionals, public relations firms, and media experts to communicate newsworthy information and gain publicity. Press releases will help keep a company name and its products in the public spotlight. Editors may receive hundreds of press releases a day. Quick judgments are made based on a release's headline, first few paragraphs, and format. If it doesn't look like news, an editor might not even read it. A writer who knows what is newsworthy is more likely to create a press release that will be picked up by the media. How can you determine what is newsworthy? Start by identifying things that interest others. A good release will use a "hook," or story angle, to make a topic relevant, timely, and interesting. To grab an editor's attention, a press release might be written to:

- Introduce a new or improved product
- Describe a new service or new merchandising
- React to other late-breaking news
- Counter negative problems
- Offer an educational brochure or publication
- Publicize a campaign kickoff or completion
- Report research or survey results
- Present new information
- Promote a public appearance, media interview, speech, or trade show activities
- Announce meetings, anniversaries, special events, or awards
- Disclose staff changes, such as promotions and appointments, or employee activities

- Announce the formation of a private practice or relocation to new or improved facilities

TYPES OF RELEASES

There are two basic types of releases: straight news and feature. A straight news release reports a serious subject in a serious manner – it gets right to the point. The lead, or first paragraph, contains a summary of the essentials – the who, what, when, where, why, and how of the story. The remainder of the release uses facts and other details to expand the lead. Announcements of the results of a scientific study, campaign kickoff or conclusion, new product or service, or personnel changes are examples of straight news releases.

A feature news release may deal with either a serious or a light topic. It is written in a relaxed, informal style; its tone may be light and entertaining. The feature news release lead teases the reader instead of summarizing the main points; it reaches its point in the third or fourth paragraph. Feature press releases use the human interest factor to draw attention to a product, service, or company.

FORMAT GUIDELINES

A professional press release follows a standard format, although many writers take liberty with certain components. Use the following guidelines to write a professional press release:

1. *Paper.* Use 8½-by-11-inch, 16- to 20-pound white bond paper or company letterhead. Use only one side of the paper. Type neatly.

2. *Length.* Keep the release as short as possible.

3. *Spacing.* Double-space all copy.

4. *Margins.* Leave a one-inch margin on each side of the page and at the bottom. Leave three to four inches at the top of the first page. Indent the first line of each paragraph five or ten spaces.

5. *Release date.* Type FOR IMMEDIATE RELEASE or FOR RELEASE + a specific date a few spaces above the first paragraph in the upper left corner. A release may also be embargoed, or held, until a certain date or time if you have a good reason for asking an editor to do so. In such a case, the heading might read FOR RELEASE AFTER 10 AM, MAY 18, 1995. A dateline – a first line telling where the story originated – may also be used. For example: New York, October 1, 1995 – The art of writing a press release . . .

6. *Identification.* Place the name and telephone number (including area code) of the person to contact for more information in the upper right corner of the first page.

7. *Photographs.* If there are pictures with your release, use the phrase "With Art" and include a brief description of each photo.

8. *Headline.* Headlines are optional, and many editors compose their own. Nonetheless, use a headline on your release unless you know an editor dislikes headlines. A short headline that tells the whole story can capture

an editor's attention. Center and underline the release headline, leaving at least two inches between the headline and the start of the text.

9. *Style.* A straight news release follows the inverted pyramid style. The lead, or first paragraph, contains key facts – the who, what, when, where, why, and how of the story. Subsequent paragraphs back up the lead with facts, placing less-important details last. A feature release uses the lead to tease the reader, rather than summarizing the main points, and reaches the point in the third or fourth paragraph.

10. *Technical words.* Translate jargon and technical words into everyday language. If technical terms are necessary, define them. Use simple words as often as possible.

11. *Quotes.* Quotes are used to lend personal authority to a statement made in the release. If a quote is used, identify the spokesperson by name and title. Quotes must be taken directly from a person or approved by the source.

12. *Sentences and paragraphs.* Keep sentences short and simple, twenty words or less. End lines with complete words to prevent typesetting errors. Paragraphs should also be short and limited to four or five lines.

13. *Active voice.* Every word counts. Use the active voice to make a stronger statement with fewer words. Cut out extra words and phrases to clarify the message.

14. *Page numbers.* If the release is more than one page, place the page number in the upper left corner (excluding the first page). Also use a header of one or two words so pages can be easily identified. Try to end each page with a completed paragraph, or at least a completed sentence. For press releases longer than one page, type "more" at the bottom of each page, except the last page. Always end the release with the symbols # # # or the digits **-30-** or **-O-**.

15. *Editing.* Always edit the release. If possible, let the draft sit overnight. Review it the next day from a fresh perspective.

16. *Proofreading.* Accuracy is critical. Check for spelling errors and grammatical mistakes. Use a word processor spell checker and check by eye. A publicist who makes mistakes will be considered unreliable by editors and reporters.

17. *Correcting errors.* If an error is discovered after the release has gone out, issue a correction immediately to every recipient.

18. *More information.* If the story has more information than will fit in a release, enclose a fact sheet or backgrounder. A fact sheet or backgrounder supplements a press release with additional information and is used when the release alone cannot tell the whole story. For example, a press release from The New York State Dietetic Association announcing its March 1993 Hunger Alert Day was distributed with a fact sheet detailing local area activities and participating organizations.

SUMMARY

A press release is the standard communication tool in public relations and working with the media. Write your rough draft and then let other people read it for impact

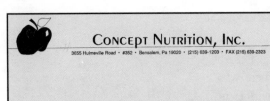

CONCEPT NUTRITION, INC.

3655 Hulmeville Road • #352 • Bensalem, Pa 19020 • (215) 639-1203 • FAX (215) 639-2323

1/29/93
NEWS
FOR IMMEDIATE RELEASE

For Further Information
Contact: Lauren Swann
(215) 639-1203

LOCAL NUTRITIONIST AUTHORS SOUL FOOD HISTORY FOR
NATIONAL COUNCIL OF NEGRO WOMEN HERITAGE COOKBOOK

The Black Family Dinner Quilt Cookbook, released this month, features a
nutrition section -- authored by Bensalem resident Lauren Swann, MS, RD --
which explores the rich cultural food customs African-Americans brought to our
country. From slave times to the present, traditional practices which
nourished African-Americans are explored and recognized as the mealtime
celebrations which physically and spiritually strengthen and unify African-
Americans.

As Nutrition Consultant, Swann was also recipe editor and developed the
educational recommendations to tastefully improve the healthfulness of soul
food cuisine. "It is interesting that the roots of African-American diets are
very much in line with today's Dietary Guidelines," says Swann, "Africans
enjoyed a diet abundant in fruits, vegetables and whole grains and continued
this habit through slave times because meat was stringently rationed by their
masters."

Endorsed by former Health & Human Services Secretary Louis Sullivan, MD, The
Black Family Dinner Quilt Cookbook is dedicated to Dr. Dorothy Height,
National Council of Negro Women (NCNW) President, in recognition of her 60

-MORE-

1/29/93 Local Nutritionist Authors Soul Food History for Heritage Cookbook 2

years of public service contributions for justice and equality. The
Black Family Dinner Quilt Cookbook features Food Memories™ from
prominent African-Americans and is a sequel to last year's Black Family
Reunion Cookbook which sold over 100,000 copies.

Lauren Swann, a registered dietitian and president of Concept Nutrition,
Inc. consulting services, became involved with the project after
publishing Soul Food: Heart of Black America in the Philadelphia
Inquirer. The Black Family Dinner Quilt Cookbook can be ordered by
calling (215) 639-1203. Proceeds from the book are donated to NCNW to
support their programs aiding African-American females and their
families.

# # #

The New York State Dietetic Association, Inc.

48 Howard Street
Albany, New York 12207
(518) 463-2415

FOR IMMEDIATE RELEASE

CONTACT: Agnes Kolor, R.D.
(914) 735-8622

Mona Boyd Browne, R.D.
(212) 678-6937

New York Dietitians Organize Statewide
Hunger Alert Day -- March 20, 1993

Albany, New York, February 22, 1993 -- The New York State Dietetic Association
today announced its plans to coordinate a statewide **Hunger Alert Day '93** in
observance of March National Nutrition Month. The event, to be held at local
supermarkets throughout the state between 9:00 a.m. and 3:00 p.m., has been
organized to collect donated food for use at community food banks and hunger
programs.

"Hunger Alert Day '93 enables dietitians, supermarkets, hunger relief organizations
and community groups to work together to help feed the hungry in our own
neighborhoods," explains Eden Kalman, R.D., President of The New York State Dietetic
Association. Volunteers will be collecting food outside more than 70 supermarkets
chains, including D'Agostino, Grand Union, P & C, and Price Chopper.

The New York State Dietetic Association is a professional organization of more
than 5,000 registered dietitians (R.D.), dietetic technicians, registered (D.T.R.) and other
qualified nutrition professionals in New York.

# # #

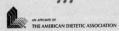

AN AFFILIATE OF
THE AMERICAN DIETETIC ASSOCIATION

Sample Press Releases (enlarged in Appendix)

(Reprinted with permission.)

---

and clarity. Consider hiring a person with marketing or public relations background who has experience writing press releases to review or rewrite your work.

Bibliography

Aronson M, Spetner D. *The Public Relations Writer's Handbook*. New York, NY: Lexington Books; 1993.

Communicating the Science of Food and Nutrition: What Can You Do to Help? Washington, DC: The Sugar Association.

Doty DI. *Publicity and Public Relations*. Hauppauge, NY: Barron's Educational Series, Inc.; 1990.

Yale DR. *The Publicity Handbook: How to Maximize Publicity for Products, Services and Organizations*. Lincolnwood, IL: NTC Business Books; 1991.

How to Write a Query or Pitch Letter

Neva Hudiburgh Cochran, MS, RD, Nutrition Consultant and Media Spokesperson, The American Dietetic Association, Dallas, Texas

Selling your idea for a story to the media or to a publisher is best achieved through a tool called a query or pitch letter. While the characteristics of the two are similar, they have somewhat different purposes. A query letter is used when you want to write your own story, article, or book, usually for a fee or royalty. A pitch letter, similar to a press release, sells an idea to the print and broadcast media in which you would be quoted as an expert, but someone else writes the article or produces the story. This option is usually used when you do not have the time, skills, or money to write the article or produce the radio or TV story, or when you want the credibility of the media's producing the story for their readers, viewers, or listeners.

Since editors or reporters formulate their impressions of you and your idea from such a letter, it is important that it look and sound as professional as possible. Ideally, the letter is one to two single-spaced typed pages on good-quality stationery. It should be long enough to develop your idea but short enough to be read quickly.

SIX STEPS TO A BEST-SELLING LETTER

1. Begin a query or pitch letter with an attention-grabbing opening sentence. For example, "Kids are nuts about peanut butter," or "Americans eat 4.7 billion pounds of crunchy snacks a year – an average of nineteen pounds per person."

2. Then summarize your idea in one paragraph to pique the editor's interest so he or she will want to know more.

3. Follow with an explanation of why the editor's audience would be interested in the story.

4. Once the groundwork is laid, give a few colorful details about the story and include photos or visual ideas, if you have them. The art possibilities alone will sometimes sell an idea.

5. Include information about yourself and why you are qualified to write or be interviewed about the topic. If you plan to write the story yourself, include names of experts you plan to interview as well as one or two samples of previously published articles.

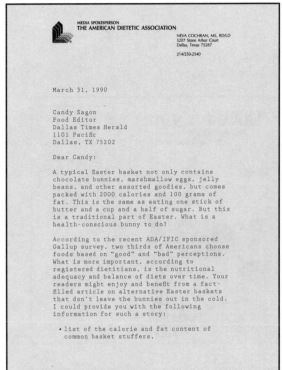

Sample Pitch Letter. (enlarged in Appendix)

(Reprinted with permission.)

6. Conclude your letter by telling the editor how to reach you if he or she is interested in the idea, and if you plan to follow up by telephone. Always include your telephone number and a business card.

It is acceptable to send simultaneous query or pitch letters to several editors, producers, or reporters. However, if more than one expresses interest in your idea, you will need to use different angles for the articles or interviews, particularly if the publications or broadcast outlets are in direct competition. For example, an idea for low-fat entrees could focus on the pros and cons of prepackaged frozen dinners for one story and on healthy meals that can be made ahead and frozen for another. If more than one book publisher is interested, you can choose the one that appears to be most capable or the one that gives the best offer.

An example follows of a successful letter used by this author to pitch a story idea about a healthy Easter basket to promote the theme of balance, variety, and moderation as the keys to a healthy diet. The letter was sent to five newspaper food editors, a radio reporter, and a television noon news anchor. The results were amazing. Three newspapers published stories, and both the radio and television stations broadcast interviews. In addition, a wire service picked up one of the newspaper articles, which resulted in nationwide publication. As a result, a radio reporter in another state conducted an interview on the story by phone.

Buoyed by the success of this pitch, a few months later, the healthy Easter basket was changed to a healthy July Fourth picnic basket. Similarly successful results occurred, including another wire-service pickup, with subsequent telephone interviews aired on radio stations in three different states.

Resulting Newspaper Articles
(Reprinted with permission.)

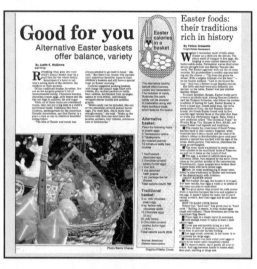

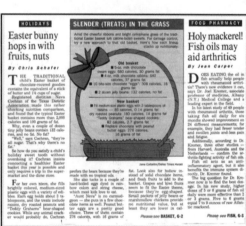

HOW TO START

Before writing a query or pitch letter, familiarize yourself with your target publication or program. Determining its audience, format, style, and choice of topics can give you insight into the types of stories that would have appeal. Also identify the appropriate editor or reporter for your particular idea. Obtain the name from the masthead or by calling the publication or station. It is important that the letter be sent to the right person and that the idea meet the needs and interests of the intended readers, viewers, or listeners.

According to Mindy Hermann, a registered dietitian and ADA Ambassador who frequently writes for magazines, "No doesn't always mean 'no.' It sometimes just means 'not now.' Don't get impatient." She adds, "There is often a long lag time between the time they get your letter and when they get back to you." Mindy got her start by writing to a magazine about a recent nutrition article she was not pleased with and expressing interest in writing for the magazine. Although they did not use her as a writer, over a period of time, she was interviewed for articles and wrote a few brief question-and-answer columns. Finally, the magazine suggested her as a writer to another publication. "I certainly did not tell them I had never written an article for a magazine," she says. This was the break she needed to establish herself as a nutrition writer and secure assignments from other publications.

While not all query or pitch letters will result in an immediate assignment or interview, a well-written letter may prompt an editor to call about another story idea or an opportunity to do an interview. Letters are often filed for future reference, and a request may come months later. By continuing to send your best ideas to the media or publishers, you begin to establish rapport, which one day may lead to a good working relationship.

Chapter 25

How to Develop a Press Kit

Amelia Catakis, MBA, RD, LD, Marriott Corporation, Washington, DC

You just wrote an exciting, informative press release. But there's more information that needs to be shared. What should you do? You need a press kit! Besides the press release, what else should you include? Whatever it takes to grab the attention of the recipients! The press kit is used to interest the media in doing an interview or article on the subject or person being promoted.

THE OUTSIDE FOLDER

First, you need a distinctive, quality folder that has pockets inside and that may or may not have a logo or message on the outside. It shouldn't be too flashy, nor should it look like a term paper. If your resources are limited, a folder made of good paper stock will do nicely.

CONTENTS

The contents must be considered carefully because many media people in larger markets receive hundreds of press releases and press kits per week. (*Time* magazine once reported that it received over 1,500 press kits per week.) The enclosed material should be easy to scan and read, and the purpose for the kit must be obvious. Materials usually included in a press kit are

- The press release
- Simple fact sheets
- Any background papers, which give more detail
- Copies of news articles supporting your press release (such as articles substantiating the problem you've identified or showing the person you're promoting featured in *People* magazine)
- Clear reprints of appropriate articles from reputable professional journals, if appropriate
- A brief biography and photograph of the main spokesperson

Always have a contact name and phone numbers. It doesn't hurt to clip or staple a business card to the press kit.

GETTING THE KIT TO THE MEDIA AND GETTING A STORY

When press kits are distributed to reporters at a press conference or a media event, the material in the kit should follow the gathering's agenda. Many times, however, press kits are delivered or mailed to reporters and writers who cover the subject of your message, such as a food editor or book reviewer. A properly prepared press kit will grab their attention and interest, which, one hopes, will create the desired follow-up.

Don't leave your marketing to chance. Follow up with phone calls to the kit's recipients, but be sensitive to the possibilities that they may not have much time to talk, especially around deadlines, and that some people do not want phone calls.

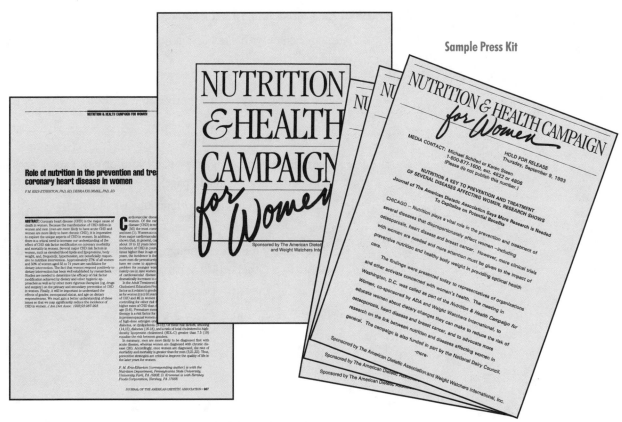

However, if you do speak to some of them, ask if they plan to do a story or interview. Have a sales pitch ready about how well the children's nutrition campaign is going, or how well the book is selling, or how the governor has now signed a declaration naming May Blueberry Month, or that you only have one more media interview time slot left for the date you are in that town.

SAMPLE PRESS KIT FOR A CORPORATE PROMOTION

Marriott School Services accounts sent this press kit to their local media to announce their plans for National Nutrition Month, 1993.

Outside: Folder was plain white with the Marriott logo

Inside: Right side

- Press release (2 pages) announcing the activities
- Fact sheet (2 pages) with details about the division
- Sample from implementation guide (4 pages) for food-service managers.

(These were typed on appropriate letterhead)

Left side

- Sample materials to be used: lunch bag, USDA Food Pyramid mobile, nutrition trading cards

SAMPLE PRESS KIT FOR A MEDIA TOUR TO SELL A BOOK

Folder: Attractive color with a public relations company logo or your own logo, or plain

Inside: Right side

- Press release on you, the author, and the book – why is it unique? (1-2 pages)

- Your biography (1 page)

- Sample news clipping on you and your unique experiences or something else of note (1 page)

- Sample questions the reporter could ask (1 page)

Left side

- The book, if it is small enough; otherwise, your black-and-white photo or another article of particular interest

How to Write a Personal CV, Résumé, and Bio

Chapter 26

*Michele M. Fairchild, MA, RD, Yale – New Haven Hospital,
New Haven, Connecticut*

Whether you are in the market for a conventional position or are entering the arena of private practice as an entrepreneur, you are about to find yourself in the business of selling . . . yourself and your abilities! Promoting yourself through your curriculum vitae (CV), résumé, or personal biography is a form of sales, packaged uniquely for your targeted audience, with the primary objective of promoting your abilities. You use these tools for visibility, to rise above the mass of competition. They distinguish you from all others who profess to offer services like yours.

Remember that promotion should create a positive image for you and your service. It should make your universe of clients and prospects aware that you exist, and are ready and willing to perform your service for their benefit.

YOUR CAREER: THE FOUNDATION

Good, successful careers do not just happen. They take careful exploration, assessment of options and opportunities, trial and error, and dedication to produce a product that is in demand – *you*. If you seek a future as a food-service manager, clinical director, or entrepreneur in your own private practice, consider what you wish to do, then determine what you will need in the way of documentable and provable experience. Pursue those opportunities or assignments that will provide the most desirable personal experience. Be active in professional and trade association activities, for they will enable you to develop key business skills while expanding your sphere of influence. Consider preparing articles for publication and papers for presentation at professional meetings. Consider pursuing high-profile jobs at major medical centers, at cutting-edge wellness programs, for sports teams, at culinary schools, or with well-known health organizations or food companies.

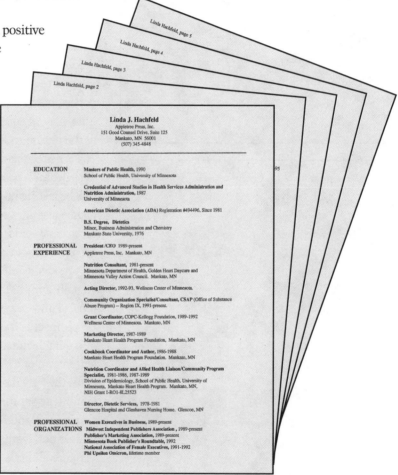

Figure 26-1. Sample Curriculum Vitae (enlarged in Appendix)
Reprinted with permission.

YOUR CURRICULUM VITAE

A curriculum vitae (CV) is a comprehensive listing of your education, job experience, awards, professional memberships, leadership activities, grants, publications, speeches, honors, and the like. As shown in Figure 26-1, it presents a more

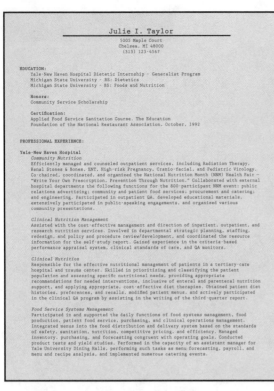

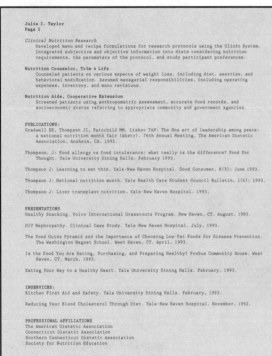

Figure 26-2. Sample Résumé (enlarged in Appendix)

complete listing than a résumé does, and may entail many pages. The format usually follows reverse chronological order, with the most recent additions listed first under each category. The CV is used primarily in academia, in government, in securing grants, and whenever very extensive, detailed information about a person's career is needed. Keep your CV on your word processor and update it as new additions occur. Glean information for your résumé from your CV.

YOUR RÉSUMÉ – A GIFT-WRAPPED PACKAGE

The style, composition, content, and appearance of your résumé will change to suit different purposes and different audiences. If you are targeting a job in business and industry, you would probably focus on past experience in business, career objectives, and what you can offer toward those objectives. If you are pursuing academic employment, you would focus on academic work, areas of research, teaching, advanced degree work, published papers, books, seminar presentations, and lectures. If you are an independent contractor, you must place yourself in the position of the person to whom you will send your résumé.

The recipient of your résumé will be making a serious business decision based on your résumé. Therefore, first impressions will be lasting impressions! If your résumé fails to pass the first-glance test, it may never be read, or, if it is read, its poor presentation may seriously detract from its content. (See Figure 26-2 for a sample of a well-presented résumé.)

Ask yourself a few important questions: Is your résumé visually appealing? Is it neat? Is it readable? Are there typos? Is it labeled and categorized to guide the reader through its content?

Impact is the secret – clearly stated, briefly presented, and quickly noted impact! Start your résumé with an impact statement, one that epitomizes the service you offer and delineates the benefits a user of your service can expect. Make it a statement or promise of direct and immediate professional or commercial interest to the reader. Be careful not to oversell, and do not overpromise. Too much hype will detract from your credibility.

It is important to keep the momentum going when addressing your capabilities. Present your areas of capability in short, concise, but clear statements, either in narrative paragraph form or as a list of bulleted items. Remember, concentrate only on the items that are directly relevant to the service you are offering.

If your readers were attracted by your impact statement and capabilities, they will look for evidence to support your claims, so present your educational training and employment history, complete with dates, places, company names, job titles, and, when appropriate, areas of responsibility, accomplishments, recognitions, and awards. As part of this section, you could consider inserting your professional affiliations and activities.

The challenge for anyone writing a résumé is to keep it within two typewritten pages, for readers have very limited attention spans, and a thick document is all too often laid aside. Once you have met this initial challenge, the next critical element is the printing of your résumé. No expense should be spared in this area. Good-quality bond with clear black lettering will put the finishing touches on your résumé and communicate a sophistication and style that will distinguish your résumé from the rest.

In summary, whether you are using a traditional résumé or a broadcast letter format (a narrative letter with descriptors of successes strategically positioned by paragraph), you should cover the standard categories of information. Include your name, address, telephone number, professional experience, education, awards, and professional affiliations and activities.

YOUR PROFESSIONAL BIOGRAPHY

A professional bio is a promotional vehicle that carries your business message, tells of your experience or qualifications, and, most importantly, announces to the recipient what benefits can be derived from dealing with you. A bio is a substitute for a conventional résumé whose format requires you to be more inventive, more attentive to details, more determined, and bolder than ever before. Because a professional bio generally does not exceed one typed page, it can be a challenge to write, design, and lay out. To make it succinct enough, you must also carefully target your audience. The following should be considered in developing your bio:

- Who are you (with examples of prestigious or highly visible career activities)
- What you can do for clients
- How to contact you

If you are in private practice, a professional bio is an important calling card. If you speak professionally, consider attaching a publicity photo. Include your professional bio in marketing packets to perspective clients to reinforce your expertise, and emphasize your accomplishments with a professional publicity photo to complete the upscale presentation of your service. See Figures 26-3 for samples of professional bios.

SUMMARY

Curricula vitae, résumés, and professional bios are tactics of selling yourself through past deeds and descriptive words. Their objective is to attract work, whether you are a consultant or an employee. There are numerous very talented people in the world, many of whom can do what you do and do it equally well. However, if you create the right documents to present your service where the demand and opportunity are the greatest, you will unequivocally be the person chosen for the job!

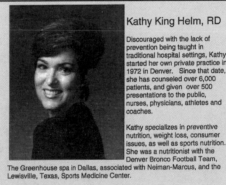

Figure 26-3. Sample Bio and Media Bio (enlarged in Appendix)
Reprinted with permission.

Chapter 27

How to Market Using Direct Mail

Kathy King Helm, RD, Private Practitioner, Lake Dallas, Texas

Each year American businesses spend over $21 billion on direct marketing (1). This type of marketing is more selective than any other mass medium. If readers open your direct mail piece, you have their full attention for a few seconds or minutes. In that time, your marketing piece educates and encourages them to take action – via a toll-free number, product order blank, coupon, and the like.

The fact that direct marketing can be very successful is contributing to saturation of the market. According to estimates, as much as 30 percent of the mail consumers receive is thrown in the waste basket *unopened*. Readers are more likely to open mail when they recognize a name or address on the outside, if an outside message attracts attention, or if the piece is unusual, like a catalog or a three-dimensional tube. The appearance of the mail piece, the message, the messenger, and the mailing list are all crucial components.

Anyone who has ever tried direct mail can tell you that you can waste a lot of money and time if you don't do it right. Although direct mail may seem like a hit-or-miss operation, that is not true. Instead it is a statistical, tactical, and creative medium. The challenge is to offer the right product to the right target market in exactly the right way. And you can avoid costly errors if you test your campaign before you roll it out.

Selling a nutrition gizmo to dietetics professionals using ADA's mailing labels isn't nearly so risky as selling a nutrition gizmo to the public. But there is a big difference in sales potential: if 10 percent of all ADA members buy a gizmo, you will sell 6,500, and if .5 percent of the public buys it, you will sell approximately 1,375,000 gizmos.

The exciting thing is that you may already have something a target market will buy enthusiastically. Do you sell patients an original tape on weight loss or a cookbook on low-fat cooking for one? Look around, you may see a colleague marketing a wonderful product with wide appeal to a very narrow market. Products with narrow appeal usually will stay small. The mail-order expert Julian Simon points out, "Successful items with wide appeal cannot remain small. Big competitors will find you out, horn into the field with their versions of the product, and steal your market." (2)

FINANCIAL CONSIDERATIONS

The typical response rate for direct mail, if you hit the right target market, is 1 to 2 percent, which is higher than all other forms of advertising. There are several strategies for deciding how much to spend on a direct mail campaign (after you have tested your direct mail piece):

- Set a budget for how much money you are willing to spend and send only that number of mailings.

- Determine the geographical range of your target market and budget enough money to mail to that area of practice.

As you try your strategy, keep a record of the response rate. Then expand to new areas, send to new prospects in the same area, mail only to former customers, or regroup and rethink your mail piece and strategies.

Calculate your break-even point by dividing the cost of the campaign by the average cost of the service or product you are selling. For example, if you spend $4,000 on direct mail promotion and you charge $125 per person for your symposium, it will take 32 registrations to break even.

SEVEN STEPS OF A SUCCESSFUL DIRECT MAIL CAMPAIGN

Step 1: Identify Your Target Market. Who will use your product with the least hesitation? Who is already familiar with its concept or function? Who buys the product locally? Describe your buyer using two factors:

- Demographics, which tell about the external aspects of people's lifestyles – age, sex, income, education level, marital status, and the like

- Psychographics, which tell about internal aspects, such as what people buy and how they live

Step 2: Research Mailing Lists. As you might guess, the mailing list is one of the most important elements of a successful direct mail campaign. No matter what you have to sell, only a percentage of your target market will buy it. You want to identify the mailing list(s) with the highest percentage of potential buyers. For example, from ADA's mailing list of all members, purchase only names of active dietitians in one Dietetic Practice Group (DPG) or in one area of practice (community, management, and so on). Reduce those lists further by buying only names in certain states.

You can create your own customer list from such sources as:

- Business cards
- Directories of members
- Voter registration lists
- *Yellow Pages*
- Zip code directories

Or you can purchase lists from state dietetic associations, list brokers, managers, or compilers (1). *List compilers* create lists from the same sources you would use, such as the ones above. However, they cross-reference lists so a name appears only once. They also may have demographic information that you lack, such as the names of all women in town who married last year and drive expensive cars. You might say, "Who cares?" But you might create a healthy culinary program for newlyweds who like to entertain. The disadvantage with this source is the lists. Compilers' lists may be a year old, and addresses may not be current.

A *list broker* is an independent agent who represents and rents lists from other businesses, such as credit card companies, catalogue retailers, magazine publishers, and the like. The lists are usually up to date. Some brokers specialize in certain kinds of lists, such as health-care accounts, consumer lists, and executive lists, and some customize lists from the lists they already have. Brokers are often experts in direct mail and are good resources to know.

A *list manager* works for the company that owns the list, deleting old names and keeping the list up-to-date. According to the Small Business Association, you can contact a list manager directly or go through a broker to get the list you want (1).

Step 3: Determine Your Offer. Decide what you plan to offer your best buyer. What can you offer in the way of value added – bonus, discount, service support, guarantee, warranty, or whatever – that will make your consumers want to buy your product when they see your direct mail piece?

Step 4: Choose Your Format. Some types of mailing offer better readership than others, while some are much more expensive to produce – like sweepstakes. You may use letters, invitations, lettergrams, card decks (showing a different product on each card), sweepstakes, tubes, boxes, food samples, or many other forms. (There are many good books about mail order and direct mail. Visit your library, contact the Direct Marketing Association [212-768-7277], or go to your local bookstore.) As mentioned earlier, dimensional mail has the highest opening rate of any type of mailing. Lettergrams tend to be frequently read, but that may change with overuse. Card decks work well in business-to-business promotion. Sweepstakes are expensive to run due to management and legal costs, and they are illegal in some states. Make sure whatever you choose is compatible with your product image, target market's expectations, and your offer. Use flair, creativity, good taste, and consistency.

Step 5: Create Your Package. Several basic elements are found in the typical direct mail package (1, 2, 3):

- The *envelope* must say the right things or the reader may never see your creative work inside. First, personalize the address – use the recipient's name. Don't address it to "Mayfield Clinic Physician" or "Manager." That's as bad as one marked "Current Resident" or "Occupant." Some direct mailers even try to avoid using labels by renting names on software and having a computer print personalized envelopes and letters.

Some consultants suggest that using a real postage stamp on the outside of expensive direct mail packages (when the image is very upscale) instead of a printed stamp helps to avoid the appearance and image of bulk mail or junk mail. Of course, it costs less to send each piece by bulk mail than by first class. However, the post office will charge you about $75 for a bulk mail permit and another $75 for the right to print the bulk stamp on the outside of your mail piece instead of buying bulk stamps. The fee is worth it because it takes more time (and cost, if you hire someone) to add the stamps later.

Write a teaser on the outside of the envelope that will make the reader want to open it. They come in the mail all the time: "10 Reasons You Should Eat a Carrot a Day," or "Are Your Patients Asking Nutrition Questions You Can't Answer?" A teaser usually asks a question, presents a problem or solution, or offers something for free. Gear your teaser to your readers' point of view. In other words, don't say, "Dietitian Desires To Expand in Cleveland Area," but rather, "Free Nutrition Service to First 10 Who Reply."

- The *sell letter* should highlight your most important benefit in its headline or first paragraph. Use short words and sentences, but don't be afraid to write a letter of one or two pages (1). According to John Caples, the author of *Tested Advertising Methods*, "Long copy sells better than short copy." (3) Personalize the heading and some content for very special leads or potential referral agents. Use the ten most powerful words in direct mail: Introducing, New, Now, You, Win, Guarantee, Free, Easy, Save, Today.

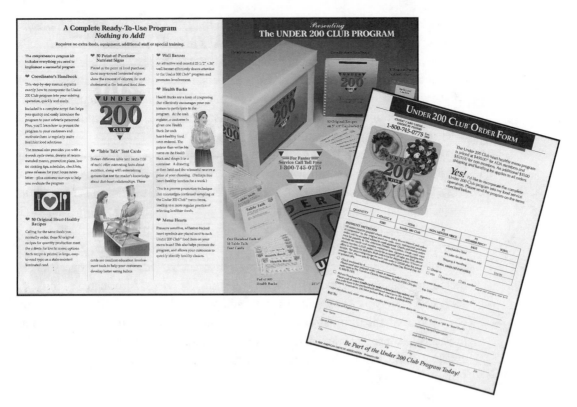

Under 200 Club Flyer

- The *brochure*, if you use one, should be easy to read and present all the information a prospect needs to make a decision and place an order (1). The brochure should be attractive and appropriate for the package, not out of date with an address marked through. Write your brochure to sell your product, not just educate the reader.

- The *lift note* is commonly used in sweepstakes and subscription renewals. It may say on the outside, "Read this if you have decided NOT to renew." A lift note can increase response by as much as 10 percent (1). Mailers use it to urge action, to overcome objections, or to introduce third-party endorsements and testimonials. It should be different in color or size from the rest of the mailing so it stands out.

- The *business reply envelope* is especially useful when you are requesting payment, a phone number, or a credit card number. A prepaid postcard might suffice if you only want the reader to indicate interest or answer a short survey.

You can readily see why some companies shrink-wrap a deck of product cards and apply a label. It's a lot easier and less time-consuming!

Step 6: Market Test Your Campaign. This is the one step that separates the winners from the losers. The goal of market testing is to avoid major losses by checking your mailing list, target market, timing, and package components before you roll out your full campaign. You can test on two levels (1):

- *Tactical*, or those things recipients don't see, such as your lists, choice of target market, and timing

- *Approach*, those things the recipient does see, such as your copy, format, and offer

Testing is one area in which an expert in direct mail or a list manager can be invaluable. Sometimes, to check a mailing list, I send a first-class mailing to a random sample of names to see whether the recipients receive the packages. If a list is old for that target market (students and military personnel move a lot), many packages will be returned, and you will know your overall list may not be worth using. (Bulk mail is not forwarded to new addresses, nor is it returned to you, so you cannot delete outdated names from your list.)

Step 7: Send Your Mail. As you can see from the earlier discussion, direct mail has many functions. You can send direct mail in creative boxes to many people at a time. Or you can personalize each package and send only a few dozen per month to people you plan to pursue as referral agents.

If you send only a few packages per month, you can handle the mailing yourself. But if you send out hundreds or thousands of packages, consider using a mailing service. Before choosing a mailing house, get bids from several operations, including local handicapped groups that offer such services. Although a mailing service will cost you $20 to $40 per thousand pieces (plus postage), depending upon what you send, the ultimate savings can be immeasurable, because a large bulk mail project can jeopardize your mental health and tranquility. Applying labels, stuffing envelopes, and dividing by zip codes is extremely repetitious and time-consuming. I ruined many holiday vacations before I discovered mailing services.

SUMMARY

One of direct mail's major advantages over other media is the ease with which it can be tested. Use this advantage and don't make costly mistakes. Read extensively on mail order and direct marketing. Do your homework so that you know the pitfalls and solutions.

Keep your message simple, honest, and attractive to the buyer. Offer something in the package that will turn the prospect into a buyer.

References

1. Bell Atlantic. *PROMOTION: Solving the Puzzle.* Arlington, VA: Small Business Video Library; 1990.

2. Simon J. *How To Start and Operate a Mail-Order Business.* 5th ed. New York, NY: McGraw-Hill; 1993.

3. Caples J. *Tested Advertising Methods.* 4th ed. Englewood Cliffs, NJ: Prentice-Hall; 1974.

Additional Resources

Standard Rate & Data Service, 3004 Glenview Road, Wilmette, IL 60091, 708-441-2141. (Publishes sources of lists.)

US Government Printing Offices, Superintendent of Documents, Washington, DC, 20402, 202-783-3238.

Direct Marketing Association, 11 West 42nd Street, New York, NY 10036, 212-768-7277. (Offers a wealth of catalogues of list brokers, books, videos, etc.)

The American Dietetic Association, 216 W. Jackson, Chicago, IL 60606, 800-877-1600. (Ask for mailing label sales.)

How to Market at Conventions, Trade Shows, and Health Fairs

Chapter 28

Ruth Fischer, MS, President, NutriSmart, Inc., Rochester, New York

E xhibiting at conventions, trade shows, and health fairs is one of many potentially effective strategies to choose from in marketing your product or service. Since exhibiting is labor-intensive, costly, and time-consuming, it is important to make the most of your exhibit. You must decide where, why, when, and what to exhibit before you decide *how* to exhibit effectively.

WHY TO EXHIBIT

An exhibit is a very visual, dynamic, and interactive way to reach target markets. The reasons for exhibiting are numerous and include both sales and public relations objectives. Purposes for an exhibit are:

- Introduction of a new product or service
- Increased name recognition for your company and its products
- Selling of a product or service
- Demonstration of a product or service
- Participation in a community event or project

WHEN TO EXHIBIT

Your product or service, target markets, and marketing objectives help you determine which exhibiting opportunities you should pursue. For example, if you have a catering service in Omaha, is there any reason for you to exhibit at the national ADA Annual Meeting and Exhibition? Probably not, if you consider only your primary business. However, if you just published a catering cookbook and you want to teach other dietitians or dietetic technicians how to cater at your regional seminars, it could be a wise choice.

Other considerations when deciding whether or not to exhibit at a show are

- Whether it fits into your marketing plan
- Whether it reaches your primary target audience
- Reputation of the show and its management
- Past attendance
- Media or other marketing support
- Number of exhibit hours without competing programs
- Dates and competing events in the region (important if attracting the public)
- Location of available booths in relation to flow of traffic
- Types of exhibitors in surrounding booths
- Cost of booth space, rental costs of furnishings, labor costs, whether a percentage of revenues must return to the show, and whether refunds are

available if less than the minimum guaranteed number attends (Few shows ask for a percentage or guaranteed attendance.)

- Cost-effectiveness

WHAT TO EXHIBIT

When deciding what to include in your exhibit, check your marketing objectives and reasons for exhibiting at the particular convention, trade show, or health fair. To be the most effective, an exhibit needs a focused message – just being represented isn't enough to justify the time and expense. Once you determine your central message, it is much easier to develop a dynamic, memorable, and effective exhibit.

THE ANATOMY OF AN EXHIBIT

The Message

The message is the core, or heart, of what you want your exhibit to demonstrate. Spend time developing your key message. Make it clear, catchy, and memorable.

Our company developed an exhibit for our new product line – Ready T' Run™ Comprehensive Packaged Programs. The main messages we want to communicate are that the new materials are effective and ready to use. The message line was Ready T' Run™ – Workshops That Work℠!

Your message should be unique to your product or service.

Key Descriptors

With the heart in place, it is possible to build the skeleton. The parts of the skeleton are the key attributes you want buyers of your service to know and remember. In our sample exhibit, the parts of the skeleton are

- Topics Available
- Where They Work
- How They Work
- Why They Work

Choose your key descriptors carefully. For an exhibit, they should be short, like the examples above.

Features

Add other body parts once the frame is in place. For example, bulleted descriptions under your key attributes can explain the features of your program or service and help the target audience understand your message. We clarified our attribute How They Work with its parts or features:

- Colorful Overheads
- Entertaining Props
- Energizing Participant Packets
- Practical Instructor's Guide
- Strategic Marketing Support

Company Identification

The head of the exhibit is your company identification. Make sure your name and logo are prominent, distinctive, and legible, and still complement the design and character of your exhibit. You want your name and logo to make a statement and become recognizable to your customers.

The Exhibit Board

The exhibit board is like the skin or covering that holds everything together. It serves as the background for your exhibit and helps define your exhibit's shape, size, and texture. The exhibit board plays a large role in determining the professionalism of your exhibit. Remember – a poorly designed exhibit projects a poor image, no matter what the quality of your product or service!

Consider buying or leasing a modular table top exhibit board. Although such displays are not inexpensive, their versatility and durability make them a reasonable investment. For most of us, it is important that the exhibit board be light-weight and easily transportable.

Commercial display boards are two-sided and come in your choice of colors. Select two colors that combine with many colors and accent your logo. Basic, adaptable colors allow you a broader spectrum of options when planning the materials to attach to your board. Many portable, modular exhibits come with a carrying or shipping case that protects them and makes them easier to store. Also, many commercial display boards include optional lighting, shelves, brochure pockets, and other customized features that you can purchase as your budget allows.

Dressing Up Your Exhibit

How you design and arrange your exhibit is like choosing what to wear. The style, design, and look of the exhibit should be appropriate for the occasion. Just as you would not wear jeans, a T-shirt, and sneakers to an important interview, your exhibit shouldn't look like just any old thing thrown together. Your exhibit may be your one chance to interest a prospective client in your product or service, so you don't want to give the wrong first impression. When planning your exhibit design, consider these tips:

- Make the artwork, graphic design, and typefaces pleasing, appropriate, and complementary to your overall look.

- Be sure that printing is large and easy to read.

- Keep messages positive and upbeat.

- Avoid clutter.

- Use color to add interest.

- Plan something special about your exhibit to set it apart and make it memorable.

- Consider using photographs, especially colored photographs, to show your product or service in use.

Adding Accessories

Although what appears on the exhibit board sets the tone for your exhibit, the handouts and other tabletop accessories are just as important as the jewelry, scarf, tie, or shoes you add to your outfit. To tell your story best, a few carefully chosen accessories are often better than too many.

Some tips for a tasteful presentation are

- Develop or choose no more than four brochures or other pieces of literature to support your exhibit. Have them focus on the product or service you are trying to sell through your exhibit. I'm sure you have all been to exhibits that displayed every piece of print material the exhibitor ever produced. You may have picked them up to read later, but probably discarded them or they got lost in the mass of information. The only thing that was memorable was the clutter, not the product. Do not be tempted to overmerchandise.

- Consider developing display notebooks for samples of your program materials or literature that further explains your services. Design the notebook to complement your exhibit and include materials that show and discuss the unique features of your product or service. The notebooks should be compact, easy to handle, and helpful in keeping your exhibit neat and manageable. Mark the notebook "Sample materials. For display only!" The notebook will help stop exhibit attendees from walking away with your precious exhibit-support materials.

- Plan a hook to get people to visit your exhibit. Something action-oriented helps attract potential customers to your booth. Successful exhibits can use one or more techniques. Some examples are to offer a prize or drawing, serve food, conduct a survey, or run a computer program, slide series, or promotional video.

Layout

Don't set up barriers between your booth and your audience. Instead, place the tables to allow for easy entry and exit. Make them perpendicular to the aisle, not parallel.

Location

Studies show that people stop or slow down at every fourth exhibit. Study the floor plan of the exhibit area before you choose your booth location and stay away from anchor (very large) exhibits that will attract a lot of traffic. Instead, choose a booth in a high-traffic area on the path going to or away from the anchor.

PEOPLE ARE MOST IMPORTANT

All who work at your booth are salespeople for your company and its products and services. They need to communicate the same image and message as the exhibit itself. Professionalism, appearance, and friendliness are key to making a positive impression.

If people are working at your exhibit who have not had experience in exhibiting, prepare them for what to expect. Exhibiting is a tiring job. With all your other designing and planning, don't forget to train the people who provide that all-important personal representation of your company. Teach everyone how to identify A accounts (top prospects), B, and C ones. Keep the business cards or lead forms in a safe place, not in a bowl on a table. Take the cards or forms back to your room at the end of each day for safekeeping.

When working a booth:

- Know your products and services. Anticipate questions that potential clients may ask. Be prepared.

- Be cheerful, enthusiastic, and outgoing. Make potential clients feel comfortable when talking with you.

- Remember that people attending conventions, trade shows, and health fairs are often looking for new ideas, products, and services. That is what you sell.

- Think of yourself as a professional salesperson. You are there to make contacts and sell your product or service.

- Dress comfortably, but appropriately; you will be on your feet for long periods of time.

- Plan enough staffing to appropriately handle the number of potential visitors. The size of the show, the length of the exhibit hours, and the size of your booth as well as your budget will determine the size staff you need.

- Try to find out the peak times for viewers; this will help you anticipate demand and plan breaks. It is important to stay fresh.

- Enjoy meeting new people and potential customers!

FOLLOW-UP

If you do not sell a product from your booth, use your booth to find qualified decision makers who may buy your product at a later date. These prospects are only as good as your follow-up. Prepare your follow-up materials before you go to the show so that they are not delayed. The A group of prospects should be contacted by phone, personal visit, or mailed packet within a week; the B group should be contacted within two weeks; and the C group should be mailed something, although follow-up can wait until the A and B groups have been contacted. On average, 80 percent of your business from the show will come from Group A, according to the Small Business Administration.

Trade Show Booth

FINAL WORDS OF WISDOM

After considering all these points, the final thing to do is to ask yourself once again if your company should be participating at this particular convention, trade show, or health fair. To make the best use of your time and marketing budget, be very careful in choosing which exhibiting opportunities you pursue.

Chapter 29

How to Write a Marketing Brochure

Tara Liskov, MS, RD, Yale-New Haven Hospital, New Haven, Connecticut

The objectives of a marketing brochure are fourfold: (1) it must capture the attention of the target audience, (2) it must be informative and factual, (3) it must present the information as benefits to the client from the client's point of view, and finally, (4) it must call the reader to action. In other words, instead of having a brochure that states, "Our services include low-fat diets and grocery shopping tours," it might say, "Are low-fat diets ruining your social life? They don't have to! Call now to sign up for our next culinary class!"

STEP ONE

The first step in preparing a great brochure is to determine your target audience and what it wants to hear. Physicians and other health-care professionals, sports teams, business and industry, fitness centers, speakers' bureaus, and prospective patients are examples of audiences you might be interested in targeting for possible business.

If physicians and other health-care providers are your target, place emphasis on how you can help them provide excellent care for their patients and what you can provide (that is, scope of services, type of counseling – group or individual, and areas of expertise). This target group wants to know that you are qualified and trustworthy, so a paragraph on your credentials and experience will help serve this purpose. Use quotes to show that other physicians are pleased with your work.

In a brochure directed to sports teams, discuss how your handling of sports nutrition problems can help players and teams win. Possible services include body-fat analysis, nutrition and exercise profiles, nutrition traveling tips, individualized counseling, and group lectures. Give sport-specific examples of how you have helped others. End with a call to action.

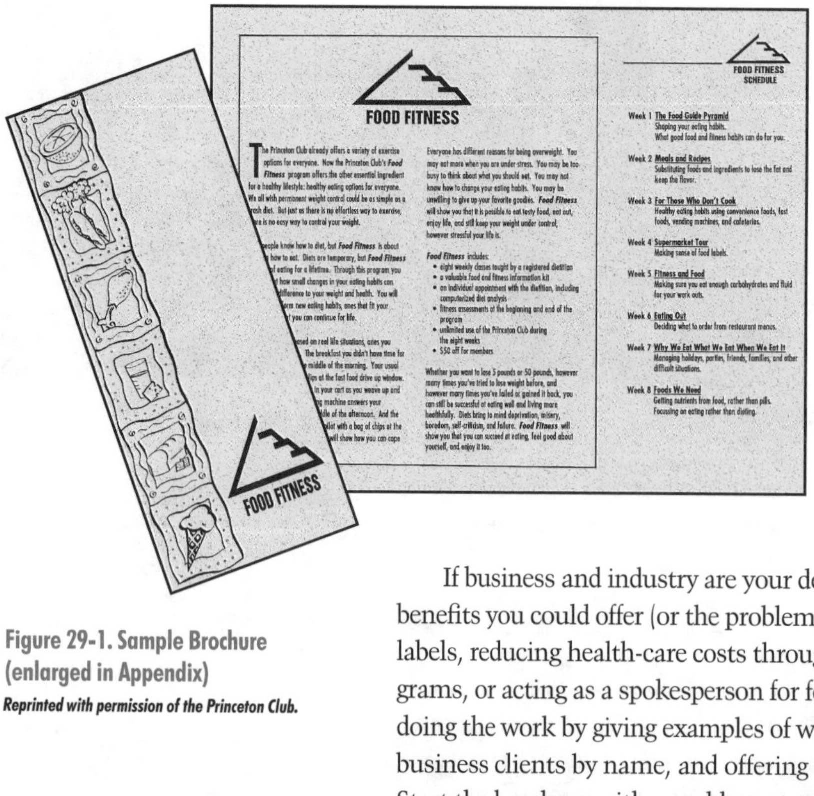

If business and industry are your desired target audiences, clearly identify the benefits you could offer (or the problems you could solve), such as calculating food labels, reducing health-care costs through nutrition lectures and weight-loss programs, or acting as a spokesperson for food products. Explain your credentials for doing the work by giving examples of work for other clients, listing other satisfied business clients by name, and offering several quotes from satisfied customers. Start the brochure with a problem statement like, "Do you have the time and energy to prepare exciting, healthy food for your next dinner party? Leave the food preparation and clean-up to To Your Health Caterers."

Figure 29-1. Sample Brochure (enlarged in Appendix)
Reprinted with permission of the Princeton Club.

Write the tone of the text to fit the target audience. Consider hiring a professional public relations expert or other person skilled in such writing to edit your work. You want your reader to feel comfortable with your practice just from reading your brochure (see Figure 29-1).

STEP TWO

Once you have determined your target audience, you must establish your credibility. If your brochure focuses on you as an individual, highlight personal achievements and accomplishments. A brief description of your academic credentials and a summary of work experiences will help to establish your credibility. Also consider listing any highlights from your bio that will be of interest to your target market.

If your brochure is intended to highlight a program that employs several individuals, highlight the successes of the program and briefly describe each speaker and his or her credentials. If the speakers will vary each time the program is given, generically describe the credentials of all the individuals (for example, "all counselors are registered dietitians and hold advanced degrees in nutrition or related fields").

STEP THREE

Convince the reader that you and your services or programs are successful. Present testimonials and quotes (with written permission from the authors). Cite your success rate or rate of business growth. List satisfied business customers. State how many clients have been seen in the last year or since the business began. Be tasteful and tactful. Don't oversell or you risk sounding desperate.

STEP FOUR

A great brochure must show that you are available and convenient to reach. Give your phone and fax numbers, and office hours, and if your location is hard to find, consider adding a small map.

If your location has adequate parking, make that clear in the brochure. If, however, you are located in an area with inadequate parking, you should try to improve the parking situation for your clients. (For example, look into parking validation or discounts, or offer suggestions for free parking, if that is of great interest to prospective clients.)

STEP FIVE

Once you have developed the text of your brochure, you must then choose the format, style, and paper quality. Again, consider hiring a consultant for graphic art ideas, or use the print shop staff, if available. Keep samples of your favorite brochures to show the kind of layout, colors, or style you like or want.

If you are marketing primarily to an audience that will refer business to you or may hire you as a business consultant, add a perforated Rolodex card at the bottom of one brochure panel, as shown in Figure 29-2. A detachable card increases the probability that prospects will file your business information with other important telephone numbers for present or future reference, as opposed to discarding it.

Figure 29-2. Flyer with Rolodex Card

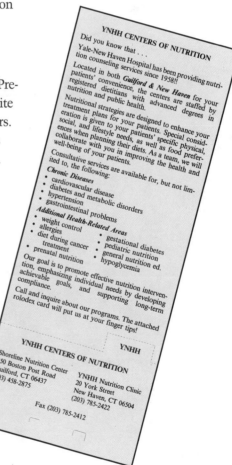

Your brochure can take any number of forms, but it should reflect to some degree your personality and style or that of your institution. Consider using bullets and different type faces, shading, or boxes to emphasize various kinds of information. Err on the side of brevity instead of wordy paragraphs and long explanations. Leave open spaces to highlight your message. Choose words that interest and excite readers and encourage them to want more.

Some dietitians use their photos in their brochures with good success. The major consideration is the quality and attractiveness of the photo. You should look alert, intelligent, well groomed, and professional. Very dark photos do not reproduce well, and home snapshots may not look professional enough for your target market. Considering the cost of starting a business today, it pays to go to a professional photographer (or to an artist for a line drawing) and work with that person until you get what you want.

Choose the highest-quality paper stock you can afford that fits your purposes. Good paper can add richness and subtly imply high-quality services. To save money, print larger quantities at a time. If you want to avoid dating a brochure with exact times for classes or other information that may change, consider leaving empty space and applying laser-printed labels with the up-to-date information, or print the information, but cover it with a label if it changes. It can be an effective marketing tool to leave your brochures in physicians' offices, fitness centers, corporate wellness offices, and wherever else clients may see it.

SUMMARY

In summary, your brochure should:

1. Emphasize benefits to the client as the most important information
2. Establish your credibility
3. Highlight your successes
4. Show your convenience and availability
5. Use the best and most effective wording, format, and style to attract customers to your door.

Then you will be well on your way to having a great brochure!

Chapter 30

How to Write Effectively to Physicians

Linda Gay, MS, RD, Clinical Dietitian, Yale-New Haven Hospital, New Haven, Connecticut

Written communication to physicians is important when establishing rapport and updating patient-care records. This form of communication is not meant to take the place of face-to-face meetings, but to facilitate their occurrence. The American Dietetic Association's Physicians' Nutrition Initiative offers training and reference materials to help dietetics professionals learn how to market themselves to physicians.

FEATURES OF A PROMOTION LETTER

A promotion letter introduces you and your services to a prospective client. This type of letter can help get your foot in the door at physicians' offices when you open a private practice, outpatient office, or any new service that you want to promote. It is well known that physicians refer their patients to people they know and respect. It is important to take the time to get to know physicians in your area and be known.

Individualization

The heading and content of one basic letter can be adapted to each prospective physician. Considering the unbelievable amounts of mail people receive today and the fact that 30 percent of all unsolicited mail goes unopened, letters should not be addressed to "Dear Local Physician" or "Dearborn Clinic Medical Team." Take the time to individualize each letter and address.

Before you compose a promotion letter for physicians, you should first analyze the situation from two points of view, yours and the physician's. Ask yourself these questions: What is the physician interested in? Does he or she have a specialty? What can you do for his or her patients? Why would the physician choose to refer a patient to you rather than to another registered dietitian? Your letter should target these key points.

Content

A short, well-written letter should briefly describe:

- How the physician can use your services for her or his patients
- What services you offer specific to that physician's interests or patients' needs
- Your credentials and experience (or enclose a professional bio or profile)
- How to schedule an appointment (your brochure with phone number, hours, location, parking, and the like may also be enclosed)

Close your letter by suggesting a face-to-face, five-minute interview in the physician's office or lunch – your treat. (Figure 30-1 shows a sample introductory letter.)

If you feel it is more effective, or if your letter is too long, send a separate professional bio or profile that outlines your educational background and your experience.

Figure 30-1. Sample Introductory Letter (enlarged in Appendix)

Jane Jones, MS, RD
Ambulatory Nutrition Specialist
828 North Forrest Avenue • New Haven, CT 06504

September 12, 1995

John Smith, MD
Obstetrics and Gynecology
2 Church Street
New Haven, CT 06504

Dear Dr. Smith:

The Yale-New Haven Hospital Centers of Nutrition would like to extend its services to your OB-GYN patients. I have enclosed a package of information that describes our staff and services. Our program emphasizes a medically oriented approach providing in-depth initial nutrition assessment and long-term counseling. Patients are seen either individually or with family members. We welcome clients of all ages, and invite you to send your referrals for individualized nutrition care.

Some problems commonly encountered in our practice include prenatal nutrition, gestational diabetes, diabetes, hyperlipidemia, hypertension, obesity, diverticulosis, and food intolerance. Our centers are staffed by registered dietitians with advanced degrees in nutrition or public health. We work closely with the referring physician and endeavor to send timely correspondence reporting on patient progress.

I would be pleased to meet with you, your associates, and your staff at your convenience to discuss our program further and answer any questions you may have.

Sincerely,

Jane Jones

Jane Jones, MS, RD
Ambulatory Nutrition Specialist

Jane Jones, MS, RD
Ambulatory Nutrition Specialist
828 North Forrest Avenue • New Haven, CT 06504

January 13, 1996

John Smith, MD
Obstetrics and Gynecology
2 Church Street
New Haven, CT 06504

Dear Dr. Smith:

Eating is an integral part of the holidays and weight loss is a challenge for the New Year. With counseling and literature from the Centers of Nutrition, your patients can enjoy traditions, holiday feasts, and celebrations without the extra calories, fat, and sugar.

At the Yale-New Haven Hospital Centers of Nutrition, we would like to concentrate our efforts during the New Year 1996 on reaching patients who, because of obesity, have an increased risk for high blood pressure, diabetes, and heart disease.

I have enclosed copies of our monthly consumer newsletter and would like to make these available to your patients. If you would like additional copies, please give me a call at 555-5555 or 555-3333.

I would also like to thank you for your continued support of the Yale-New Haven Hospital Centers of Nutrition. We remain committed to providing your patients with meaningful dietary counseling, whether it be for existing medical conditions or to promote wellness.

Sincerely,

Jane Jones

Jane Jones, MS, RD
Ambulatory Nutrition Specialist

Figure 30-2. Sample Follow-up Promotion Letter (enlarged in Appendix)

This will provide the physician with more detailed information about you and help establish your credibility faster. If you have several nutrition counselors in your practice, include a professional profile of each staff member. Do not repeat the same information in the promotion letter as you list in the bio, it only needs to be explained once.

Private practitioners often use letters from referring physicians along with introductory promotion letters to help open new doors. Even if you move from one state to another, you can become established faster if you use referral letters from former physician colleagues who knew you and respected your work.

As part of your introductory package, you could include a brochure. Since convenience is an important consideration, you might want to provide a brochure with a perforated Rolodex card. The brochure would allow you to describe your facility and its services, while the detachable card would help ensure that your phone number is stored in a handy place. You should also include your business card.

Keep a record of when you mailed your promotional letters and plan to call for an interview or lunch within one to two weeks.

BUILDING RELATIONSHIPS

Getting to know the office staff is an effective way to increase business as well. Should Dr. Smith tell one of her staff members to refer a patient to the dietitian, you want to be sure that you are the one who receives that call!

When Yale-New Haven Hospital Centers of Nutrition opened its first satellite office, we needed to increase our visibility with area physicians. After sending a promotion letter and following up with a call, we scheduled luncheons with the office staffs in several of the larger practices. No matter how busy the practice, staff members still need to eat, so we found this a perfect way to get their attention. The office staffs were appreciative of the meal, and we were able to describe our services in a relaxed environment.

Once you have attracted referrals from physicians, you need to foster the relationships. Physicians will appreciate timely feedback that outlines their patients' progress. You could offer a quarterly newsletter or consumer-oriented literature for distribution in their offices. Promotion letters for new services or products can be combined with follow-up communiqués, as illustrated in Figure 30-2. In this way, you are providing information for the physicians to distribute to their patients while at the same time reminding them of your services. Of course, you will include your name, address, and telephone number on each piece of material. Patients might ask their physicians about your services or refer themselves directly. (See the case study on thanking your referral sources.)

In summary, the important points to remember when writing an effective promotion letter are:

1. Be sure to target the interests of the physician.
2. Establish your credibility.
3. Describe the particulars of your practice.
4. Include a business card or personalized Rolodex card.
5. Remember to follow up with a phone call to verify that addressees have received the information.

Case Study: THANKING YOUR REFERRAL SOURCE – A GREAT WAY TO MARKET YOURSELF

L. Kathleen Mahan, RD, Consulting Nutritionist, Seattle, Washington, and Co-Author of Food, Nutrition and Diet Therapy, *8th ed.*

A follow-up letter to the referral source, often a physician, can be an extremely effective and efficient way to market your practice. I have had a consulting practice for sixteen years, and my associates and I have always operated separately from our referral sources. For this reason, follow-up letters are an extremely important way to communicate about the nutritional care of clients. But I have also found it to be a wonderful marketing and rapport-building tool.

For a follow-up letter to be an effective marketing tool, it must

1. Begin with a thank you for the referral
2. Be succinct – absolutely no more than two pages
3. Be clear and easy to read or scan quickly, which is best achieved by grouping information and using headings
4. Be timely – mailed and on its way within three days of seeing a patient
5. Have your name or your practice's name in bold letters so that even when sitting on a physician's desk, it is quickly recognized as coming from you
6. Include several of your business cards, which make it easy for the physician and nurse to refer the next patient, possibly that very day. (If they respect your skills and abilities, nurses who work for physicians refer patients to you more often than their bosses do.)
7. Include a closing that encourages the physician to call you if any questions or items need to be discussed

Copies should also be sent to the primary health-care provider, even if that person did not refer the patient. What a way to reach another physician and show that the referring physician trusts you and your work!

Sending a follow-up letter that reflects the preceding ideas makes communication about patient care double as a marketing tool. It requires no more time or expense than preparing a standard report, but the thank you included in a letter builds tremendous rapport with the referral source.

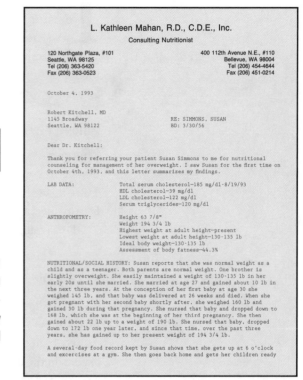

Follow-up Letter to Referring Physician (enlarged in Appendix)

Chapter 31

How to Market a Newsletter

Betty Goldblatt, MPH, RD, Executive Editor, Environmental Nutrition Newsletter, *New York, New York*

In starting a newsletter, it is important to have a strong idea of what the newsletter is all about. To clarify this to yourself, and eventually to copywriters and prospective subscribers, develop a statement of what the newsletter is – its editorial platform, its special market niche, and what makes it unique. Having a clear concept of what you are all about is a key element in achieving success.

NATIONAL NEWSLETTERS FOR THE PUBLIC THROUGH DIRECT MAIL

This discussion pertains to subscription newsletters that take no advertising. Such newsletters are marketed to a selected population of health-minded consumers. The consumers are identified by list brokers whose business it is to rent subscriber lists to direct marketers.

First of all, there are two sides to selling newsletter subscriptions:

- The actual marketing program, direct mail being the proven best type
- The continuing selling of the newsletter through the editorial product

The editorial product and the direct mail package go together. The promises made in the subscription offer must be fulfilled by the newsletter. Developing a direct mail package that accurately portrays a publication is a job best left for experts in the direct mail copywriting field. The initial expense is high, but a package that works is the key element in gaining initial subscribers who will pay for their subscriptions and renew for years to come. Subscribers who find that the promises of the direct mail package aren't met by the product will not pay for their initial subscription and will not renew.

List-marketing firms have two divisions – brokerage and management. List brokers market their client lists to prospective renters and try to keep the lists in use. They charge for names on a per-thousand basis, with a minimum number per order. Charges are paid by the list renter.

To find a list broker or list manager in your area or suited to your specific needs, consult *Direct Marketing Market Place*, National Register Publishing, New Providence, NJ, updated annually. It is available at most large public libraries.

After reaching a subscription base of approximately 10,000, a newsletter owner can have the subscriber list managed (or rented). The manager offers the list to prospective renters.

FINDING OUTSIDE HELP

If you are thinking of starting a newsletter and have no experience in the newsletter-marketing field, the Newsletter Publishers Association (NPA) is an excellent resource. This is a national not-for-profit trade association of newsletter publishers and suppliers. The association holds an annual international conference that covers all aspects of the industry and publishes the biweekly newsletter *Hotline*. There are nine chapters located throughout the United States that meet monthly to enable members to network and learn more about the complex newsletter-marketing and publishing field.

WRITING FOR THE PUBLIC MARKET

Writing style for the consumer market is very different from writing for professional journals. When writing for consumers, use a friendly, direct style. It's best to limit professional jargon, but it's all right to use technical terms because subscribers to nutrition newsletters are quite well read in the nutrition field. Offer readers practical advice. Get continuous feedback from readers to determine if you are staying on course and meeting their needs and expectations. Use the feedback to determine a reader profile that will enable you to write with your specific audience in mind.

The design of your newsletter needs to be reader-friendly, inviting the reader to continue on to the end. To make the newsletter easy to read,

- Use catchy headlines and titles for the articles

- Break up articles with frequent subheadings

- Consider adding summarizing statements in the margins, or highlight key statements in the text with a different typeface

- Use a type size that is appropriate to your audience – larger for children or elderly people

- Use illustrations or cartoons to add life and human interest to articles

- Consider introducing several articles on the front page, with continuing text in the following pages

A sample newsletter is shown in Figure 31-1.

If you are not a professional writer but think you would like to become one, test your writing skills before going into your own newsletter publishing business. Write some articles and see if you can get them published. Otherwise, seek out experienced professional writers to work with you. A great idea that is poorly written will have less potential for success.

FINANCIAL CONSIDERATIONS

The goal in marketing a newsletter is to earn a profit substantial enough to make all your efforts worthwhile. Newsletter publishing is a challenge and a very expensive undertaking. Marketing expertise and a large commitment of capital are essential. A business plan that includes a comprehensive marketing plan is the first step. Costs include mailing, fulfilling subscription orders, and securing renewals, as well as the monthly costs of editorial salaries and expenses, and overhead. Such costs very quickly mount into the tens of thousands of dollars. Growth from start-up to profit typically takes from three to five years, so an owner must be able to sustain the extended negative cash flow.

An ideal situation is to combine a nutritionist's expertise with the talents of writers, professional marketers, and copywriters, plus an organization that has funds

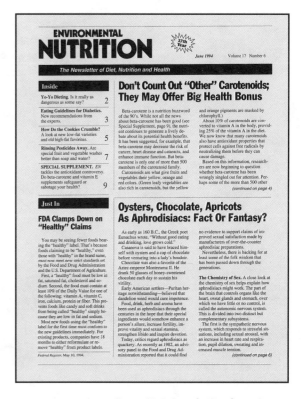

Figure 31-1. Sample Newsletter Cover

to invest and is willing to carry the loss during development. This may mean giving up some control to an investor, but it can greatly increase the chances for success.

OTHER MARKETING OPTIONS

Newsletters can be marketed through means other than direct mail. One less-expensive option is through a "ride along" in another product's selling package – typically a single sheet of paper with a subscription offer. This method is much less effective than a complete direct mail package, but is much less costly.

Another way to market a newsletter is to offer it as a generic product to organizations such as wellness programs, fitness centers, and medical clinics. The organization prints the newsletter on its own masthead and distributes it through its own means. The same editorial product can thus be sold to many different companies.

Various ways of using print advertising to sell newsletter subscriptions have been tried over the years, but they have never proven to be worthwhile. Advertising in newspapers and magazines is very costly. A more cost-effective way to reach consumers through the print media would be to write an article for a newspaper, get paid for it, and mention the newsletter's name and address in the piece. Interested persons will write in and ask for a sample and how to subscribe.

Resource

Goss F. *Success in Newsletter Publishing, A Practical Guide*. 4th ed. Arlington, VA: Newsletter Publishers Association; 1993.

How to Create and Use Focus Groups

Chapter 32

Ruth B. Fischer, MS, President, NutriSmart, Inc.,
Rochester, New York

A focus group is a qualitative information-gathering technique that typically brings together eight to twelve individuals for one to two hours to discuss a predetermined topic. It is a loosely structured discussion between a researcher and respondents that focuses on psychological characteristics that affect consumer behavior.

Focus groups are a social marketing-research method frequently used by marketers and advertisers to obtain consumer information useful in designing a product or packaging, measuring advertising effectiveness, or determining product pricing. The technique can also be useful in designing, marketing, evaluating, and pricing dietetic and health-education products and services. It is often used before going to a large-scale survey.

WHAT CAN A FOCUS GROUP DO?

Through in-depth interviewing techniques with a small group of people, a focus group examines general concerns about a product or service and can help identify

- Product focus
- Consumer reactions to potential products and services
- Consumer resistance to products and services
- Potential reasons for buying

WHY USE A FOCUS GROUP?

Frequently, when designing and marketing nutrition and dietetic programs and services, we place emphasis on the knowledge or the behavior *we* want clients to have. Programs and services focus on our message. It concerns, disappoints, and sometimes baffles us when

- Clients drop out of our programs
- Classes fail to fill
- Lack of business forces staff cutbacks
- People believe our workshops or printed materials are confusing or boring
- We feel our programs and services lack administration and colleague support

Commercial marketers learned they need to know and understand what makes consumers want to buy their products and what results in consumer satisfaction. They use focus groups to understand what potential consumers want, why they buy, and what constitutes satisfaction. In other words, they are client-driven.

Unfortunately, too often we train dietetics professionals and other nutrition educators to be content-driven, rather than focusing on what is needed to satisfy the customer and make our sale. Being client-driven does not negate the importance of the content, but merely emphasizes the need for packaging the message appropriately.

WHEN SHOULD YOU USE A FOCUS GROUP?

The focus group is not appropriate for every market research situation. It is important to remember that the data are qualitative rather than quantitative. In some situations it may be better to do mail or telephone surveys with larger databases.

However, the focus group helps us better understand both our internal (administrator and colleagues) and external (patients or clients) markets. If used effectively, it helps determine:

- The best marketing approach for our programs and services
- The kinds of instructional materials that might be easiest to use and most helpful for a targeted client group
- How a program or service might be altered to better meet the needs of a client group
- The cost of programs and services
- The hot buttons for gaining support and referrals from our colleagues

Focus groups yield a great amount of detail from a small number of consumers. The format of the focus group allows you to understand consumers from their point of view.

UNDERSTANDING CONSUMER BEHAVIOR

Understanding the process by which consumers make decisions helps in the designing, planning, and conducting of a focus group. The consumer behavior model, as shown in Figure 32-1, can be helpful in adapting the focus group technique to your unique purpose.

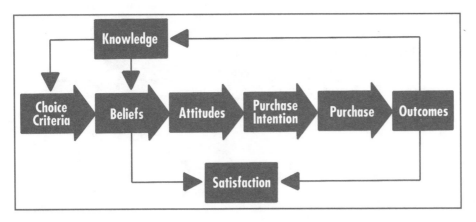

Figure 32-1. Consumer Behavior Model

Reprinted with permission from JE Nelson, The Practice of Marketing Research (Boston: Kent Publishing Co., 1982), p. 200.

Knowledge influences both consumer choice criteria and beliefs. *Choice criteria* are attributes of consumption alternatives that consumers use to make comparisons. Obviously, the choice criteria will differ depending on the product or service offered and the knowledge the individual brings to the process. For example, selecting which grocery store to frequent may include such attributes as distance, price, store size, store layout, cleanliness, quality and variety of produce, other service departments, carryout service, friendliness of employees, and consumer information available.

Beliefs reflect the consumer's views of a consumption alternative's performance on various choice criteria. For example, a consumer might believe that Store A has better prices and is closer and that Store B has more variety of produce and is always clean.

Choice criteria and beliefs combine to form attitudes. *Attitude* is a consumer's overall like or dislike for an alternative. The attitude is a learned predisposition to respond consistently to a given alternative. An attitude toward supermarket shopping might be "I like a clean store." An attitude differs from the action more specifically characterized by the purchase intention of "I will only shop in a clean store."

Choice criteria, beliefs, and attitudes are extremely important in determining consumers' intent to purchase a product or service. When researching the market for your product or service, it is important to determine:

- What attributes consumers include in their choice criteria
- How consumers rate each attribute's importance
- How beliefs differ among potential consumer segments

Thus, attitude leads to or influences *purchase intention*. Purchase intention is how likely a consumer is to buy within a certain time frame. Purchase intention is also helpful in forecasting future product demand.

Purchase is the act of buying. It is the only visible behavior in the model. The consumer shops at Store B because variety of produce and store cleanliness are more important to this consumer than price and distance.

In the consumer behavior model, *outcomes* are the mental results of buying. Two outcomes are of most interest to us as we market our programs and services: knowledge and satisfaction. If consumer *knowledge* changes, the result may be a change in consumer behavior. *Satisfaction* is also important. Satisfaction results from the consumer's comparison of prepurchase beliefs with the postpurchase performance. For example, if the consumer shops at Store B in the belief that the produce is better but is disappointed by the quality and selection, he or she may decide to shop elsewhere. On the other hand, if the consumer likes the quality and variety of the produce, the product performance satisfies the consumer, who will likely be a repeat shopper.

Understanding consumer behavior relative to the product or service you plan to offer should influence the development of the product or service and the strategies for selling it. Try to relate the consumer behavior model to the consumer's choice of a weight-management program or another product or service important to your practice.

STRENGTHS OF USING FOCUS GROUPS

A focus group results in rich and varied data expressed by consumers in their own words. By interviewing several consumers at one time, you save time and money. Another strength is the interactive process of the small group as members respond to questions. The benefits that you can expect to see from the group interaction process are:

- *Synergism*, the group's ability to produce results in greater quantity and diversity than the sum of separate individual efforts
- *Snowballing*, the group's ability to take a small point made by one member, add to it, and reveal significant insights
- *Stimulation*, the elements of general excitement, enthusiasm, and even competition created by a group of similar consumers or other members
- *Security*, the feeling of safety in numbers that allows a member to discuss sensitive topics with group support

- *Spontaneity*, the idea that after the moderator asks a question, only interested members respond, making answers more meaningful, less forced, and less conventional

For example, holding a focus group on what type of weight-management program to offer and when to offer it might be very productive before your hospital makes a decision on implementation. The group discussion generates more information than interviewing individuals separately. A point made by one participant might trigger a very important comment from another member of the group, and so on, providing you with additional insight about the type of program to select.

The discussion excites the participants and makes them comfortable about sharing their feelings and needs. You might learn very different perceptions of what potential participants feel works best for them. Discuss the similarities and allow disagreements. Individuals in the group feel less pressure to respond to each question than they might in a personal interview.

Give some thought to the strengths of using focus groups and how they provide information to the planning or evaluation stage in your company or organization.

WEAKNESSES OF USING FOCUS GROUPS

The focus group technique is so popular that sometimes we use it when other information-gathering strategies are more valuable or appropriate. It does not replace quantitative data collection. Use it as only one tool in the decision-making process and not as the sole justification for a decision affecting your company's product or services.

Some problems in using focus groups occur when

- The quality of the facilitator is inadequate or inappropriate
- The group is shy and reluctant to participate in the discussion
- The sample group is too small
- The members are not randomly selected from the target population, thus adding bias to the results
- The people who participate in the group are only those who can afford to spend one to two hours at the research location

Also, it must be kept in mind that it is important to avoid situations that inhibit consumer reaction during the focus group meeting.

SETTING UP A FOCUS GROUP

Participants of focus groups are usually specifically invited because they represent either the characteristics of the target market or the average consumer of the product or service. Participants may or may not be paid for their time, but if one is paid, all should be paid. Often gift certificates, product samples, or gifts are given instead of cash payments.

Look for participants who are willing to speak up and become actively involved in the discussions but will not dominate the group. Imbalance may also occur when group members acquiesce to a more experienced member's opinion instead of offering their own. A good facilitator will help resolve problems at the time of the session, but some problems can be anticipated and avoided.

Dietitians who are affiliated with hospitals or industry probably have people within their organization who can assist in implementing a focus group. If you do not have this luxury, seek help from the business or marketing department of a local college or university. It isn't necessary to use expensive market research companies to get a focus group conducted professionally and effectively.

Although a focus group interview is informal and relatively unstructured, the facilitator typically uses a framework to guide the process. Use product samples or program materials as props to assist the focus group in reacting and responding to your product or service and your competitors'. Frequently, focus groups are audio- or videotaped, but inform participants about either of these procedures and ask for their consent.

A comfortable environment is important to the success of a focus group. Some people use special rooms with one-way mirrors so that clients can observe the focus group without being seen. This minimizes distraction for focus group participants, but they should still be informed about the observers.

The All-Important Facilitator

The facilitator is the key person in determining the success of the focus group process. The facilitator should

- Have a pleasant appearance and voice
- Enjoy meeting and interacting with people
- Have a genuine interest in the researched project
- Be sensitive to the needs of both the members of the focus group and the client desiring the information
- Be a quick thinker and a good listener

Have the facilitator meet with you and other key people in the management group. Clearly define your research questions and what you hope to learn from the focus group. This will greatly assist the facilitator in preparing key open-ended questions to keep the group process flowing and help assure that you meet your goals.

The facilitator must be skilled in leading the group process. The facilitator needs to

- *Provide a comfortable environment*. If the participants do not feel at ease, the discussion will not flow and people will not open up to share their thoughts and feelings.
- *Allow focus group members to do the talking, follow their own train of thought, and use their own words*. Charge the facilitator with the task of keeping the respondents speaking and expressing their feelings about the research topic. The facilitator should not excessively control the environment or prompt speakers to use phrases that are not their own.
- *Summarize the respondents' statements*. Another important function of the facilitator is to summarize the respondents' statements to capture the essence of their thoughts. Restating the responses may also stimulate others in the group to comment.
- *Ask probing or investigative questions*. Well-phrased questions clarify the meaning of what respondents say or allow new topics to be explored. They

can also keep the discussion moving when it slows down. However, it should be noted that moments of silence are acceptable. Silence allows respondents to think about what has just been said and to pull their own thoughts together. It is during silent moments that the less-assertive group members may feel more comfortable about speaking up.

- *Have a topic outline available.* An outline makes sure the facilitator covers all topics during the focus group. It is important to design the focus group to be free-flowing and spontaneous. Too much structure will impede the flow of useful information.

- *Avoid making evaluative comments.* A focus group discussion is not an evaluative process, but rather an opportunity to brainstorm and gain a wide variety of information. The facilitator should not lead participants to believe that one answer is better than another. Analyze what was said after the meeting is completed and the respondents have left.

SUMMARY

The focus group is a powerful tool that can help dietetics professionals and nutrition educators more effectively position their products and services to meet the needs of their target markets. Although it is a useful tool, it is not a panacea, and should not be misused or overused. On the other hand, don't be intimidated by the cost and relative complexity of using focus groups.

References

Kurtz DL, Boone LE. *Marketing.* 2nd ed. New York, NY: Dryden Press; 1981.

Nelson JE. *The Practice of Marketing Research.* Boston, MA: Kent Publishing Company; 1982.

Case Study: **FOCUS LUNCHEONS – A MARKETING TOOL FOR BUSINESS**

Karolyn Christopher, MS, RD, LD, Vice President, The Norton Group, Missouri City, Texas, and Former Nutritional Sales and Systems Manager, Sysco Food Services, Inc., Houston, Texas

Focus groups can explore what the customer's product awareness is or what the customer wants to know. Given this basic principle, I began to consider using focus groups shortly after I arrived at my new position in Houston at Sysco food brokerage. We wanted to learn if everything about each product met the customers' needs, and if not, what changes customers would like to see.

I first considered holding a traditional focus group in a meeting room with one-way mirrors and a single leader to channel the questions. Midway through this possibly tedious event, I would serve a quick meal from a carryout restaurant. For their participation, I would pay group members a predetermined amount of money. This process sounded plain and impersonal to me. Therefore, I decided to develop a program that would increase sales, answer key marketing and manufacturing questions, address issues that directly affect the customer, and provide an atmosphere that was fun and rewarding.

HOW FOCUS LUNCHEONS WERE BORN

Being new to the area, I quickly set out to determine which of Sysco's product areas needed increased movement and recognition. After researching computer printouts and making personal calls on health-care accounts, I made a list of key products that needed direction and input from our customers. Initially, the list contained twelve product lines consisting of food and nonfood items.

I requested a meeting with the director of the marketing department to discuss my plan. This served two purposes: (1) to get any suggestions that he might have, and (2) to make him aware of what I was about to do and to include him in the process of developing the concept. (Note: It is always wise to keep your superiors informed and involved in new projects. If you're as fortunate as I have been, your superior will allow you freedom to develop your own strategies and handle your own programs. Everyone shares the success. There is clear understanding of what "we" all want as an outcome of the focus luncheons.)

STEP-BY-STEP HOW-TO

The organization of the program, the style of the event, the setting, the types of questions, the cost, and the wrap-up can be summarized into a five-step process.

Step 1: Make List of Participants

From many sources, as well as my own experience, I have found that ten to twelve participants will provide the type of interaction that is necessary to get the results we need. I try to keep my client attendees to six and include among the other four to six someone from the marketing and sales department of the company, perhaps a representative from the corporate office, at least one or two people from the manufacturing company, and myself. A total of twelve participants, and no more, come to this event.

I qualify each and every person on my list of clients by asking the following questions:

1. Does the person need the product(s) that I want to present?

2. Is the person working in an area in which this product would be useful?

3. Is the person a key decision maker about this product?

4. Does the person have knowledge of what customers want?

5. Is the person willing to come and share information in a group setting?

These questions are important to getting the proper mix of people at the focus luncheon. The correct answer for each question is yes.

Step 2: Issue Invitation

It is a good idea to call and talk personally with the people you want to attend. This establishes a personal connection with you and gives you the opportunity to discuss the concept of the focus luncheon. After the conversation and verbal commitment, mail a formal confirmation letter or note. Include the starting and ending time, date, address (including a map if the location is unfamiliar to participants), name of the room in the hotel or building, and telephone number of the meeting location. Ask for at least a week's notice if the attendee has to cancel, and give the name of an assistant or secretary who can take messages for you.

Step 3: Plan Product Presentation

Either you or someone from the manufacturing company should present the product at the luncheon. My focus luncheons all had a manufacturer's representative do the presentation. I recommend meeting with this person previous to the luncheon to review your objectives. If a manufacturer's representative will be making the presentation at your focus luncheon, ask him or her to observe the following guidelines:

1. Because this is not a sales presentation, don't discuss direct pricing. (Sometimes salespeople have difficulty in understanding this concept since sales is the reason for their existence.)

2. Present concise product information *after* asking the group questions about the product line. Participants should learn in a nutshell what the basic purpose of the product is.

3. Discuss the product as it is used in the participants' work setting.

Following are sample questions we asked during our focus luncheons:

1. Does the product meet the needs of the customer?

2. Is the labeling appropriate?

3. Are directions clear?

4. Is the box size appropriate for the usage?

5. What are future applications for the product?

Finally, ask the group to use their personal experience to suggest changes in the product. This is just a sample of questions to address. It is helpful to have your agenda and questions on a flip chart or other visual aid so that you can, at a quick glance, continue to keep your session on track.

Step 4: Plan Social Aspects

We've been talking about a focus luncheon, but not once have we talked about *the lunch*. It should be nice. Personally, I feel that we in the food-service and health-care businesses are always taking care of others, and now it is time to sit back, converse, enjoy a lovely luncheon, and learn.

We meet at 11:30 A.M., and serve the luncheon at 11:45 A.M. or 12:00 P.M. It is a sit-down lunch, served with style on an oval table that will seat twelve. We place flowers, notepads, and pencils on the table. We don't allow smoking, which seems appropriate since most of the discussions revolves around health and health-directed products. Each participant gets a token gift provided by the manufacturer who presents the product. This is not an expensive gift, something less than $25.00, such as a golf shirt, a calculator, a small thermos to keep foods hot or cold, or a basket of samples from the company that represents the featured product.

The luncheon serves another purpose besides providing nourishment. It allows group members to get to know each other before we really start to talk about the product(s). It is very important to have a seating schedule with preprinted place cards for the attendees. The planned seating allows people to make new acquaintances, and it ensures that customers visit with someone other than their peers.

Step 5: Close of Focus Luncheon

The time frame is from 11:30 A.M. to 2:30 P.M., the schedule is key, and ending on time is important. There is always focus luncheon follow-up: notes and leads that are taken at the focus luncheon need to handled promptly.

THE RESULTS

After the focus luncheon, our results show improved relationships between the attendees and the manufacturer, the product(s), and the company I represent. We find answers to product-related questions and the participants leave with the opinion that the sponsors of the event really care and respect their opinion. We do. We make changes and take new directions based on their comments. Focus luncheons have become so popular with both our customers and the manufacturers that I have had no trouble finding sponsors for the monthly event.

NOTE OF ADVICE

Choosing the people for the focus luncheon is very important. Spend time to select individuals who will provide you with honest, usable information and are willing to take three hours out of their busy schedule to help you. Be certain to thank each attendee personally. Follow through on any promises to make follow-up visits after the focus luncheon.

How to Self-Publish and Market Your Book

Chapter 33

Linda Hachfeld, MPH, RD, CEO, Appletree Press,
Mankato, Minnesota

You've written a book (actually a manuscript), and you're not sure where to go from here. You could send the manuscript to a publisher, but you've enjoyed writing it and have title ideas. You are excited about how the book could be designed and have a good idea of where it could be sold and who will buy it. Currently, you are wondering, "Why not do it myself?" You may be on the threshold of becoming a self-publisher, but there are many considerations before you make that decision.

Self-publishing has been around for a long time. Although a new, and perhaps untried, track for registered dietitians, self-publishing is a well-worn path traveled by such notable authors as Walt Whitman, Beatrix Potter, and Samuel Clemens (Mark Twain). That's right, these famous individuals put such titles as *Leaves of Grass, The Tale of Peter Rabbit,* and *Huckleberry Finn* into print themselves. More recently, Ken Blanchard's *One-Minute Manager* and Earthworks Group/Earthworks Press's *50 Simple Things You Can Do to Save the Earth* are self-published books that appeared on best-seller lists.

It is clear that a number of authors have published their own work, often with great financial success. Indeed, many went on to have their work, once in print, picked up by major publishing houses, and while these success stories are inspiring, self-publishing is not for everyone, nor should every manuscript be published. In fact, less than 10 percent of the manuscripts written each year are ever published.

This chapter will explain why you might consider self-publishing and describe some of the marketing challenges, risks, and rewards. First, let's look at a few facts about the general world of publishing, a sort-of "Did You Know":

- More than *47,000 books* (original and reprint) are published each year.
- According to R.R. Bowker, the book-publishing industry in the United States consists of nearly *32,000 firms,* with some *5,000 new publishers* starting each year.
- Sales amount to nearly *$9 billion* a year for the over *860,000 active titles* listed in *Books in Print.*
- Altogether, more than *60,000 people* are employed in book publishing in the United States.
- More than *100 new book titles* are published each day.
- The average life expectancy of a nonfiction book is about *43 months.*
- Books go out-of-print at a rate of roughly *3,000 a year.*
- It is estimated that some *350,000 book-length manuscripts* are written each year, but only *32,000 go into print.*
- Out of every *10* new books published, *3* will sell well, *4* will break even, and *3* will be losers.

ARE YOUR EXPECTATIONS REASONABLE?

A book publisher will pay to have your manuscript reviewed, edited, typeset, printed, bound, distributed, and marketed. The publisher essentially takes the financial risk that your book will do well in the marketplace. You, of course, have a lot of time, effort, and reputation at stake in any book published under your name. Why not hire a literary agent, if one will take your book, and negotiate the best advance and contract you can, then go on with your life and wait for the royalties to come in?

Why self-publish? For a great many people, the primary reason for self-publication is control. If you sell your manuscript to a publisher, matters are pretty much out of your hands. Someone else takes over making the decisions about your work. The title, color, size, and finished content are determined by someone else (although you have the chance to proof pages). More importantly, the amount of money and time dedicated to promoting your work is also determined by someone else. Let's face it, you may not like the idea that other people will make decisions about the original work you created. But are you willing to financially support the risk involved, and are you qualified to make all the decisions?

Before venturing into self-publication, you must consider your expectations. What do you want to achieve from the publication of your book? If you self-publish, be prepared to devote a great deal of time to the promotion and marketing of your work. Do you have the time to write press releases; research and contact magazines, newspapers, radio and television shows; and make follow-up phone calls? Do you want to fulfill orders (that means boxing, labeling, sending, and invoicing) to customers? Are you resourceful in understanding your market and where to find them? Do you want to sell to the trade (bookstores, distributors, and wholesalers), and can you accept industry price standards, meaning that discounts from the retail cover price will range from 40 to 60 percent?

Another reason many consider self-publication is the expectation of making more money. Typically, for a paperback, an author will receive a royalty of 6 to 8 percent of the net receipts for the first 10,000 to 30,000 copies and 8 to 10 percent of the net receipts thereafter. The standard hardcover royalty is about 10 percent. But remember the earlier figures – seven out of ten books break even or lose money, whether self-published or published by someone else. If your paperback book is published at a retail price of $12.95, your expected royalties can be figured as follows:

5,000 copies @ 6% royalty at full retail price	$3,885
5,000 copies @ 6% royalty with a 50% discount to distributor	$1,943
5,000 copies @ 6% royalty with a 42% discount to retailer	$2,253
Projected royalty income total on 15,000 copies	$8,081

You need to decide if this is acceptable; if not, you may want to consider self-publishing. You may also discover that an established publisher is willing to pay a higher percentage in royalties or willing to give you, the author, more latitude in making decisions about the finished book. In this case, you will want to rework the figures before making a decision to commit to a publisher or to self-publish.

WHAT IS SELF-PUBLISHING?

Becoming a publisher of your own written work means taking ultimate responsibility for the whole process of preparing, producing, selling, physically distributing, and collecting money for your work, as well as for all the business functions that inevitably relate to the funding of your business. The decision to publish your own work is a decision to undertake everything any other publisher might do in behalf of your work.

You are embarking on an entrepreneurial venture, which means you are entering a new industry and will need to run it as a business. If you are the entire staff of your new company, you will find that you will perform many jobs, some of which you will welcome and enjoy, others of which may be tedious and objectionable, yet necessary to your success. Here is a list of how you will spend your time as a self-publisher or independent publisher.

- *Writer/acquiring editor:* Write the books to be published and, perhaps, acquire other writers' books for publication.

- *Managing editor:* Oversee preparation of manuscript: copyedit; select typeface and illustrations; prepare specification sheets for obtaining bids from printers; hire typesetters, keyliners, artists, book designers; check proofs at each phase of production; determine print run for your book and where you will store your inventory.

- *Financial/business manager:* Obtain the funds to finance the publishing operation, prepare budgets with projected income and expenses, keep financial records, establish accounts, deal with vendors, track and monitor all expenses and revenues; in short, establish the management information system that will enable you to take the financial pulse of your company. You will need this information to determine whether your company is self-sustaining, losing money, or making money.

- *Fulfillment manager:* Make sure books are delivered where they need to go; determine how you will ship your books; establish freight company accounts, keep records of all sales and shipments; pack books for shipping; prepare invoices, shipping labels, and billings; establish a system in which all the "little details" are accounted for, from having the right size box and the right amount of packing material to completing an order on a timely basis.

- *Marketing/promotion/sales director:* Develop a market for your book, make decisions about where to sell your book, set price, and plan how you will make sales happen; write press releases to garner publicity; write ad copy for different markets; meet with book-industry folks, such as sales representatives, bookstore managers, and distributors; and spend a great deal of time on the telephone making the above-listed contacts and promoting your book to news, food, and health editors of magazines, radio programs, and television shows.

MARKETING A SELF-PUBLISHED BOOK

Marketing should be taken into account from the very inception of your book idea. Consumers and their needs should influence the content, style, wording, cover, price, distribution, and promotion of your book.

Before the book is printed, you should call R. R. Bowker (800-521-8110) to order an ISBN (International Standardized Book Number) to be printed on the back cover of your book. The fee is $100 for a 15- to 21-day turnaround and $151.50 for a 72-hour response. An ISBN makes it easier for bookstores to order your book and ensures inclusion in *Books in Print*, a reference available at all libraries and bookstores.

If your book is for the public, to gain exposure, you will have to send out book samples with press releases, pitch interview ideas to the media, and attend industry and public book fairs. There are at least five distribution channels you can use:

1. Wholesalers warehouse the book and fill orders from bookstores, but do no promotion. You pay them 50 to 55 percent of the retail price for their services, and they sell to stores at a 40 to 43 percent discount, which leaves them 10 to 15 percent for warehousing your book.

2. Distributors will market your book to retail stores through their catalogues and sales staff. They work on consignment – that is, they don't buy the books. They usually sell them for 42 percent off the retail price and split the remaining 58 percent 30/70, with you getting the 70 percent to cover printing, paper, and binding (PPB) and your profit. On a book that retails for $10, that would mean $4.06 to you.

3. A retail bookstore will ask for a 40 to 43 percent discount. College bookstores will ask for 30 percent discount on orders of 1 to 15 copies and 40 percent on larger orders, but it's all negotiable. Many stores may ask for the right to return unsold copies, but the returns are often in poor shape because price tags or careless handling ruin the covers.

4. A toll-free 800 phone number service can take orders for your book and sell it through mail order.

5. ADA's Product Marketplace, a booth at the Annual Meeting, and privately owned book catalogues can be useful in marketing your book to other health professionals for their libraries and patients.

In addition, books for the professional market can be promoted and sold through ads in the *Journal of the American Dietetic Association*, and in state and DPG newsletters. Order forms can be sent to target groups by direct mail and distributed at speeches and meetings. Booth space can be rented at conventions and seminars. And several dietitians offer group mailings and catalogues that can promote your book.

RISKS AND REWARDS

The list of self-publishing activities may look overwhelming, but no one does everything at once. What's important to realize is the scope and range of activities in which you will become engaged. Now let's move on to the risks and rewards of self-publishing.

The risks of self-publishing can be captured in two words: *time* and *money*. As you can tell from the list of activities a self-publisher performs, the job is enormously time-consuming. Only you can answer the question, "Do I really have the time to devote to the promotion of my book?"

Another valid question to ask yourself is, "Can I, or do I want to, wear all the hats of a self-publisher?" If writing is your love and you truly want to do more of it, will you have enough time to write *and* run a business? This brings to mind a quotation from James Healey that captures the essence of running your own business: "An entrepreneur spends sixteen hours a day to avoid having to work for someone else for eight hours."

Perhaps the book will do so well that you will have the means to hire support staff or pay someone else for the services you are willing to give up. It can happen, as it did for me in starting and operating Appletree Press, Inc. Now approaching my fifth anniversary in the publishing industry, I added full-time staff after eighteen months of operation and now can hire necessary talent by the project.

This brings us to the other risky part of becoming a self-publisher – money. You will need money to produce and launch your book. In this industry, you will spend a great deal of money up front in the hope of earning it back through sales of a finished product. It is risky, and it is a key factor that prevents many from self-publishing.

THE REWARDS OF SELF-PUBLISHING

If you were to ask a number of self-publishers if they would do it again and what they gain from self-publishing, you would get responses similar to the following:

"Absolutely!"

"It is an unending learning experience. It's so exhilarating to make decisions that will make or break your business. What a great feeling to know you are important to the existence of a business!"

"I enjoyed it at the time, but I don't ever want to spend that much effort again on so many chores I don't enjoy. I'll let a publisher do it next time."

"The recognition. People see me as an expert, and it has opened doors for speaking engagements and even writing another book."

It's obvious that on a personal level, realizing your book in print is a reward in and of itself. Books are irresistible to many people, and the author is one of the first to marvel at how the blank page has been transformed into something that has lasting presence.

The book you've produced is also of value to other people, and they are willing to spend money to get it. The financial rewards may be a means of building your own company, realizing a dream, or launching you into something more lucrative. It could be your route to success, as it was for Thomas Peters. His book, *In Search of Excellence*, sold a decently successful 15,000 copies when it was self-published, and when it was picked up by Harper & Row, it sold over a million copies in hardcover!

In conclusion, I would like to share the following references, which I use in my day-to-day operations. I referred to them in writing this chapter, and I heartily recommend them as balanced views of what you need to consider in self-publishing. May your book be a best seller!

Bibliography

Bell P. *The Pre-Publishing Handbook*. Eden Prairie, MN: Cat's-Paw Press; 1992.

Brownstone D, Franck I. *The Self-Publishing Handbook*. New York, NY: New American Library; 1985.

Poynter D. *The Self-Publishing Manual.* 5th ed. Santa Barbara, CA: Para Publishing; 1989.

Other Important Industry References

Books in Print by R. R. Bowker. Subject Guide lists 860,000 active titles by subject headings. The absolutely essential starting place when evaluating the uniqueness of a prospective new title. Check your library.

Literary Market Place (LMP) by R. R. Bowker. The who's who in American publishing today. It includes 15,000 major listings and 30,000 contact names; provides address sections for reviewers, subsidiary rights buyers, wholesalers, printers, fulfillment houses, artists, and publishing houses; and identifies subject interests of over 2,500 publishers. Check your library.

Case Study: **HOW MY CATALOGUE BUSINESS BEGAN**

Pat Stein, MS, RD, Owner, Nutrition Counseling/ Educational Services Catalogue, Olathe, Kansas

I n 1980, I left my position as an outpatient clinic dietitian and Assistant Professor at the University of Kansas Medical Center to establish a private practice, one of the first in the Kansas City area. It quickly became apparent that my competition was national weight-loss companies and that they provided their clients with slick, professionally printed instructional materials. I was using material that was photocopied from a typed master. In a survey, I found that the hospitals in town were using similar quality materials, so I decided to write and publish a professionally typeset book and throw away the typed masters.

To obtain a reasonable cost per book, it was necessary to print larger quantities than I was accustomed to making when I used photocopies. The first printing of The "Can Have" Diet was 1,000 copies. To market what was, for me, this astronomical number of books, I visited most of the chief clinical dietitians in the area, trying to convince them that their clients needed my book. Sales were primarily local for the next few years. Then in 1987, I decided that the book deserved a wider market and printed 5,000 copies. I approached two people who were in the business of marketing client education materials to a national audience and was turned down by both!

With 5,000 books to sell and only my own practice and a few local hospitals to use them, it was clear I needed to start a direct marketing campaign. I developed an attractive self-mailing flier, which included another book I had co-written, *Anorexia Nervosa: Finding the Lifeline*. Initially, we mailed only to the dietitians in my state of Kansas and in neighboring Missouri, about 2,000 people. The sales were good enough to warrant more attempts, but it became clear that even with a good response, the two rather inexpensive books could not cover my costs and generate a good profit. My husband, Ira, suggested that the next mailing piece include the titles of the books I kept on hand for clients to purchase — a grand total of seventeen items.

For this mailing, we branched out to more surrounding states and added the Consulting Nutritionists and Sports, Cardiovascular and Wellness Nutritionists dietetic practice groups to the mailing list — about 10,000 people in all. Again, sales looked promising, but we were still performing a public service.

Then Ira and I decided to go for broke and mailed a twelve-page, four-color catalogue on glossy paper to 50,000 people. We netted $100.00 profit for the first six months of that year.

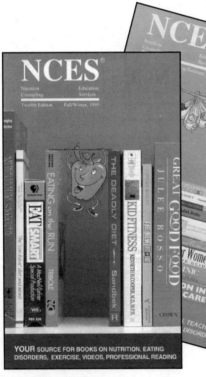

Sample Catalogue Covers

Now, five years later, we are mailing a 32-page, four-color catalogue on less-expensive glossy paper to 255,000 people twice a year. The catalogue contains over 300 books and other items related to nutrition, exercise, eating disorders, and general health. These range from books and videos suitable for laypersons, to slide shows and other kinds of educational programs, professional textbooks, and home study courses for the health professional. We now print 15,000 to 20,000 copies of *The "Can Have" Diet and More!* each time it is revised.

The catalogue business is not for the faint of heart. We continued performing a public service for most of the next five years and only realized some return on our money and labor during the last two years. About two years ago, we built and moved into our own office-warehouse building. Our staff has expanded from one part-time book packer, my husband, and me to include another registered dietitian and two more full-time persons.

Our catalogue provides a marketing vehicle for many dietitians who have developed books or other teaching tools. With the cost of producing and mailing each catalogue at about $100,000, we have to believe there will be a market for a particular item before we will consider listing it in the catalogue. People who have items or books they wish to have considered for listing in the catalogue send us copies. If we believe an item has accurate, interesting information that others will buy, we will negotiate a discounted purchase price with the individual or company. As I found out, self-published books can be difficult to market, even when they are printed in a thoroughly professional manner, but our catalogue business helps self-publishers and potential buyers find each other.

Chapter 34

How to Write a Proposal

Linda McDonald, MS, RD, LD, Nutrition Consultant, Houston, Texas

The purpose of a proposal is to sell yourself to a prospective client. A proposal is a marketing tool, and it had better be a good one. There is just one winner in a proposal competition – the rest are losers.

WHY WRITE A PROPOSAL?

In business you write a proposal for many reasons. For example:

- There is a need or problem that can't be fulfilled or answered by the present staff of the company.

- Clients may request proposals to compare consultants, to verify that a consultant understands the problem, or because they are required to advertise for consultants through RFPs (Request for Proposals). RFPs are often required by government agencies and public companies.

- You may suggest a written proposal to document the specifics of a verbal agreement, to explain an idea or unique service that would benefit a particular company, or to agree on specifics as the basis for a contract.

- You may use a proposal to sell yourself – to detail how your services are superior to those of your competitors.

- You may write a proposal to provide private counseling for a physician's patients, weight-control classes for a corporate wellness program, consulting for a nursing home, public relations support for a food company, a book for a publisher, or computer nutrient analysis of menu items for a restaurant.

KINDS OF PROPOSALS

Sole-Source Proposals

A sole-source proposal is one for which there is no competition. The client has complete confidence in you and does not wish to consider anyone else, but requests a proposal to make sure you are in agreement on the specifics: expected outcomes, time frame, compensation, tasks, and so on. An example might be a proposal to a physician for providing private counseling to patients.

Unsolicited Proposal

An unsolicited proposal may result from your insight or knowledge of a client's needs, or as a follow-up to a sales lead or interview. For example, you may send a proposal letter to a restaurant that has nutritious items on their menu and propose providing computer nutrient analysis.

Long Versus Short Proposals

Proposals can take several forms, ranging from a formal RFP that is 100 pages long for a major project, like remodeling an institutional kitchen, to a simple letter that is one or two pages long. You can also make a verbal proposal and follow up with a letter. Herman Holtz suggests in *How to Succeed as an Independent Consultant* (1), that small projects, in the range of $2,000 to $15,000 dollars, usually require only simple, informal proposals, or a letter proposal. Above $15,000, a formal proposal of 25 to 50 pages is suggested. Proposals take valuable time and effort, so whether you respond at all and how much time you put into the project will depend on the benefits to your business, both financial and image-building, and your chances for winning. Winning will depend on preparing a successful proposal.

HOW TO PREPARE A SUCCESSFUL PROPOSAL

Do Your Homework

The secret of writing a winning proposal is to give the impression of being supportive without being overbearing. You want to show that you are knowledgeable, efficient, professional, and empathetic to the potential client's needs and position. Focus on what you can do for the client and not just on your credentials and experience.

Before you write a proposal, it is essential that you do your homework and assess some basic issues. These include knowing your client, the problem, and the solution. Next, select the type of proposal that is appropriate, draft a tentative outline, develop a plan of action, and do the necessary research. Questions to ask include:

- Exactly what is the need or problem?
- Has the assignment previously been attempted?
- Who will you be reporting to?
- Who will be making the decision on the proposal?
- Who needs to be interviewed?
- What kind of personality does the company have?
- Have you been involved in similar situations in the past?
- Who are your competitors? What are their strengths and weaknesses?
- Is there a planned budget?
- Will you be expected to do this work, or can it be done by staff or a subcontractor?

Many sources are available for collecting information for your proposal. Interview senior management and employees of the company; ask for an annual report, company brochures, and sales literature; talk to other suppliers, consultants, and vendors; and visit your local library and newspaper.

In *How to Succeed as an Independent Consultant* (1), Herman Holtz states that a proposal must have great impact if it is to do its job well. To provide that necessary impact, he contends that the following qualities must be apparent to the client:

- *Competence.* The client must sense your power as a consultant who brings complete technical and professional competence to the job.
- *Dependable.* The client must feel that you are completely reliable and will never fail to carry the job through to a successful conclusion.

- *Accurate.* The proposal must convey the sense that you are careful to be absolutely precise and accurate in every action and in every step you take.

Following are the keys to accomplishing this effect: (1, 2, 3)

- *Details.* A presentation that cites specific facts and details, particularly quantified data, is much more likely to impress a reader and be credible. Anyone can generalize.

- *Interesting statistics.* Study your facts to see what impressive numbers you can develop (such as total number of contracts you have fulfilled or total dollar amount of contracts resulting from similar proposals). If your numbers are startling enough, see if you can work them into the introduction.

- *Clear language.* Be direct; leave no doubt about your meaning.

- *Quiet confidence.* Hype sounds defensive, as though you are trying to compensate for weakness. Avoid adjectives and superlatives that convey this weakness; instead use a quiet, confident tone that conveys strength (1).

- *In Control.* Clients want a consultant who seems to know exactly what to do. They want you to relieve them of worry and tedious, time-consuming involvement. Be sure to reflect confidence in what you propose to do. However, make it clear that you know the client is still in control.

- *Thoroughness.* Carelessness and lack of attention to detail can lose you the contract.

You don't have to tell the client how you are going to accomplish your job – that's your competitive edge. Ron Tepper (2) states that one of the most difficult decisions is how creative to get in a presentation without fearing that someone will steal your ideas. He continues by saying that a consultant should present unique, curiosity-stirring ideas that the client knows will meet the company's objectives, but that implementation should not be detailed.

In *Writing Business Proposals and Reports* (3), Susan Brock suggests testing for the "I" perspective. She states that proposals will be more effective if you use *you* more than you use *I*. To test for the "I" perspective, compare the number of times you use the words: *me, us, I,* and *we* versus the words *you, your,* and *yours.* The more often you use the latter words, the more likely your writing will convey your concern for your reader's needs. Compare the following:

I can provide the best nutrition counseling by using *my* unique experience and skills.

Your patients will benefit from knowledgeable and unique nutrition counseling services in the convenience of *your* office.

Our calculator is the best buy and most complete on the market for calculating nutrient intakes and exchanges.

You will have more time to spend with *your* patients when you use our time-saving, user-friendly calculator.

Don't make the proposal an intimidating legal document. Make it reader-friendly. Don't ramble. Don't confuse readers who are not used to dietetic jargon or acronyms. Use colorful terms, and write in a practical, how-to manner so that everyone understands what you mean.

STRUCTURE OF A PROPOSAL

A proposal should contain the following elements: (2)

1. *Overview or summary.* Provide an overview in a cover letter, an abstract, or the first paragraph of a letter proposal. A cover letter should state the purpose of your proposal, offer to answer questions either by phone or in person, request the assignment, and express thanks for the opportunity to submit the proposal.

2. *Objectives.* Describe your understanding of the client's problems or needs.

3. *Solutions.* Describe your unique approach to solving the problem or serving the client's needs. What strategies will you use, and how will you implement the strategies and approach you are promising? Keep strategies general rather than specific so that you maintain your competitive edge.

4. *Information about you.* Explain why the client should select you. What are your experiences and qualifications? In a formal proposal, include résumés of the individuals you are proposing to staff the project. Don't put down the competition, just play up your strengths in areas where competitors are weak.

5. *Fees.* Tell what the client can expect to pay, including your fees and all expenses. There may already be a proposed budget for the project, but you must explain how you will allocate funds.

6. *Summary.* Present the key selling points of your proposal at the beginning. Then use this portion to summarize the important information so that managers can quickly get a good idea of what your approach will be.

7. *Appendix.* Include any other relevant or supporting materials that will enhance your proposal: time lines, references, sample literature, news articles, research papers, copy of the Ethics Code of ADA, and the like.

Robert Kelley (4) suggests that before the proposal is due, and while it is still in rough-draft form, you call your client to go over your work so far and ask for advice. This makes the client a working collaborator in the proposal. Incorporating some of the client's advice and suggestions into the formal proposal makes the client feel that you are truly trying to address his or her problems and want to collaborate to find solutions.

Ask to present your proposal in person. Remember that your proposal is a marketing tool, so structure its physical appearance and your presentation accordingly. Proposals need not be dry or boring. Your proposal will provide an initial impression of your professional work and of your ability to communicate. A well-written and well-presented proposal can give you the competitive edge.

References

1. Holtz H. *How to Succeed as an Independent Consultant.* 2nd ed. New York, NY: John Wiley & Sons, Inc.; 1988.

2. Tepper R. *Consultant's Proposal, Fee and Contract Problem-Solver.* New York, NY: John Wiley & Sons, Inc.; 1993.

3. Brock SL. *Writing Business Proposals and Reports.* Menlo Park, CA: Crisp Publications, Inc.; 1992.

4. Kelly RE. *Consulting, the Complete Guide to a Profitable Career.* New York, NY: Charles Scribner's Sons; 1986.

Linda McDonald, MS, RD, LD, Nutrition Consultant, Houston, Texas

Being familiar with Guiltless Gourmet products, low-fat versions of high-fat snacks, I felt I could work with this company. Before making a proposal, I needed to learn more about the company, so I called Dave Foreman, Guiltless Gourmet's Marketing Manager, and asked for an appointment. I explained that I had some marketing ideas and wanted to see if they might fit into Guiltless Gourmet's future plans.

I purposely went to the first meeting with Dave without formed ideas because I wanted to hear what he had to say. My ultimate goal was to sell the company on the benefits that I could offer as a dietitian. I thought that if I could sell them on a marketing project and build a relationship with them, I could eventually obtain a monthly retainer.

I had asked Dave to include some other employees from customer service and marketing in our meeting. As we talked, I asked the following questions:

- Where were they heading: health food, grocery stores, specialty and gourmet stores, or food service?

- What was the philosophy of the company?

- What marketing techniques and tools had been most beneficial?

- Were dietitians useful in marketing their products?

- Were other dietitians using their products in seminars?

- Did they have any consumer education pieces?

- Had they been asked any questions about their products on nutrition topics such as allergies, kidney dialysis, and low-fat diets?

At our meeting, Dave suggested that I write a letter explaining some of my ideas. I sent it along with a packet of information and some of the materials I had developed for other clients. In the letter, which is reproduced at the end of this case study, I requested another meeting.

The second meeting was with Doug Foreman, President of Guiltless Gourmet, and the representative of their marketing firm. Here I made a big mistake. I thought this would be another fact-finding meeting, so I wasn't as prepared as I should have been. Doug thought I was going to make a formal proposal with estimated costs and specific product ideas.

I described how I saw myself working with their products and suggested the marketing tools outlined in my letter of May 26th. We discussed how I would work with their present staff. At that meeting, the customer service director became my ally because he recognized the need for the materials that I was proposing.

Finally, I developed proposals for five different projects. (Remember, I was hoping to start with one project.) The projects I suggested were

---

LINDA McDONALD, MS, RD, LD
11102 Lakeside Forest Lane
Houston, TX 77042-1032
Telephone 713/978-6960
Facsimile 713/978-7044

May 26, 1992

David Foreman
Guiltless Gourmet
123 Chip Drive
Austin, Texas 77000

Dear Dave:

Thank you for the opportunity to visit, meet your staff, and observe the production of Guiltless Gourmet chips. Your products are right on target for the growth in health-conscious eating, and it is obvious that Guiltless Gourmet is successful and growing. Not only are your products tasty, but they are full of good complex carbohydrates and low in fat, cholesterol, and sodium.

As discussed, your emphasis on the health-conscious consumer and the use of the health professional as a tool for marketing your products fits some ideas I have had for promoting Guiltless Gourmet. Your products have proved useful when I have presented topics such as Low Fat Snacking, Holiday Survival Skills, and Heart Healthy Nibbles.

A registered and licensed dietitian can add authority and credibility to your products in our health-focused community. You can benefit from the following services:
1. Review promotional materials for accuracy of information and appropriate health-related language. This will be increasingly important as the new FDA labeling guidelines go into effect.
2. Act as a resource for your staff on health-related questions.
3. Represent Guiltless Gourmet at conventions and meetings and provide a network of qualified health professionals for local market areas.
4. Develop health-related promotional materials and programs, such as
   Guiltless Snacking Brochure – A marketing piece that includes snacking tips, comparison charts of Guiltless Gourmet products with regular products, recipes, and nutrient information for products.
   Recipes – Encourage the use of Guiltless Gourmet products with unique and tasty recipes for dishes such as taco pie, layered dips, casseroles, soups, Mexican favorites, and sauces.
   Guiltless Snacking Seminar – A Speaker's Kit for health professionals that can use Guiltless Gourmet products in seminars and classes. Kit will include lesson plan, handouts, tips for conducting tastings, and marketing tips.

Dave, you know that I have been excited about your products since the start of Guiltless Gourmet. I would welcome the opportunity to work with you as a consultant and suggest that we start with one project on a trial basis. Just let me know which project you are interested in and I will prepare a proposal.

Enclosed are sample materials developed for Tenneco Corporation's Fitness program. You are already familiar with my participation in the Houston Gourmet books. The enclosed resume will give you more information on my education and business experience.

Please call if you have any questions or need additional information. I look forward to working with Guiltless Gourmet and will call next week to discuss this with you further.

Sincerely,

Linda McDonald

Linda McDonald

LINDA McDONALD, MS, RD, LD
11102 Lakeside Forest Lane
Houston, TX 77042-1032
Telephone 713/978-6960
Facsimile 713/978-7044

PROPOSAL

Date: June 1, 1992

To: Dave Foreman
Director of Marketing
Guiltless Gourmet

From: Linda McDonald, MS, RD, LD

Proposal: Develop Recipes for Guiltless Gourmet Products

Objective: Encourage use of Guiltless Gourmet Products by providing recipes for point-of-purchase promotions, educational programs, packaging, and marketing literature.

Format: 3"x5" cards or pads. Graphic representation to be determined by marketing firm.

Contents: Eight recipes, nutrient analysis, and dietary exchanges.

Suggested
Recipes: Party/Snack Layered Dip
                      Nachos
                      Mexican Potato Skins
         Soups   Tortilla Soup
                      Bean Soup
                      Potato Cheese Soup
         Entrees   Taco Pie
                      Chicken Casserole
                      Pasta Sauce
                      Omelette
         Salads   Taco Salad
                      Dressings

Procedure: 1. Submit recipe ideas for approval
           2. Develop recipes
           3. Test recipes
           4. Computer-analyze recipes
           5. Work with marketing firm on graphic presentation.

Time: One month

Cost: $1000 plus out-of-pocket expenses

(enlarged in Appendix)

1. A snack brochure
2. Eight recipes highlighting Guiltless Gourmet products
3. A speaker's kit
4. My representing Guiltless Gourmet at the ADA Annual Meeting and Exhibition
5. A monthly retainer to provide marketing and technical assistance to their staff

All five were accepted. However, the fifth was contingent on successful completion of the first four projects. I am currently under contract with Guiltless Gourmet on a monthly retainer.

Chapter 35

How to Market Yourself as a Speaker

Dick Huiras, Speaker, Author, President, HuMark Enterprises, Houston, Texas

Speaking as a part-time or full-time career is very rewarding, not only because of the feedback from your audience, but also because it increases your self-esteem and leads to financial gain. The following suggestions are given for individuals who enjoy the art of speaking, have some talent in speaking, and want to reach their target markets more effectively.

MARKETING YOURSELF

As a professional speaker, you must always be looking for opportunities to market yourself. Writing books or articles for lay and professional publications helps you become known and improves your name recognition with audiences. Appearing in the media serves a similar function, plus it sometimes offers a little notoriety. Networking with professional groups and becoming an active member of organizations such as The American Dietetic Association, the American Society of Association Executives, or the National Association of Meeting Planners gets your name in front of people who are influential in selecting speakers.

If you want to speak to dietetics-related groups, send a letter with your speech topics to local, regional, or state presidents or program planners, or to home economics, wellness, food-service, or clinical organization officers. Include copies of or quotes from positive letters from other satisfied program planners or attendees.

You may also send out a black-and-white glossy 5″ X 7″ photo along with your updated résumé or professional bio. Always have your name on your handouts and offer business cards or brochures to listeners, usually at the end of your presentation. Offer your book or other product as a door prize, if it's appropriate. After your presentation, send a gracious letter to your hosts and keep in contact with holiday greetings.

When you first start your speaking career, you should expect to do a certain amount of speaking (usually free) to local clubs and organizations. Few of these meetings will result in paid engagements, but they are great arenas for improving your presentation style, building your confidence, and finding out what your audience likes to hear. The old adage still holds true – you must always crawl before you walk, and you will practice walking long before you become a star or make a lot of money at speaking. If people like to hear you speak, they will look for opportunities to have you return. That's why it's so important to entertain as well as to inform your audience.

USING REFERRAL AGENTS

As a speaker, your can spend your time and effort doing one of two things: pursuing speaking engagements, or making money at speaking. It is a full-time job to make connections with groups and meeting planners. Negotiations on speaking fees and expenses can take hours or even days. For these reasons, you may consider seeking someone to represent you to organizations and conventions: Speakers bureaus and agents serve that purpose. But before you run out to find professional representation, realize that bureaus and agents expect you to already be a very good speaker with experience and recognized expertise before they will represent you. Some may want you to be a published author of a recent well-known book or have some other claim to fame.

Speakers Bureaus

Before listing with a speakers bureau, spend time researching several different ones. Also, most bureaus will want to interview you or hear you in action before they will agree to represent you. Many bureaus will handle all topics and all levels of speakers, while others are very selective of topics and speakers' abilities. Check with the local chapter of the meeting planners' association in your area to assess the confidence level and trust they have with the bureaus you are considering. It is your reputation on the line.

Speakers bureaus usually promote you only with the materials you give to them and will not assist you in developing more current or exciting promotional materials. Their fees for representing you will range from 25 to 30 percent of your speaking fees.

It is the policy of most speakers bureaus to find the best speaker for an engagement rather than to concentrate solely on promoting you as a speaker, which is understandable. However, this means you may have to sell yourself and your topics to bureau personnel to ensure that they appreciate what you can do. You can help make their job easier if you have clever titles for your presentations and include several distinctive topics that make you stand out from the crowd.

Agents

A professional agent will focus on selling you as a speaker at major business and other functions (depending on your topics), while allowing you to do what you do best – speak. However, you must have a certain level of ability and flair as a speaker to attract an agent.

A reputable agent will charge either a set retainer fee to represent you or a percentage of your speaking fees. The agent will represent you and negotiate the highest possible speaking fee with a client, collect from the client, and then pay you, usually within the first week following the engagement.

In most situations, an agent will assist you in designing any brochures or marketing materials you will use for your promotion. He or she will guide you in improving your handouts or slides and creating a mailing list.

Based on past experience, the agent will evaluate you as a package. He or she will look at your strengths in knowledge, presentation, dress, makeup, and many other areas that make you stand out as a great speaker. If you need to build on any of these strengths, the agent might give you names of appropriate specialists or tell you how to find them.

Negotiations on speaking fees and expenses can take hours or even days. Good agents have integrity, confidence, the trust of their clients, and a reputation in the industry for promoting quality talent.

Agents can often accomplish things that you yourself could not. For example, I was considering speaking at an annual meeting of a state organization. The organization was small and had a very limited budget for speakers. The fee they offered was much below my standard fee, which included airfare and, if necessary, one night's lodging. My agent sold them on my ability as a speaker, but told them that I would be very reluctant to accept the engagement. Because most organizations have extra money in separate accounts for different activities, they found the additional money I required in their lodging and general expense accounts.

A third party will often promote you better and more forcefully than you will promote yourself. If you hate to ask for money or aggressively promote yourself, but are a good speaker with a clever message, an agent may work for you. Look in your *Yellow Pages*, check your library, or call speakers' organizations to find names.

PROMOTION PIECES EVERY SPEAKER MUST HAVE

Brochures

You should have two types of brochures. The most important brochure is the *presentation brochure*. The more sophisticated and professional this brochure is, the better it paves the way to a higher speaking fee. First impressions make all the difference. This brochure should include:

1. A recent photograph of you taken by a professional photographer
2. A short biography
3. A complete listing of the topics you speak on and a short description of each topic
4. A list of groups, organizations, and companies who have hired you to give presentations
5. Testimonials from some of the people who have attended your presentations (Your credibility is enhanced when you quote people who have hired you, are well known locally or nationally, or are experts in the topics you present.)
6. Your name, address, and phone number

You should also have a *one-page brochure* that is suitable for using on a fax machine. It should contain information on the topics you present and notable information on you as the speaker. This brochure should be used only if a meeting planner requests that you fax information. (Many agents require this type of information sheet as a reminder of your availability as a speaker, not as a first introduction to a meeting planner.)

Video

If you plan to market yourself to large companies or national organizations, you need a VHS videotape to compete in today's market. This tape should be ten to fifteen minutes in length, with four or five segments from different presentations. When editing the tape, pick only the footage that shows you at your best, plus enthusiastic reactions from audiences. Be sure to eliminate audience members who may be sleeping, yawning, or leaving the room for *any* reason. The best audience representations are those in which only laughing or applause is heard.

DO'S AND DON'TS

Whether you are marketing yourself or using a bureau or agent, the do's and don'ts remain the same. These are the areas in which most speakers make their biggest mistakes and, consequently, experience failure in the world of speaking.

Do's

1. *Homework.* Get to know as much as possible about each group or organization you address. Some good information to know is why and how the organization was formed, its mission statement, its length of time in existence, any outstanding local or national credits, and who the major players are within the organization. Your interest in the organization will set up a positive impression and future recommendations.

2. *Site.* Once you have been hired, ask permission to view the room in which you will be speaking, if it is local, or request a description of the room layout. Identify how large the room is; the configuration of tables and chairs, such as U-shaped, open classroom, or theater, and whether there will be a head table; and if a microphone is required. Check where the projector, overhead, video player, or screen will be, if you need them. This will eliminate any problems or embarrassment on the day of the presentation.

3. *Attendance.* If the group is having a social hour or meeting before you speak, ask if you may attend. This is a great time to get to know the members and find out more about the organization. It will show that you have a real interest in them besides just speaking.

4. *Customization and Personalization.* When you know about a group, you can customize your information so that the audience will better relate to your presentation. Nothing is more boring than always hearing about someone else, and nothing is more interesting than hearing about yourself.

5. *Award dinners.* Make an appointment to meet with the organization to discuss the type of award, its reason, and the honoree. During the social hour, spend time with the honored guest to gain personal insight and additional information for use in your presentation.

6. *Themes.* If the organization is using a theme to promote their meeting, find out why they chose the theme and incorporate it into your presentation. For example, if the theme is the Old West, you might want to use some southwestern graphics on your overheads, or draw an analogy between your topic and the Old West.

7. *Purpose.* If there is a particular purpose for the meeting, such as to provide information, education, or entertainment, it is important to adjust your presentation accordingly. For instance, if the meeting is dealing with governmental regulations, it would not be in your best interest to use examples about basket weaving or cross-country skiing. The success of any meeting depends on the the ability of the meeting planner to keep a common theme throughout a program.

Don'ts

1. *Dress code.* This is not the time to make a fashion statement, unless, of course, it is an integral part of your presentation and is expected. In business meetings, you should present yourself as an expert and professional. Men should wear business suits with understated ties. Women should wear something that is in good taste and not distracting. Audiences want to hear your words of wisdom, not be dazzled by your wardrobe. Bright, loud, and flamboyant costumes and colors are out, unless required by your topic.

2. *Hygiene.* Look clean and meticulous. Be sure your hair is professionally cut and styled. Your clothing should be neatly pressed and fresh from the cleaners. Do not wear overbearing cologne or aftershave, which can be very offensive to your audience.

3. *Speaking.* Never speak totally off-the-cuff. Have your speech planned and rehearsed ahead of time so that it flows and never becomes confusing to the audience. Type your speech or outline in large, easy-to-see print. Speak loudly enough to project to the rear of the audience. Audiences do not want to strain to hear a speaker and risk missing important information. Do not talk too much about yourself, which can become very boring even if you have lived a full and exciting life. Never, never tell off-color or ethnic jokes. Also stay far away from sexist remarks or stories, or you will surely never be invited back or recommended to speak again. Joke telling is an art that should be used very carefully. Learn to use humor in your speeches; it is a favorite of everyone.

THE SELLING GAME

Most professional speakers make it a point to write and publish a book, and produce audiotapes and videos for retail sales. When you speak to a group for free, it is almost a foregone conclusion that you will be invited to sell your materials and give yourself a short commercial. However, be sure to clarify this and negotiate it up front.

When you speak for a fee, do not presume that the meeting planner will allow you to sell your materials. You are there to present your topic, not to make a profit on your book. When you contact the meeting planner to discuss the topic and the audience, give him or her a token copy of your book or tape, and offer to donate a copy as a door prize or to raise funds at a silent auction. The planner can then decide if it is appropriate for you to sell materials or even pass out order blanks. Many planners will allow you to set up a table in the back of the meeting room or an adjacent hall after the meeting to give audience members the opportunity to purchase a book or tape. Remember, they are doing this for the members, not as a favor to you.

If a meeting planner will not allow you to sell your book or tapes, you might give one away as a door prize. Have the audience members put their business cards in a bowl, and at the end of the speech have someone draw one card for the door prize. Keep all the cards, though. You can use them to develop a mailing list to promote future tapes, books, and speaking engagements.

Many speakers will, as their last statement, make themselves available for ten to fifteen minutes after their presentation. You will generally get people who have a genuine interest in your materials or wish to hire you for future engagements.

Now that you have the marketing tools, success can be yours in the world of public speaking.

Resource

Carol Posey, American Speakers Association, Houston, Texas. Phone interview, August 1993.

Chapter 36

How to Market Nutrition in Supermarkets

Nelda Mercer, MS, RD, Director of Preventive Nutrition, MedSport, Ann Arbor, Michigan

The main challenge no longer is to determine what eating patterns to recommend to the public (although, admittedly, there is more to be learned), but also how to inform and encourage an entire population to eat so as to improve its chance for a healthier life (1).

The time could not be better for dietetics professionals to take advantage of the heightened consumer awareness of the role of nutrition in health. According to a 1993 report by the Food Marketing Institute (2), shoppers continue to see substantial room for improvement in their diets. Two out of three shoppers think their diets could be healthier and are very concerned about the nutritional content of the foods they eat. In addition, this report noted that nutrition is second only to taste, and outweighs price and product safety, when consumers choose the food they buy. Consumer research further shows that concern about fat is at an all-time high. Cholesterol now appears to be taking a back seat to fat. Calorie, sodium, and sugar contents of foods rank next in line as key dietary concerns for today's consumer.

The average traffic count in a successful supermarket can be upwards of 10,000 to 12,000 customers per week. Survey data suggest that the customer visits the supermarket an average of 2.2 times per week (2). Since consumers make 80 percent of their food-purchasing decisions at the grocery store shelf (3), what better place than the supermarket to educate consumers in making healthy food choices that can positively affect the health and well-being of their families? In the 24 minutes it takes the average shopper to complete food selections (4), supermarkets can, and do, act as sources of nutrition information through advertisements and promotions, food labels, and product information at the point of purchase.

For more than a decade, supermarkets across the country have provided nutrition-information programs. The programs vary widely in scope, focus and origin. Some consist only of nutrition-information materials provided to customers at the point of purchase, such as brochures or leaflets. Others are more elaborate in scope, using shelf labels, videos, cooking demonstrations, supermarket tours, recipe cards, brochures, bag stuffers, employee buttons, in-store nutrition counseling, and other techniques (4, 5, 6, 7, 8). Advertising budgets for such programs also vary widely, covering everything from in-store posters and store announcements to radio, television, and newspaper ads.

KEY INFORMATION ABOUT THE SUPERMARKET INDUSTRY

The supermarket business is a highly competitive business. Retailers often work on a 1 to 2 percent profit. The way a supermarket owner makes a profit is through volume. In many instances, volume reflects customer loyalty. The key elements that make up customer loyalty stem from the customer's perception of the extent to which the store provides good service, quality, variety, and price; offers value-added services; and keeps the customer's best health interest in mind. Successful marketing strategies must take these key elements into account.

In addition, the goodwill a nutrition program can generate enhances the supermarket's positioning in the community. Such goodwill can go a long way in ensuring customer loyalty. A lifetime customer may be worth $100,000 to a retailer (9), which is why retailers make an effort to understand and anticipate the needs and desires of their customers.

Data from focus groups conducted for a Michigan supermarket revealed that the customers liked and appreciated the store's "aggressive" nutrition program, which they viewed as a value-added service. Customers felt that the store had their best interest in mind and that their health needs were important to the store owners. The nutrition program, which was sponsored by The University of Michigan MedSport, Preventive Cardiology Program, did much to enhance the store image as a supermarket with a conscience. Store owners have commented that providing these programs in their supermarkets gives them a competitive edge over larger chain stores in their service areas. As one store owner put it, "The program gives us one more means with which to compete other than price (10)."

A customer survey conducted at the same Michigan supermarket was designed to test customer awareness and utilization of the nutrition-education shelf-labeling program that had been in existence for the previous eighteen months. Results of the survey showed that 73 percent of the customers surveyed were aware of the program. A substantial percentage (42 percent) of respondents said that the program influenced the foods they purchased, and 40 percent who were aware of the program reported that it positively influenced where they shopped (11). Research findings such as these will help support your proposal. In addition, it will be to your advantage to know and point out to retailers the benefits their stores can gain from nutrition programs, including improvements in customer loyalty, customer satisfaction, corporate image, market performance, and effectiveness of advertising and promotion (12).

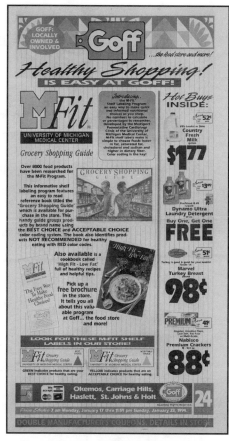

Grocery Store Ad with MedSport Tie-In.
Reprinted with permission of MedSport and Goff Stores.

PLANNING A PROGRAM THAT WORKS

Before starting to plan and develop a supermarket nutrition program, it is wise to review what previous programs have accomplished and what their administrators have learned. Others' experiences can be very valuable to you as you set out to determine what type of program is best suited to your particular demographic area and will meet the needs of the community. Good planning is the key to success. The Food Marketing Institute has published an excellent summary of supermarket nutrition programs that includes details regarding the focus, format, evaluation method, and research results for a variety of programs (13).

The following elements contribute to the overall effectiveness of a supermarket nutrition program (14):

- The program develops messages that are relevant to the consumers' interests and concerns.
- The program uses point-of-purchase shelf labels as cuing devices to direct consumers to healthful foods.

- The program provides practical nutrition information from credible sources.

- The program is highly visible and is distinguishable from commercial food advertising.

- The program generates awareness through mass media advertising and community ties.

- The program has been in existence for more than one year.

- Supermarket personnel work effectively with the program.

To elaborate on the last point, the importance of having trained, well-informed supermarket employees cannot be overstated. Training all employees, from management to store level, is essential. It is the responsibility of each employee, whether a shelf stocker, cashier, deli food server, meat or seafood counter attendant, produce manager, store manager, or store owner, to implement the nutrition program in the supermarket environment. Adequately informed personnel will ensure that the program will maintain visibility and exposure to the customer. If the program receives only sporadic exposure, or if employees lack sufficient knowledge to promote the program to customers, the program will be ineffective and lose customer acceptance. Although educational videos can be expensive to produce, they provide a simple method for training store personnel and eventually prove to be cost-effective. Training manuals can also be used effectively. An effective training manual includes the following materials (13):

1. A letter from management stating their commitment to the program

2. A letter from any health partner, restating the goals of the program

3. A brief description of the program

4. A brief description of how you will be tracking and evaluating the program, with sample monitoring forms

5. Timelines, dates, and responsibilities for implementation

6. Drawings or samples of program elements, and information on installing display elements and reordering materials

7. A list of commonly asked questions and appropriate answers to help store personnel respond to basic questions consumers might have

8. A list of community nutrition resources for more in-depth responses

9. A list of corporate, on-site, or other retail personnel whom store employees can contact for clarification

In addition, successful nutrition programs take advantage of every marketing opportunity that may present itself. Following consumer trends is an important factor to consider. For example, an interesting trend to note and follow is that currently one out of seven shoppers (15 percent) purchases take-out food from a supermarket. This practice is up from 10 percent in 1986 (2). A smart nutrition program will take advantage of this trend and market healthy take-out selections from the deli, self-service soup and salad bars, and in-store bakery. More than 40 percent of bakery operators reported placing greater merchandising emphasis on healthy bakery items last year (15). Programs such as chef training and certification, similar to those designed for restaurant programs (16), and adapted for the supermarket chef or food-production personnel, have been quite successful in Michigan super-markets. Retailers favorably view this program as another means of setting their store apart from the competition as a provider of a value-added service.

MARKETING YOUR SUPERMARKET NUTRITION PROGRAM

Once your nutrition program has been adequately planned and all the key elements have been developed, it is time to sell your program to an appropriate supermarket retailer. At this point, developing a marketing plan is essential. (Chapter 20 will help guide you through this process.) It is important to take the time to learn as much as you can about the particular supermarket or chain that you are targeting. In other words, you need to do your homework. When possible, start out by obtaining the company's annual report. Learn about the company's mission statement. In response to fierce competition from warehouse clubs and supercenters, successful supermarket retailers have analyzed their strengths and concentrated on their niches. This is where your proposed nutrition program will either fit in or be doomed. Doing your homework ahead of time will allow you to identify a supermarket retailer who will be receptive and whose goals are in sync with yours.

Success is also determined by presentation. It cannot be overstated that your business savvy and the first impression you make with the supermarket retailer will determine your effectiveness. Chapters in this book that deal with the how-to's of personal marketing, writing a personal biography or résumé, writing a proposal, setting prices, and negotiating an agreement will provide you with the basic skills to get you off to the right start.

After your program has been accepted by a supermarket retailer, it is time to move forward in identifying and implementing your marketing strategies. The following ten steps will help guide you through this process:

1. Work with the supermarket's marketing director, merchandising manager, or consumer affairs specialist to decide on marketing strategies.

2. Set a kickoff date for the program. You may need to coordinate kickoffs at several store locations.

3. Several weeks before the kickoff, inform the media (local newspapers, radio stations, and TV stations, including cable TV). Press releases are an effective way of informing the media. (See Chapter 23 for how to write a press release.)

4. Arrange a press conference with interested media on the day of the kickoff. This will bring good exposure for the program and provide free advertising. It is recommended that you, or the health organization you represent, take the lead in the press conference and that the retail partner take a supporting role. This will give the program credibility and decrease the likelihood that the program will be viewed as an attempt by the retailer to seek publicity (13).

5. Press kits should accompany all press releases and should be passed out at all press conferences. A press kit should include (13):

   • Background information on the program

   • A list of presenters and participants

   • Biographies of speakers

- A press release with quotes from key industry and health leaders
- Program materials, such as recipes, brochures, and newsletters

6. Send letters to area hospitals or health centers offering to speak to the nutrition staff about the program. This serves two purposes: first, it informs local dietitians of the program and encourages them to support it and recommend it to their patients; second, it promotes the supermarket as a provider of a value-added service.

7. Market your program to dietitians, nutritionists, and health professionals in the community by inviting them to a pre-event tour and tasting. This type of public relations not only will brief these professionals on your program but also will help to win their acceptance and support. This will further enhance the program's credibility.

8. Market your program in the store with point-of-service materials, such as shelf labels, shelf talkers, employee (associate) buttons, posters, bag stuffers, banners, triaramas, brochures, videos, nutrition information kiosks, newsletters, recipe cards, and weekly store ads.

9. Depending on the store's advertising budget, use other forms of advertising, such as radio and TV commercials, billboards, newspaper ads, and fliers to keep the program alive. Advertising must be continual because success depends on the store's ability to keep the program highly visible.

10. Create a service image in the community. Keeping your program visible in the community, school, and home can be accomplished through special in-store events. For example, offer supermarket tours targeting special groups, such as senior citizens, children, scouting groups, and service organizations. Sponsoring cooking classes taught through area hospitals or outpatient facilities will also result in positive public relations. Unpaid community-service advertising, direct mail, in-store or hospital newsletters, bulletins, and community forums are all excellent, cost-effective means of promoting your program.

Although the concept of providing nutrition programs in supermarkets is not new, the timing for these programs is still right. With the signing of the Nutrition Labeling and Education Act (NLEA) of 1990 and the new mandatory food-labeling laws that resulted (17), nutrition remains very much in the forefront of consumers' minds and stores' marketing plans. Well-designed supermarket nutrition programs can play an integral part in translating the NLEA and the national dietary guidelines into good food choices for consumers. The future success of supermarkets will depend on their ability to identify and take advantage of consumer trends that will improve their market share and allow them to compete with the giants of their industry. Fast thinking and wise programming are the answer, and a nutrition program can be part of the solution.

References

1. Improving America's diet and health, from *Recommendations to Action*. Food and Nutrition Board, Institute of Medicine, Committee on Dietary Guidelines Implementation; 1991.

2. Food Marketing Institute. *Trends in the United States, Consumer Attitudes and the Supermarket 1993*. Washington, DC: Food Marketing Institute; 1993.

3. Point of Purchase Advertising Institute Inc., 2 Executive Park, Fort Lee, NJ 07024.

4. Food Marketing Institute. *How Consumers Are Shopping the Supermarket*. Washington, DC: Food Marketing Institute; 1991.

5. Light L, Tenney J, Portnoy B, et al. Eat for health: a nutrition and cancer control supermarket intervention. *Public Health Rep.* September-October 1989; 104(5):443-450.

6. Ernst ND, Frommer P, Moskowitz J, et al. Nutrition education at the point of purchase: the foods for health project evaluated. *Prev Med.* 1986; 151:60-73.

7. Mullis RM, Hunt MK, Foster M, et al. The Shop Smart for Your Heart grocery program. *J Nutr Educ* 1987; 19(5):225-228.

8. Mercer NM. *M-Fit Supermarket Shelf Labeling Program*. University of Michigan MedSport, Preventive Cardiology Program, PO Box 363, Ann Arbor, MI 48106.

9. McNeal JU. *American Demographics*. June 1993.

10. Busch J, Owner/President, Busch's ValuLand, Ann Arbor, Michigan, *M-Fit Supermarket Shelf Labeling Program*.

11. Mercer NM, Rhodes KS, Bookstein LC, et al. Evaluation of consumer acceptance of a point of purchase nutrition education supermarket shelf labeling program. *J Am Diet Assoc.* 93(9):A61 (September 1993, suppl.).

12. Grim CJ. Researching consumers through consumer education materials and toll free numbers: a summary of recent research part III. *MOBIUS*. Summer 1988:5-8.

13. Food Marketing Institute. *Nutrition Information in the Supermarket: How to Plan, Implement and Track Programs That Work*. Washington, DC: Food Marketing Institute; 1993.

14. Light L, Portnoy B, Blair JE, et al. Nutrition education in supermarkets. *Family & Community Health*. May 1989; 12(1):43-52.

15. Bakery update 1993 – product trends. *Progressive Grocer*. March 1993; 72(3):102.

16. Mercer NM, Burt ER, Rhodes KS, et al. A chef certification program for healthy dining. *J Am Diet Assoc.* 90(9):A94 (September 1990 suppl.).

17. *Federal Register*. January 6, 1993; 58(3). Microfiche.

Chapter 37

How Students Can Assist in Marketing Your Business

Anne B. Kelly, RD, Director of Materials Development,
NutriSmart, Inc., Rochester, New York

Over the past several years, I have been a student volunteer, a student in a practicum program, and a supervisor of students as part of my job. After experiencing both sides of the student-employer equation, I am an advocate of using students – dietetics, diet technician, marketing, business, journalism, graphic design, and others – to assist in marketing a business.

Students can be excellent helpers, whether your practice is in nutrition education, consulting, food service, or clinical dietetics. They are eager, talented, young professionals who want meaningful and practical experience in business. Most students (and their professors) look for opportunities to put their new knowledge to work.

It is important when starting or expanding a new project or business to have sufficient personnel to carry out the tasks. Students can serve this purpose while helping you contain costs. Although not a substitute for full-time employees, hiring lower-cost student help or becoming a rotation site for interns can benefit both you and the student. Part-time or temporary employees can be expensive, and it is often difficult to find people with the right job skills.

To make the experience beneficial to both parties, not just your business or department, avoid hiring students just to do filing, copying, and errands. After completing a practicum with NutriSmart, Inc., Jennifer Tirone, a marketing student in Buffalo, New York, commented: "In class I learned all the elements of developing a marketing plan. As part of my class assignments I had worked with hypothetical situations. One of the most valuable experiences I received during my practicum was being part of the development of a real marketing plan. I was able to work through the project from stage one to the very end. It was exciting to see how planning really does make a difference in developing a marketing strategy that works!"

Many students are assets when it comes to creative thinking and brainstorming sessions. They do not know the ways that "things have always been done." Fresh ideas and new points of view generate other ways of carrying out tasks.

Students learn the latest information, so they help a company stay competitive. Also, by keeping in contact with colleges and universities in your area, you have additional access to the newest information and technology.

Working with student employees is a good public relations tool for your company or department. Sometimes it is possible to work on joint projects with area colleges and universities, or to receive media coverage for your efforts because you involve students in worthwhile projects.

The popularity of your business or department attracts the best candidates for potential future employment. If your company or department needs to expand, some of your student helpers may be candidates for full-time employment. The hiring process can be expensive and time-consuming. By hiring a former student worker, you hire a known commodity, and you reduce training costs. Your new employee has a jump start on meeting your job needs.

WHAT KIND OF ASSISTANCE DO YOU NEED?

Before recruiting students, look at what job functions need to be performed and who can best perform them. A marketing or business major may be a perfect match for conducting market research, assessments, and basic competitive analyses. A student with teaching or educational experience may be ideal for assisting in the development of educational materials. A graphic arts student may provide valuable input for the layout and design of brochures or advertisements.

Develop a marketing strategy and know your business needs before offering a student an opportunity with your company. Different projects often require different skills. Look closely at the marketing tasks. Students can help do such things as

- Sell and display at health fairs, exhibits, and conferences,
- Assist in material development and design,
- Develop brochures, newspaper advertisements, news articles, and other written materials,
- Conduct background research on potential clients, grant sources, and competitors,
- Assist with sales calls, especially telephone follow-ups that use a script,
- Establish a mailing list database, and
- Make progress with your move to computerization.

By considering the projects you want to accomplish and the kinds of skills required to complete the project, you may find that journalism, marketing, computer, or health education students as well as dietetics students may be helpful.

Student employees may come from either the undergraduate or the graduate level. In addition to working for you for the long term, they may also be available for very specific short-term needs. Many courses require students to develop brochures or exhibits, conduct market research, and the like. In many cases these are team projects, and students can help you at the same time that they fulfill class assignments.

For example, our company wanted to do a market research study on expanding a product line into a national market. We knew hiring a market research firm would be cost-prohibitive. We didn't want to make an expensive mistake, yet we didn't have the time internally to conduct the study. We also wanted an unbiased source to evaluate the data.

The solution came from working with an advanced marketing course instructor at a local university. To fulfill part of their course requirement, the business students jumped at the opportunity to develop an in-depth marketing plan for a real company. The team was a powerhouse – a nurse educator, a sports journalist, an accountant, and a professional sales representative. The result was a detailed analysis covering everything from target markets to trends analysis. The report was extensive and professional. A professional market research firm charges several thousand dollars for the same type of report.

We had a similar relationship with a graphic arts major. The student created original graphics for our educational materials and, at the same time, built up her professional portfolio.

HOW TO FIND STUDENTS

Some colleges and universities have co-op programs that work very effectively with the business community. You can contact department deans to meet interested students or schedule interviews with the university's placement and internship office. Individual instructors can also be helpful in recommending students to fit your needs. Frequently, faculty members are looking for business leaders who are willing to speak to classes about their businesses. Our company gives a presentation on entrepreneurship every spring for the community nutrition course at our local university. As a result of our presentation, many students choose to do their practicum with our company.

Having an opportunity to interview and select candidates is preferable to receiving assigned students. And it is helpful to prepare the same kind of job description you would for any position. Listing job functions and required skills clarifies expectations for both you and the student.

Plan your interview questions carefully to ensure that you learn as much as possible about the students' interests, internship goals, and career plans. During the interview, listen to what they hope to obtain from the experience and make sure it fits your business plan. Some qualities to look for in students are

- Good interpersonal skills,
- Above-average oral and written communication abilities,
- Motivation,
- Self-starting ability, but willingness to take instruction and advice,
- Computer experience,
- Conscientiousness,
- Dependability,
- Independence, but ability to be a team player,
- Willingness to look up information without feeling threatened, and
- Defined career goals.

One point to remember is that the best student is not always the best candidate or the hardest worker. You need individuals who not only are book smart, but also have the ability to apply information in real business situations.

Discuss problems, should they arise, with the student and/or a faculty sponsor. It is wise to have a termination policy for students, just in case a relationship is not mutually beneficial.

Ruth Fischer, President of NutriSmart, states: "One reason I hired Jenny, besides her being a business major, was that she was a competitive cyclist in the Rochester area and active in fitness. We contracted with a local company to design an exercise and nutrition component for their wellness program. We needed additional help in marketing the project. Although Jenny didn't have the scientific background in nutrition and exercise, she had the interest in them and was eager to learn. Her skills complemented those of other staff members. She conducted library research and developed worksheet drafts, brochure prototypes, and marketing materials for our senior staff to review and edit. She did revisions on the computer that enabled us to achieve final product without totally tying up staff time."

MAKING IT WORK

Remember to be patient and positive throughout the student-employment experience. Establish an environment of mutual respect for each other's position, abilities, and problems. To create the best situation, put on your mentor's cap.

When working with students, be aware of their goals and expectations. Be specific about your goals and their job functions and responsibilities. Consider meeting once or twice a week to review their work and answer questions. You, your staff, and the students must keep the working situation in perspective and keep communication flowing. Make the students feel a part of the company by including them in meetings and discussions about current projects. Let them gain from your experience and remain open to their eagerness to share their perspective.

Other aspects to consider are orientation and training, establishing payment policies, and scheduling formal or informal evaluation sessions. Expose students to your business plan, project development, and critical decision making. This helps students understand your company culture and the complexities of your business. When they feel a part of the team, they commit to your business, have a more realistic view of the business world, and help you market your business better!

However numerous the advantages, using students to market your business may have its drawbacks. Once you are aware of the pitfalls, set realistic expectations, anticipate possible problems, and prepare ahead of time to avoid them. Hiring a student or volunteer may mean

- More people to supervise,
- Less experienced help,
- More delegating of work, and
- More time spent mentoring and coaching.

The elements for a successful relationship with a student worker are

- Careful planning of needs and projects,
- Matching the appropriate student with identified tasks,
- Setting realistic goals within an allotted time frame,
- Being able to interview, orient, and support the student,
- Keeping communication open,
- Being positive, and
- Establishing mutual respect.

Employing students to help market your business can be successful if both parties want to make it work!

Chapter 38

How to Market Through Networking
Sharon O'Melia Howard, MS, RD, Private Practitioner,
Kennett Square, Pennsylvania

Why do dietetics professionals need to network? We may be trained to be nutrition experts, but we have a lot to learn about the real world of business, as intrapreneurs and entrepreneurs. Networking can enable you to

- Meet people with new resources and perspectives,
- Share your expertise and knowledge,
- Boost your business, get referrals, and find new opportunities or careers,
- Improve your professional image in your field or community,
- Find qualified business advisers, employees, and mentors,
- Learn new business and problem-solving skills, and
- Reduce feelings of isolation and gain emotional support.

A PERSONAL EXAMPLE

As a dietitian in private practice, I often feel isolated from other professionals because most of my days are spent in one-on-one contact with clients. To illustrate how networking works and the potential it can offer you, let me share this personal example.

A client of mine mentioned she was the editor of a newsletter for a local organization for businesswomen called Women's Referral Network. The group meets monthly to network over lunch and listen to a speaker on a topic of interest to women in business. This struck me as a great opportunity to learn how other women solve business problems, increase my professional visibility outside of dietetics, and maybe even make new friends!

I was introduced to the group by my client. I quickly became involved with the program committee and accepted the opportunity to speak about nutrition and women's health at one of the luncheons, which was attended by 150 women. From my networking at the luncheons and my speech, I attracted new private clients, found a new office to sublease, hired a firm to do my mailings, obtained a part-time secretary, and was asked to work with the caterer to provide light, low-fat meals for our meetings.

More opportunities followed. I met an enterprising woman at one luncheon who was starting a news magazine for women entrepreneurs. As we chatted, I mentioned that I occasionally wrote for local newspapers and would love the opportunity to write for her. Not long after that she offered me a regular column in her magazine. Her business grew substantially, and she now offers business seminars. Because of my column, I receive complementary registration for her wonderful programs, where I meet dynamic businesspeople in the Philadelphia area. As a result of their advice and examples, I have improved my business practices.

My involvement in the business world landed me a job teaching entrepreneurism to dietitians in a graduate school. My magazine editor friend and now mentor, benefits from having my students attend her seminars and subscribe to her magazine. This story has no ending – it's exciting to know that being open and willing to participate can bring many unpredictable benefits in return.

WHO SHOULD BE IN YOUR NETWORK?

Your network can move in many directions, like a spider's web or the spoke of a wheel with you at the hub. Select your directions carefully and evaluate your steps as you go, because you have only so much time and energy. Develop networks where you can make a contribution and realize long-term benefits for your business.

You already have many people and contacts in your network: friends, family, their friends and colleagues, community and religious groups, dietetic associations, clients, physicians, employers, co-workers, cultural and hobby groups, neighbors, local and national business or political organizations, and the like.

HOW DO YOU NETWORK?

1. *Write your personal and professional goals*. As you clarify these on paper, you will find it easier to select the directions to pursue.

2. *Get an attitude*. Develop a positive attitude to make the effort to get to know others. Networking should become a habit. You never know where or when a business opportunity may arise.

3. *Have a plan*. Based on your time and energy, decide how many networking opportunities you can attend or create each month. Attend local and national meetings to meet people as well as to hear speakers. Call an acquaintance for lunch.

4. *Improve interpersonal skills*. Set a goal for each large function you attend. Collect ten business cards and give out ten of yours. Be sure to greet people openly and be able to describe what you do in twenty words. As you elicit information from another person, think about what you do that can benefit him or her. Be resourceful and genuinely interested.

5. *Follow up your contacts*. Send an informal, friendly letter to all your new business card contacts within three days. Mention ideas that might be interesting to pursue. If you have a reason to meet, suggest it, and call within two weeks to schedule it. Enclose any materials or articles that may be of interest to the person. Keep a file of the business cards, arranged either by event, state, country, or alphabet.

6. *Persevere*. People do not always remember casual acquaintances. It often takes several meetings before someone will remember you. Salespeople know that 82 percent of their sales are made after the fifth call. You may need to attend five events or meetings before you reap benefits from your efforts. Be visible, be a good listener, and be yourself.

7. *Say thank you*. Send short notes to let others know you appreciate their efforts. One very successful businesswoman told me that in five years not one woman has thanked her for leads and special favors, but men have reciprocated with business leads and helpful feedback. Women need to see the benefit in helping other women in their businesses and careers. Men have been doing this very well for some time.

Communication channels become less formal as jobs become less secure and opportunities are more entrepreneurial. Networks for the purpose of job searches become crucial. Many consultants report that 70 to 80 percent of their jobs come through networking rather than from sending out résumés and answering ads.

Networking is fun, potentially profitable, and effective!

Glossary

advertising. A paid promotional strategy that draws attention to a product, service, or company to elicit a response (a purchase or inquiry).

anchor exhibit. On a trade show floor, a large, high-traffic booth.

audit. Certification by an objective third party (such as the ABC – The Audit Bureau of Circulation, BPA – the Business Publication Auditor, or CAC – Certified Audit Circulations) that a publication's circulation data are valid.

brand advertising. Advertising devoted to building public awareness of particular advantages or benefits and a favorable attitude toward a product.

broadcast media. Electronic media that deliver messages to mass audiences (TV and radio, for example).

business-to-business promotion. The promotion of a product or service that will be used in the operation or maintenance of a business (rather than for personal use).

card deck. A form of direct-mail marketing consisting of a package of loose or bound reply cards, each promoting a separate product or service; card decks may include multiple offers from a single company or offers from multiple companies (often grouped by category of product or service).

concentration. The strategy of focusing an advertising budget in a particular medium rather than scattering dollars across a range of media.

continuity. *See* **frequency**.

cost center. A business venture or department that must be supported by outside funds because it does not generate enough revenue to cover its expenses. A wellness program for employees that does not charge users fees is a cost center for the employer.

cost-recoverable operation. A business venture or department that is expected to break even and cover its expenses.

creative-driven advertising. Advertising that gives a higher priority to shock or entertainment value than to sales strategy and actual results.

database-driven advertising. Direct-response advertising that seeks not only an inquiry or an order but also information about the respondent that can be stored in the advertiser's database and used to continue the relationship and stimulate sales.

decision-maker. The person who has ultimate responsibility for deciding whether to go with an idea or purchase or let it pass. This can be a business owner, department head, purchasing agent, or client. *See* **influencer**.

demographics. Socioeconomic characteristics (such as age, sex, income, and marital status) pertaining to residents of a geographic unit, such as a county, zip code, town, and the like are also referred to as demographics.

dimensional mail. Mail with greater physical dimension than a flat envelope or postcard (a box or tube, for example), which traditionally has the highest opening rate of any type of direct mailing.

direct mail. A promotional strategy using a direct delivery service (such as the post office) to distribute a marketing message. *See also* **direct-order marketing** and **direct-response marketing**.

direct-order marketing. All forms of business based on selling goods or services directly to the public, without an intermediary. Such businesses obtain orders through direct-response advertising in magazines and newspapers, on television or radio, by direct mail, or in any other medium, and deliver product to the customer's address. Examples include selling by infomercial and on the Home Shopping Network.

direct-response marketing. Promotion through any medium (such as mail or phone call) that is designed to generate direct, measurable action from the recipient.

distress time. Unsold TV airtime offered at a discount to last-minute purchasers.

E.V.P. (extra-value proposition or value-added). Any supplementary service or product bundled with the sale of goods or services that makes the package so attractive that the consumer develops a favorable mindset about the product and remains loyal; for example, a consumer hot line, free recipe booklets, free in-service training for a physician's staff, or free child care at meetings.

field size. The number of characters that can be entered and stored in a field, which is an area in a computer file reserved for a particular type of data (such as the company name field or street address field in a file that contains a direct mail list).

focus group. In marketing research, a small group of selected people asked to react to packaging, price, or other components of a product or service; creatively brainstorm new uses; or share their experiences with a product or service. An experienced focus group leader is used to ask questions and manage the discussion.

frequency. In advertising, along with continuity, the number of times a prospect is exposed to a given message; also referred to as *repeat exposures*.

image advertising. Advertising designed to create, through constant repetition over a long period of time, a favorable image of the likability, reliability, or fashionability of a product or maker.

impact. The ability of an advertisement or other promotion to grab reader or audience attention and leave a lasting impression.

individualized marketing. Any integrated program of sales communications directly from the advertiser to selected members of the public, whether by means of letters, brochures, audiocassettes, videocassettes, telephone messages, computer disks, advertiser-sponsored events, or any other means of direct contact.

influencer. The person or persons who can affect the decisions made by a decision maker; the influencer may be just as important to convince as the decision maker.

integrated marketing. A holistic approach to all components of the marketing mix that seeks to do whatever is necessary to identify, contact, activate, and cultivate individual customers and increase market sales and market share; its goal is to develop a synergy between the components.

lift note. In a direct mail package, a letter within a letter, often placed in a separate envelope that stands out from the other elements, that overcomes objections and urges immediate action.

list broker. An independent agent who rents mailing lists from other sources, such as credit card companies, catalogues, and magazine circulation lists.

list compiler. A vendor who creates mailing lists from public sources, such as voter registration lists, zip code directories, and *The Thomas Register*.

list manager. An employee who works directly for a company that owns a mailing list (such as a catalogue company or magazine publisher), whose job is to maintain and update the list.

marketing. An aggregate of functions, such as market research, planning, promotion, and sales, involved in moving goods or services from the producer to the consumer.

marketing mix. Four (or more) universal elements of marketing that are often called the four Ps – product, promotion, place, and price. All are fairly controllable factors used in making decisions about marketing strategies and objectives. A product may be either tangible or intangible (such as a service); promotion is persuasive communication aimed at targeted users; place refers to where the product is available; and price encompasses both the monetary and the intangible values of the product.

marketing research. The gathering of factual information about consumer preferences for products or services to establish the extent and location of the market for a product, or to analyze the product in comparison to an alternative or the competition.

market niche (market segment). A clearly defined subgroup of customers or potential customers with common characteristics relevant to the marketing of a product; for example, one-career couples with expendable income of $40,000 to $60,000. Niche marketing is the sharp targeting of messages to reach a specific subgroup, in contrast to mass marketing, which hits everyone.

market share. The approximate percentage of all potential customers that one competitor holds or hopes to capture for a particular product.

market value. The price at which both buyers and sellers are willing to do business.

match code. A computer code placed on each element of a direct mail package (envelope, letter, order form) to ensure that all components match; a critical element in the automated assembly of personalized mailings.

merge-purge. The process of combining two or more mailing lists while eliminating duplicates or unwanted names and addresses.

mission statement. A short statement of the philosophy and fundamental nature of a business; it answers the questions "What business are we in?" and "Who do we serve?"

multichannel distribution. Creating more than one distribution channel for a product. For example, if you have always sold your homemade fruit baskets through flower shops, you might also start to advertise locally directly to the consumer and offer free or low-cost delivery in town.

narrowcasting. A term applied to cable TV to differentiate its localized reach from network TV's mass reach (broadcasting).

objectives. Concrete, measurable, realistic targets a business wants to achieve; for example, "Increase sales of gizmos by 10 percent over last year's sales," not simply "Increase sales."

pitch letter. A letter used to suggest a story idea to a print reporter or program director at a radio or television station, with you as the subject or an expert source.

plan of action. A clear road map for carrying out all the strategies in a marketing plan; it specifies who, when, how long, how much money, and what other resources are required for each tactic and coordinates them in chronological order, when necessary.

pot shot. Placing random, single ads in different newspapers and on radio or TV to see what happens.

preemptible time. A TV time slot purchased by one advertiser that can be pre-empted by any other advertiser offering a higher price for the same slot.

press release. The fundamental tool of public relations, a brief news release, written in a standard format, used to generate press coverage for an event, person, product, service, or company.

product. Anything offered in the marketplace to be exchanged for something of value, such as money, time, or commitment; it may be either a tangible good or an intangible service.

profit center. A business venture or department that generates or is expected to generate a profit. *See also* **cost center** and **cost-recoverable operation**.

psychographics. A measure of people's internal factors or habits, such as what they buy, what is important to them, and how they perceive things.

public relations. A promotional strategy that provides low-cost or no-cost publicity about a person, product, service, or company; its usual goal is to obtain news coverage, but it may also be to create goodwill (through free services, charitable work, and the like).

query letter. A letter sent to publishers, newspapers, magazines, and other media suggesting a possible story or book idea that you want to write for them.

reach. In advertising, the number of people exposed at least once to the vehicle (magazine, newsletter, radio spot) carrying an ad.

run-of-station time. TV advertising time purchased for a set period of time (one week, for example), during which the station places the spot(s) in any unsold time slots.

seeding. Deliberate placement of decoy names in a direct mail list to trace list usage and delivery; also known as *salting*.

social marketing. The design, implementation, and control of programs calculated to influence the acceptability of social ideas (such as eat more fruits and vegetables, or eat less fat); social marketing focuses on changing personal or social behavior for the benefit of the person and the public.

strategies. The general approach taken to achieve an objective; for example, "Increase gizmo sales through telemarketing, a direct mail campaign, and press releases."

strategic assumptions. Statements an organization as a whole adopts about major trends and changes in the external environment that will affect the future, and presumably, its target market and future markets.

SWOT. An acronym that stands for strengths, weaknesses, opportunities, and threats; a situational-analysis technique often used in market research.

tactics. The specific actions, decisions, and resources required to implement strategies; for example, "Hire a full-time salesperson two weeks before the product is released on the market" or "Buy client list of purchasing agents at companies in a 50-mile radius."

target market. The primary customers or potential customers for a product or service.

targeting. Channeling marketing efforts and resources to specific market segments or niches that have the highest payoff potential.

teaser copy. Brief, high-impact copy on a piece of direct mail, usually near the outside address, intended to stimulate interest and increase opening and readership.

vertical integration. A company's attempt to control its supply and distribution channels by buying its suppliers or distributors. For example, a restaurant might start growing its own herbs and organic vegetables instead of buying them from an expensive importer, and, as its herb and vegetable business grows, it might buy several other restaurants who use (or will begin using) large amounts of organic vegetables and herbs in their dishes.

vertical market. A target market that is narrow, but deep, and thus offers good potential for saturation; for example, only people with diabetes might want your diabetes cookbook, but the majority of people within that market could use it.

visibility. *See* **impact**.

Index

Y

Yadrick, Martin, 129
Yale-New Haven Hospital
   Nutritional Classification and
   Assessment Program, 124
Yancey, Jean, 2
Yellow Pages advertising, 38, 83
Young, Marty, 98

AGREEMENT FOR NUTRITION CONSULTING SERVICES

This document shall serve as a Letter of Agreement between Nutrition Consultants, Inc., 1234 Apple, Saint Paul, Minnesota, and HealthSystems, Inc., 0000 Avenue South, Minneapolis, Minnesota. The contract period is from October 15, 1995 through October 14, 1996.

Nutrition Consultants, Inc., shall be compensated for services in developing a registered dietitian referral system in the amount of $3,500.00. Reimbursable expenses in addition to the fixed fee shall include long-distance telephone calls, photocopying, postage, fax services, mailing lists, incentive awards, and other incidentals directly related to provision of services.

In addition, Nutrition Consultants, Inc., agrees to seek out promotional opportunities for HealthSystems, Inc., to assist in increasing its client base. These activities will focus on RDs, the local media, and corporations. For this ongoing service, Nutrition Consultants, Inc., will be compensated by a monthly retainer of $500.00 for the duration of this agreement.

Requested services outside the scope of this agreement will be billed at the rate of $75.00 per hour. All additional services will require advance authorization from the designated HealthSystems, Inc., representative.

A monthly activity report will be submitted, along with an invoice for direct and other authorized expenses, by the first of each month. Invoices are to be paid by the fifteenth of the month in which they are submitted. Interest in the amount of 8 percent per annum will be added to all late payments.

Nutrition Consultants, Inc., agrees to maintain current registrations, licenses, malpractice insurance, and all other requirements necessary to practice as registered dietitians in the state of Minnesota.

Both Nutrition Consultants, Inc., and HealthSystems, Inc., acknowledge that the relationship entered into by this agreement is that of independent parties and not that of employer and employee. Both parties enter into this temporary relationship for the purpose of affecting the provisions of this Letter of Agreement, and do not deem or construe to create a relationship as agents, employees, or representatives of each other.

Either party may terminate this agreement, with or without cause, at any time upon giving the other party sixty (60) days' written notice.

HealthSystems, Inc.　　　　Nutrition Consultants, Inc.

By _____　　　　By _____

Its _____　　　　Its _____
　Designated Representative　　　Designated Representative

Date _____　　　　Date _____

Figure 15-1. Letter of Agreement

AGREEMENT BETWEEN
CORPORATE HEALTH-CARE CORPORATION
AND
NUTRITION CONSULTANTS, INC.

THIS AGREEMENT, effective January 1, 1995, between Corporate Health-Care Corporation ("CHC") and Nutrition Consultants, Inc. ("NCI").

WHEREAS, CHC is a for-profit corporation organized and operated for the purposes of developing and marketing alternative health-care delivery systems and related products and services; and

WHEREAS, CHC desires to arrange for the development and implementation of health-promotion programs and NCI are duly registered dietitians and health educators who desire to develop and implement health-promotion programs for CHC;

THEREFORE, in consideration of the mutual covenants herein contained, the parties hereby agree as follows:

SECTION 1. NUTRITION CONSULTANTS, INC., OBLIGATIONS:
1.01. Food for Health Program. NCI shall develop, implement, and maintain the Food for Health Program for CHC. The Food for Health Program shall consist of, but not be limited to: (a) presentations on good nutrition; (b) the development of guidelines for healthy eating; (c) demonstrations of practical and healthy food preparation; and (d) the development of brochures and other literature on the subject of good nutrition. See Attachment A for details.
1.02. Health-Promotion Program Articles and Publications. NCI shall research, develop, and write health-promotion articles for the magazines, brochures, and other written media published by CHC. NCI shall develop and provide health-related scientific data for the magazines, brochures, and other written media published by CHC. The publication of such articles and scientific data shall be subject to the final approval of CHC.
1.03. Media Placements. NCI shall develop, implement, and coordinate media placements for the promotion of the Food for Health Program and other health-promotion programs developed by NCI or CHC. NCI shall also develop, implement, and coordinate media placements concerning general health information as a public service to local communities. NCI shall obtain final approval on all media placements prior to scheduling a media placement or committing CHC in any manner.
1.04. Liability Insurance. NCI shall procure and maintain, at their sole expense, professional liability insurance with remaining coverage satisfactory to CHC. Upon request by CHC, NCI shall provide evidence of insurance coverage. NCI shall notify CHC, in writing, to the attention of the Chief Executive Officer, within ten (10) days of changes in carriers, changes in remaining coverage, or notification to NCI of any claims against, denials of, restriction on, termination of, or changes in NCI professional liability insurance.

Figure 15-2. Formal Contract

1.05. Laws, Regulations, and Licenses. NCI shall maintain all federal, state, and local licenses, permits, and association memberships, without restriction, required to practice as registered dietitians or health educators. NCI shall notify CHC in writing, to the attention of the Chief Executive Officer, within ten (10) days of any suspension, revocation, condition, limitation, qualification, or other restriction on NCI's licenses, permits, and/or association memberships by any state in which NCI is licensed as dietitians, health educators, or other health-care professionals.

SECTION 2. CHC OBLIGATIONS

2.01. Payment for Services. CHC shall reimburse NCI for services rendered under the Agreement ("Contract Fee") an amount equal to thirty-three thousand and six hundred dollars ($33,600) in the contract year January 1, 1995, through December 31, 1996. The contract year thereafter shall be the calendar year from January 1 through December 31. CHC shall pay NCI in monthly payments of two thousand eight hundred ($2,800.00) the first business day of each month beginning with January 1, 1995, made payable to NCI.

2.02. Payment of Out-of-Pocket Expenses. CHC shall reimburse NCI for all reasonable out-of-pocket expenses, including, but not limited to, supplies, subscriptions, educational resources, travel expenses, and mileage that are incurred in connection with the provision of services under this Agreement. Said out-of-pocket expenses shall be limited to $1800.00 per annum for supplies and travel, and to $350.00 per annum for subscriptions and educational resources as determined by the budget. Said out-of-pocket expenses shall not include normal travel and mileage between NCI's place of business and CHC's corporate headquarters.

2.03. Office Space. CHC shall provide adequate work space and support staff to NCI at CHC's corporate headquarters as detailed in Attachment B.

2.04. Copyrights and Trademarks. Any health-promotion data, information, articles, publications, brochures, or programs, and any specific information connected therewith, uniquely developed or implemented by NCI for CHC shall be considered the property of CHC. CHC shall have the rights to all copyrights and trademarks for all uniquely developed health-promotion data, information, articles, publications, and programs, and the specific information connected therewith.

SECTION 3. TERM AND TERMINATION

3.01. Term. The term of this agreement shall commence on January 1, 1995 and shall continue and remain in effect through the remainder of the calendar year 1995, and for each calendar year thereafter until such time as this Agreement is terminated as hereinafter provided.

3.02. Termination. This agreement may be terminated by CHC, with or without cause, or by NCI, with or without cause, upon sixty (60) days written notice to the other party.

SECTION 4. MISCELLANEOUS

4.01. Independent Contractors. The relationship between CHC and NCI is that of independent contractors only and NCI is not an employee or agent of CHC. Nothing contained in this Agreement shall constitute or be construed to be or create a partnership, joint venture, or an association between CHC and NCI, nor shall either party, or its employees, agents, and representatives be considered employees, agents, or representatives of the other party.

4.02. Amendment. Any amendment to this Agreement proposed by CHC at least thirty (30) days prior to the effective date of such amendment is incorporated herein; provided, however, that in the event any change or modification to this Agreement is requested by any State or Federal regulatory authority as a result of a filing of this Agreement with such authority, such change or modification shall be incorporated into this Agreement from the effective date of this Agreement.

4.03. Assignment. CHC shall have the absolute right, in its sole discretion, to assign all or any of its rights or responsibilities hereunder to any corporation that is a subsidiary or affiliate of CHC. In the event of assignment, this Agreement shall be binding upon and inure to the benefit of CHC's successors and assigns. NCI shall not have the right to assign any of their rights without the prior written consent of CHC, which consent shall not be unreasonably withheld.

4.04. No Waiver of Rights. The failure of any party to insist upon the strict observation or performance of any provision of this Agreement or to exercise any right or remedy shall not impair or waive any such right or remedy. Every right and remedy given by this Agreement to the parties may be exercised from time to time and as often as appropriate.

4.05. Entire Agreement. This Agreement is the entire Agreement between the parties. No representations or agreements between the parties, oral or otherwise, has any force or effect.

4.06. Impossibility of Performance. Neither CHC nor NCI shall be deemed to be in default of this Agreement if prevented from performing for reasons beyond its control, including without limitation, governmental laws and regulation, acts of God, wars, and strikes. In such case, the parties shall negotiate in good faith with the goal and intent of preserving this Agreement and the respective rights and obligations of the parties.

4.07. Governing Law. This Agreement shall be construed in accordance with the laws of the state of Minnesota.

IN WITNESS HEREOF, the parties hereto have caused this Agreement to be executed.

CORPORATE HEALTH PLAN CORPORATION   NUTRITION CONSULTANTS, INC.
0000 Eagle Drive   1234 Apple St.
St. Paul, Minnesota XXXXX   St. Paul, Minnesota XXXXX
By _____   By _____
Its _____   Its _____
Date _____   Date _____

Figure 15-2. Formal Contract

The purpose of a break-even analysis is to determine the amount of revenue (sales) necessary to pay all expenses incurred by the business. In preparing this analysis, you must determine the cost of goods sold and all other expenses that are associated with the business. This is normally done as follows:

1. Variable expenses tend to change directly with the amount of revenue, and include such items as the cost of goods sold, hourly labor, copier/office supplies, credit card fees, and cash over/short. These are normally expressed as a percentage of revenue (a video that sells for $60.00 and costs you $30.00 will have a cost of sales of 50%; $30.00/$60.00 = .50 = 50%). These cost relationships remain essentially constant regardless of the revenue volume. If you have multiple products and/or services, it is important to determine a cost for each:

Product/Service	Cost %
Nutrition consultation	0.0%*
Cookbooks	25.0%
Videos	50.0%
Educational materials	15.0%

*The cost of this product is the registered dietitian, which is fixed and not included in the variable cost of sales.

2. Fixed expenses tend to not change directly with the amount of revenue, and include such items as the management salary, utilities, rent, and insurance. These expenses tend to change due to nonrevenue relationships (i.e., electricity is a greater expense in the summer months in Texas).

3. Segregate expenses into variable (expressed as a percent of revenue) and fixed (expressed in annual dollars) as shown in Figure 20-12.

4. Select a revenue volume for each type of goods or service that you will provide. In the early planning stage, it is often easier to think of what percent of total revenue each product will represent. If you use a total revenue number of $100, then the percent of the product and its dollar amount are the same:

Product/Service	Revenue %	Revenue $
Nutrition consultation	41.0%	$41.00
Cookbooks	20.0%	20.00
Videos	19.0%	19.00
Educational materials	20.0%	20.00
	100.0%	$100.00

Don't worry if your actual revenue volume is higher. The percentages will remain valid regardless of the revenue.

5. Calculate total expenses with the following emphasis:

Variable: Percent of expense and profit
Fixed: Total dollars

Prepared by Eric P. Jessup

Figure 20-9. Break-Even Analysis

Weight Maintenance

1800 to 2500 calories
60 to 75 grams fat
70 to 100 grams protein
250 to 350 grams carbohydrate
less than 3000 mg sodium
less than 300 mg cholesterol

Breakfast   400 to 600 calories
Lunch   500 to 700 calories
Dinner   700 to 1000 calories
Snacks   max. 200 calories per day

Weight Maintenance	DINNER				
Course	Calories	Fat	Protein	Sodium	Cholesterol
Appetizer or Soup	<150 <100	<5 gm <2 gm	<10 gm	<300 mg <300 mg	<50 mg
Salad	<100	<5 gm		<150 mg	
Entree: Main item with sauce	<225	<10 gm	<30 gm	<500 mg	<100 mg
Starch	100	<2 gm		<150 mg	
Vegetable	<50	<2 gm		<100 mg	
Dessert	<200	<4 gm		<100 mg	
Bread	<100	<2 gm		<200 mg	
Beverage	80 to 100	trace	trace		
Total	less than 1000	less than 30 gm	approx. 50 gm	less than 1500 mg	less than 150 mg

Figure 18-1. Example of Nutritional Cooking Criteria: Suggested Menu Parameters

From the attached examples, the results are
Variable expense: 19.4%
Variable profit: 80.6%

Fixed expense: $141,370

Calculation of break-even:
Total fixed expenses of   141,370
divided by variable profit percent of   80.6%
results in required revenue of   175,397

Break-even proof:
Estimated total revenue $175,397
Total variable expenses   (34,027)   19.4%
Total fixed expenses   (141,370)
Total profit before taxes $0

Prepared by Eric P. Jessup.

	10% Less		Most Likely		10% More	
Revenues						
Nutrition consultation	$ 67,500		$ 75,000		$ 82,500	
Cookbooks	22,500		25,000		27,500	
Videos	45,000		50,000		55,000	
Educational materials	67,500		75,000		82,500	
Total revenue	$202,500		$225,000		$247,500	
Cost of sales						
Cookbooks	(5,625)	25.0%	(6,250)	25.0%	(6,875)	25.0%
Videos	(22,500)	50.0%	(25,000)	50.0%	(27,500)	50.0%
Educational materials	(10,125)	15.0%	(11,250)	15.0%	(12,375)	15.0%
Total cost of sales	(38,250)	18.9%	(42,500)	18.9%	(46,750)	18.9%
Labor						
Registered dietitian	(50,000)	24.7%	(50,000)	22.2%	(50,000)	20.2%
Secretary	(20,000)	9.9%	(20,000)	8.9%	(20,000)	8.1%
Taxes & benefits	(21,000)	10.4%	(21,000)	9.3%	(21,000)	8.5%
Total labor	(91,000)	44.9%	(91,000)	40.4%	(91,000)	36.8%
Controllable expenses						
Educational supplies	(2,025)	1.0%	(2,250)	1.0%	(2,475)	1.0%
Office supplies	(2,400)	1.2%	(2,400)	1.1%	(2,400)	1.0%
Copier supplies	(1,620)	0.8%	(1,800)	0.8%	(1,980)	0.8%
Books and subscriptions	(2,000)	1.0%	(2,000)	0.9%	(2,000)	0.8%
Cash over/short	(203)	0.1%	(225)	0.1%	(248)	0.1%
Travel	(3,500)	1.7%	(3,500)	1.6%	(3,500)	1.4%
Professional fees	(2,000)	1.0%	(2,000)	0.9%	(2,000)	0.8%
Telephone	(3,600)	1.8%	(3,600)	1.6%	(3,600)	1.5%
Utilities	(2,400)	1.2%	(2,400)	1.1%	(2,400)	1.0%
Repair & maintenance	(1,200)	0.6%	(1,200)	0.5%	(1,200)	0.5%
Equipment rental	(2,400)	1.2%	(2,400)	1.1%	(2,400)	1.0%
Controllable expenses	(23,348)	11.5%	(23,775)	10.6%	(24,203)	9.8%
Controllable profit	49,902	24.6%	67,725	30.1%	85,547	34.6%
Administrative and general:						
Advertising	(8,000)	4.0%	(8,000)	3.6%	(8,000)	3.2%
Accounting service	(2,400)	1.2%	(2,400)	1.1%	(2,400)	1.0%
Total administrative and general	(10,400)	5.1%	(10,400)	4.6%	(10,400)	4.2%
Occupancy expenses:						
Rent expense	(12,000)	5.9%	(12,000)	5.3%	(12,000)	4.8%
Common area	(600)	0.3%	(600)	0.3%	(600)	0.2%
Insurance	(1,300)	0.6%	(1,300)	0.6%	(1,300)	0.5%
Depreciation	(6,570)	3.2%	(6,570)	2.9%	(6,570)	2.7%
Total occupancy expenses	(20,470)	10.1%	(20,470)	9.1%	(20,470)	8.3%
Profit before taxes	$19,032	9.4%	$36,855	16.4%	$54,677	22.1%
Add depreciation	6,570	3.2%	6,570	2.9%	6,570	2.7%
Cash flow before taxes	$25,602	12.6%	$43,425	19.3%	$61,247	24.7%

Figure 20-10. Pro Forma Income Statement

	Jan	Feb	Mar	Apr	May	Jun	Jul	Aug	Sep	Oct	Nov	Dec	Total
Revenues													
Nutrition consultation	6,370	5,753	6,370	6,164	6,370	6,164	6,370	6,370	6,164	6,370	6,164	6,371	75,000
Cookbooks	2,123	1,918	2,123	2,055	2,123	2,055	2,123	2,123	2,055	2,123	2,055	2,124	25,000
Videos	4,247	3,836	4,247	4,110	4,247	4,110	4,247	4,247	4,110	4,247	4,110	4,242	50,000
Educational materials	6,370	5,753	6,370	6,164	6,370	6,164	6,370	6,370	6,164	6,370	6,164	6,371	75,000
Total revenue	19,110	17,260	19,110	18,493	19,110	18,493	19,110	19,110	18,493	19,110	18,493	19,108	225,000
Cost of sales													
Cookbooks	(531)	(479)	(531)	(514)	(531)	(514)	(531)	(531)	(514)	(531)	(514)	(529)	(6,250)
Videos	(2,123)	(1,918)	(2,123)	(2,055)	(2,123)	(2,055)	(2,123)	(2,123)	(2,055)	(2,123)	(2,055)	(2,124)	(25,000)
Educational materials	(955)	(863)	(955)	(925)	(955)	(925)	(955)	(955)	(925)	(955)	(925)	(957)	(11,250)
Total cost of sales	(3,609)	(3,260)	(3,609)	(3,494)	(3,609)	(3,494)	(3,609)	(3,609)	(3,494)	(3,609)	(3,494)	(3,610)	(42,500)
Labor													
Registered dietitian	(4,167)	(4,167)	(4,166)	(4,167)	(4,167)	(4,166)	(4,167)	(4,167)	(4,166)	(4,167)	(4,167)	(4,166)	(50,000)
Secretary	(1,667)	(1,667)	(1,666)	(1,667)	(1,667)	(1,666)	(1,667)	(1,667)	(1,666)	(1,667)	(1,667)	(1,666)	(20,000)
Taxes and benefits	(1,750)	(1,750)	(1,750)	(1,750)	(1,750)	(1,750)	(1,750)	(1,750)	(1,750)	(1,750)	(1,750)	(1,750)	(21,000)
Total labor	(7,584)	(7,584)	(7,582)	(7,584)	(7,584)	(7,582)	(7,584)	(7,584)	(7,582)	(7,584)	(7,584)	(7,582)	(91,000)
Controllable expenses													
Educational supplies	(191)	(173)	(191)	(185)	(191)	(185)	(191)	(191)	(185)	(191)	(185)	(191)	(2,250)
Office supplies	(200)	(200)	(200)	(200)	(200)	(200)	(200)	(200)	(200)	(200)	(200)	(200)	(2,400)
Copier supplies	(153)	(138)	(153)	(148)	(153)	(148)	(153)	(153)	(148)	(153)	(148)	(152)	(1,800)
Books and subscriptions	0	0	(250)	(1,000)	0	0	(600)	0	0	0	0	(150)	(2,000)
Cash over/short	(19)	(17)	(19)	(18)	(19)	(18)	(19)	(19)	(18)	(19)	(18)	(22)	(225)
Travel	(75)	(75)	(75)	(75)	(1,000)	(75)	(75)	(1,750)	(75)	(75)	(75)	(75)	(3,500)
Professional fees	0	(1,000)	0	0	0	(500)	0	0	0	0	(500)	0	(2,000)
Telephone	(306)	(276)	(306)	(296)	(306)	(296)	(306)	(306)	(296)	(306)	(296)	(304)	(3,600)
Utilities	(204)	(184)	(204)	(197)	(204)	(197)	(204)	(204)	(197)	(204)	(197)	(204)	(2,400)
Repair and maintenance	(102)	(92)	(102)	(99)	(102)	(99)	(102)	(102)	(99)	(102)	(99)	(100)	(1,200)
Equipment rental	(200)	(200)	(200)	(200)	(200)	(200)	(200)	(200)	(200)	(200)	(200)	(200)	(2,400)
Total controllable expenses	(1,450)	(2,355)	(1,700)	(2,418)	(2,375)	(1,918)	(2,050)	(3,125)	(1,418)	(1,450)	(1,918)	(1,598)	(23,775)
Controllable profit	6,467	4,061	6,219	4,997	5,542	5,499	5,867	4,792	5,999	6,467	5,497	6,318	67,725
Administrative and general													
Advertising	(400)	(400)	(600)	(800)	(1,000)	(1,000)	(1,000)	(400)	(600)	(600)	(800)	(400)	(8,000)
Accounting service	(150)	(750)	(150)	(150)	(150)	(150)	(150)	(150)	(150)	(150)	(150)	(150)	(2,400)
Total administrative and general	(550)	(1,150)	(750)	(950)	(1,150)	(1,150)	(1,150)	(550)	(750)	(750)	(950)	(550)	(10,400)
Occupancy expenses													
Rent expense	(1,000)	(1,000)	(1,000)	(1,000)	(1,000)	(1,000)	(1,000)	(1,000)	(1,000)	(1,000)	(1,000)	(1,000)	(12,000)
Common area	(50)	(50)	(50)	(50)	(50)	(50)	(50)	(50)	(50)	(50)	(50)	(50)	(600)
Insurance	(108)	(108)	(108)	(108)	(108)	(108)	(108)	(108)	(108)	(108)	(108)	(112)	(1,300)
Depreciation	(548)	(547)	(548)	(547)	(548)	(547)	(548)	(547)	(548)	(547)	(548)	(547)	(6,570)
Total occupancy expenses	(1,706)	(1,705)	(1,706)	(1,705)	(1,706)	(1,705)	(1,706)	(1,705)	(1,706)	(1,705)	(1,706)	(1,709)	(20,470)
Profit before taxes	4,211	1,206	3,763	2,342	2,686	2,644	3,011	2,537	3,543	4,012	2,841	4,059	36,850
Add depreciation	548	547	548	547	548	547	548	547	548	547	548	547	6,570
Cash flow before taxes	4,759	1,753	4,311	2,889	3,234	3,191	3,559	3,084	4,091	4,559	3,389	4,606	43,420

Figure 20-11. Budget

Prepared by Eric P. Jessup.

The New York State Dietetic Association, Inc.

48 Howard Street
Albany, New York 12207
(518) 463-2415

FOR IMMEDIATE RELEASE   CONTACT: Agnes Kolor, R.D.
(914) 735-8622

Mona Boyd Browne, R.D.
(212) 678-6937

New York Dietitians Organize Statewide

Hunger Alert Day -- March 20, 1993

Albany, New York, February 22, 1993 -- The New York State Dietetic Association today announced its plans to coordinate a statewide **Hunger Alert Day '93** in observance of March National Nutrition Month. The event, to be held at local supermarkets throughout the state between 9:00 a.m. and 3:00 p.m., has been organized to collect donated food for use at community food banks and hunger programs.

"Hunger Alert Day '93 enables dietitians, supermarkets, hunger relief organizations and community groups to work together to help feed the hungry in our own neighborhoods," explains Eden Kalman, R.D., President of The New York State Dietetic Association. Volunteers will be collecting food outside more than 70 supermarkets chains, including D'Agostino, Grand Union, P & C, and Price Chopper.

The New York State Dietetic Association is a professional organization of more than 5,000 registered dietitians (R.D.), dietetic technicians, registered (D.T.R.) and other qualified nutrition professionals in New York.

# # #

AN AFFILIATE OF
THE AMERICAN DIETETIC ASSOCIATION

Sample Press Releases
(Reprinted with permission.)

Revenues		
Nutrition consultation		41
Cookbooks		20
Videos		19
Educational materials		20
Total revenue		$100
Variable Expenses		
Cost of sales		
Cookbooks	25.0%	(5.00)
Videos	50.0%	(9.50)
Educational materials	15.0%	(3.00)
Controllable expenses		
Educational supplies	1.0%	(1.00)
Copier supplies	0.8%	(0.80)
Cash over/short	0.1%	(0.10)
Total variable expenses	19.4%	(19.40)
Total variable profit	80.6%	80.60
Fixed Expenses		
Labor		
Registered dietitian		(50.000)
Secretary		(20.000)
Taxes and benefits		(21.000)
Controllable expenses		
Office supplies		(2.400)
Books and subscriptions		(2.000)
Travel		(3.500)
Professional fees		(2.000)
Telephone		(3.600)
Utilities		(2.400)
Repairs and maintenance		(1.200)
Equipment rental		(2.400)
Administrative and general		
Advertising		(8.000)
Accounting service		(2.400)
Occupancy expenses		
Rent expense		(12.000)
Common area		(600)
Insurance		(1.300)
Depreciation		(6.570)
Total fixed expenses		(141.370)

Prepared by Eric P. Jessup.

Figure 20-12. Expense Analysis

years of public service contributions for justice and equality. The Black Family Dinner Quilt Cookbook features Food Memories™ from prominent African-Americans and is a sequel to last year's Black Family Reunion Cookbook which sold over 100,000 copies.

Lauren Swann, a registered dietitian and president of Concept Nutrition, Inc. consulting services, became involved with the project after publishing *Soul Food: Heart of Black America* in the *Philadelphia Inquirer*. The Black Family Dinner Quilt Cookbook can be ordered by calling (215) 639-1203. Proceeds from the book are donated to NCNW to support their programs aiding African-American females and their families.

# # #

CONCEPT NUTRITION, INC.

3655 Hulmeville Road • #352 • Bensalem, Pa 19020 • (215) 639-1203 • FAX (215) 639-2323

1/29/93
NEWS
FOR IMMEDIATE RELEASE

For Further Information
Contact: Lauren Swann
(215) 639-1203

LOCAL NUTRITIONIST AUTHORS SOUL FOOD HISTORY FOR
NATIONAL COUNCIL OF NEGRO WOMEN HERITAGE COOKBOOK

The Black Family Dinner Quilt Cookbook, released this month, features a nutrition section -- authored by Bensalem resident Lauren Swann, MS, RD -- which explores the rich cultural food customs African-Americans brought to our country. From slave times to the present, traditional practices which nourished African-Americans are explored and recognized as the mealtime celebrations which physically and spiritually strengthen and unify African-Americans.

As Nutrition Consultant, Swann was also recipe editor and developed the educational recommendations to tastefully improve the healthfulness of soul food cuisine. "It is interesting that the roots of African-American diets are very much in line with today's Dietary Guidelines," says Swann, "Africans enjoyed a diet abundant in fruits, vegetables and whole grains and continued this habit through slave times because meat was stringently rationed by their masters."

Endorsed by former Health & Human Services Secretary Louis Sullivan, MD, The Black Family Dinner Quilt Cookbook is dedicated to Dr. Dorothy Height, National Council of Negro Women (NCNW) President, in recognition of her 60

-MORE-

Sample Press Releases
(Reprinted with permission.)

MEDIA SPOKESPERSON
THE AMERICAN DIETETIC ASSOCIATION

NEVA COCHRAN, MS, RD/LD
5207 Stone Arbor Court
Dallas, Texas 75287
214/250-2540

March 31, 1990

Candy Sagon
Food Editor
Dallas Times Herald
1101 Pacific
Dallas, TX 75202

Dear Candy:

A typical Easter basket not only contains chocolate bunnies, marshmallow eggs, jelly beans, and other assorted goodies, but comes packed with 2000 calories and 100 grams of fat. This is the same as eating one stick of butter and a cup and a half of sugar. But this is a traditional part of Easter. What is a health-conscious bunny to do?

According to the recent ADA/IFIC sponsored Gallup survey, two thirds of Americans choose foods based on "good" and "bad" perceptions. What is more important, according to registered dietitians, is the nutritional adequacy and balance of diets over time. Your readers might enjoy and benefit from a fact-filled article on alternative Easter baskets that don't leave the bunnies out in the cold. I could provide you with the following information for such a story:

- list of the calorie and fat content of common basket stuffers.

- alternative foods, well-liked by children, to fill an Easter basket that are lower in fat and calories but high in nutritional value.
- nonfood items that children would enjoy to round out the basket.

These items, along with a few pieces of favorite Easter candy, would make a colorful photograph and nutritious alternative (800 calories and 40 grams of fat, yet packed with nutrients) to the traditional Easter basket.

I am a registered dietitian with fourteen years experience in clinical, community, and education settings. During this time I have done over 300 media interviews. As spokesperson for The American Dietetic Association. I am available to assist you with this or any other nutrition-related story.

Please call me at 214/250-2540 if you are interested in this idea.

Sincerely,

Neva H. Cochran

Neva H. Cochran, MS, RD, LD

Sample Pitch Letter.
(Reprinted with permission.)

LEADERSHIP

ADA, SCAN Practice Group, 1985-present
Minnesota Dietetics Association, 1976-present
South Central District Dietetic Association, 1976-present
Minnesota Public Health Association, 1988-present

Board Member and Facilitator, Women Executives in Business (WEB), 1989-present

President/Chair of the Board, Midwest Independent Publishers Association (MIPA) 1993-95

Preceptor/Mentor, REACH Graduate Program, University of MN 1992-94

Executive Board Member, Challenge 2001, (Drug Prevention Program for greater Mankato community) 1992-93

Executive Board Member and Grants Chair, CHAP (Council of Health Action and Promotion for greater Mankato community) 1992-present

Chair, Women and Heart Disease Committee, AHA-MN Affiliate, 1991-93

President, American Heart Association - MN Affiliate, Mankato Division, 1990-1991

Board Member, American Heart Association - MN Affiliate, Mankato Division: President Elect, 1989-1990; Community Programs Chair, 1988-1989; Nutrition Committee chair, 1987-1988; Communications Chair, 1991-1992

Co-Author, Legislation in Senate, State of Minnesota, SF 858 — Establishment of community-based health promotion teams. Introduced by Senator E. Renneke. Bill passed May 1989.

Chair, Leadership Mankato, Health Issues and Ethics. Mankato Chamber of Commerce. March 1989.

Charter Board Member, Minnesota Dietetic Association Foundation. 1988-1991

Chair, Health Action Council (Coalition), Greater Mankato community 1989-1990

Chair, Obesity: The Dilemma, Health Professionals Conference sponsored by Health Consortium, Minnesota, 1986

Chair, Minnesota Dietetic Association, "Breaking Tradition: A Profession in Transition" annual spring meeting, 1985

Minnesota Dietetic Association:
Program Committee Chair, 1989-1990
Candidate for President, 1992, 1988
Council on Practice Chair, 1987-1988

South Central Dietetic Association:
Fundraising Chair, 1988
Public Relations, 1988
President, 1986

Continuing Education Chair, 1985-1987
Program Chair, 1985

Vice President, 1985
Secretary, 1982-1984
Charter Member, 1980

Linda J. Hachfeld
Appletree Press, Inc.
151 Good Counsel Drive, Suite 125
Mankato, MN 56001
(507) 345-4848

EDUCATION

Masters of Public Health, 1990
School of Public Health, University of Minnesota

Credential of Advanced Studies in Health Services Administration and Nutrition Administration, 1987
University of Minnesota

American Dietetic Association (ADA) Registration #494496, Since 1981

B.S. Degree, Dietetics
Minor, Business Administration and Chemistry
Mankato State University, 1976

PROFESSIONAL EXPERIENCE

President/CEO 1989-present
Appletree Press, Inc. Mankato, MN

Nutrition Consultant, 1981-present
Minnesota Department of Health, Golden Heart Daycare and Minnesota Valley Action Council. Mankato, MN

Acting Director, 1992-93, Wellness Center of Minnesota.

Community Organization Specialist/Consultant, CSAP (Office of Substance Abuse Program) – Region IX, 1991-present.

Grant Coordinator, COPC-Kellogg Foundation, 1989-1992
Wellness Center of Minnesota. Mankato, MN

Marketing Director, 1987-1989
Mankato Heart Health Program Foundation, Mankato, MN

Cookbook Coordinator and Author, 1986-1988
Mankato Heart Health Program Foundation. Mankato, MN

Nutrition Coordinator and Allied Health Liaison/Community Program Specialist, 1981-1986, 1987-1989
Division of Epidemiology, School of Public Health, University of Minnesota, Mankato Heart Health Program. Mankato, MN,
NIH Grant 1-RO1-8L25523

Director, Dietetic Services, 1978-1981
Glencoe Hospital and Glenhaven Nursing Home. Glencoe, MN

PROFESSIONAL ORGANIZATIONS

Women Executives in Business, 1989-present
Midwest Independent Publishers Association, 1989-present
Publisher's Marketing Association, 1989-present
Minnesota Book Publisher's Roundtable, 1992
National Association of Female Executives, 1991-1992
Phi Upsilon Omicron, lifetime member

Figure 26-1. Sample Curriculum Vitae
Reprinted with permission.

GRANTS

Grantwriter and Coordinator: Women's Network for Entrepreneurial Training SBDC, WEB & SEMIF (Southeastern Minnesota Initiative Fund) $12,800, 1992

Grantwriter: Challenge 2001, Minnesota Department of Human Services for $45,000, 1992

Grantwriter: Women & Heart Disease, American Heart Association, Mankato Division for <$1,000, 1991-1992

Grantwriter & Project Supervisor: Multi-Disciplinary Chemical Abuse Prevention Team, Department of Education and Office of Drug Policy for $11,000, 1990

Grantwriter: Speakers Bureau and Exercise for Heart Community Campaign Health Promotion Council for < $1,000, 1990

Grantwriter: Elementary Education Materials for School District #77 Health Promotion Council for $1200, 1989

Coordinator: Community Oriented Primary Care Project Grant, Mankato, Kellogg Foundation, National Rural Health Association for $75,000, 1989-1991

Principle Investigator, Grantwriter, and Co-Chair: Green Isle, My Health for Better Living Project, Minnesota Initiative Fund, McKnight Foundation for $4700, 1987-1988

PUBLICATIONS

Books: Hachfeld, L. **GIFTS OF THE HEART.** Appletree Press, Inc.: Mankato, MN. 1990

Hachfeld, L. and B. Eykyn. **COOKING ALA HEART.** MHHP and Appletree Press, Inc., Mankato, MN. 1988. Revised 2nd edition, 1992.

Unpublished Manuscript: **The Green Isle Project: A Health Promotion Program in Action;** University of Minnesota–School of Public Health, 1989

Articles: Hachfeld, L. "How to De-Fat Your Favorite Recipes." Health Confidential. December 1993

Interview by Debra Indorato, RD. "Sage Advice–Words of Wisdom from Successful Consulting Nutritionists." Consulting Nutritionists Newsletter, Winter, 1994

Mullis, RM, MK Hunt, M Foster, L Hachfeld, D Lansing, P Snyder, P Pirie, Environmental Support for Healthful Food Behavior: **The Shop Smart for Your Heart Grocery Labeling Program.** JOURNAL OF NUTRITION EDUCATION. October, 1987. Reprinted: NUTRITION NEWS summer 1988.

Hachfeld, L. Worksite Nutrition Intervention Project. JOURNAL OF NUTRITION EDUCATION. October, 1986.

Mullis RM, M Foster, L Hachfeld, MK Hunt, D Lansing, V Niemi, P Snyder, B Shannon; A Guide for Building Partnerships with the Food Marketing System. American Dietetics Association and the Minnesota Heart Health Program. May, 1987.

Hachfeld, L. **Food Allergies: Sublingual Provocative Testing,** ENVIRONMENTAL NUTRITION NEWSLETTER, August, 1984. Reprinted: Tummy Yummers, a CHILD CARE FOOD PROGRAM NEWS BULLETIN, Minnesota Department of Education, March, 1985

Interviewed and contributed articles: **Eat Healthy– And Love It and How One Town Got Healthy.** REDBOOK MAGAZINE, April, 1984.

Interviewed by Jane Brody, New York Times Health Columnist: **Whole Cities Organize to Fight Heart Disease.** NEW YORK TIME NEWSPAPER, September 6, 1983.

PRESENTATIONS Resetting the American Table; Mended Hearts Annual Conference, 1994, Minneapolis, MN.

Women in Business:The Entrepreneurial Spirit; Women's Rural Health Conference, 1994 and MN AHEA Convention, 1994, Mankato, MN.

Business Women In Leadership; WNET Conference, 1994, Rochester, MN.

Women and Heart Disease; American Heart Association–MN Affiliate. St. Peter Regional Treatment Center,1994; Training of Trainers, 1992 Mankato, MN and St. John's University, Collegeville, MN.

Food Trends of the Future; Keynote address to Minnesota Dietary Manager's Association, 1992 Mankato, MN.

Future of Nutrition in Heart Disease; Continuing Medical Education Seminar for Primary Care Physicians sponsored by Methodist Hospital and Park Nicollet Medical Foundation, 1991 Minneapolis, MN

Trends In Nutrition, Future Fare; Minnesota Affiliate–American Heart Association; State Women & Heart Disease Conference, 1991 Minneapolis, MN

Writing & Publishing: Weaving Your Ideas Into Words; Keynote address to Oklahoma Dietetic Association annual meeting; 1991 Stillwater, OK.

Wellness Programs in Rural Communities; Oklahoma Dietetic Association annual meeting; 1991 Stillwater, OK

Green Isle Project: My Health for Better Living Poster Session presentation; Surgeon General's Conference Agricultural Safety and Health; 1991 Des Moines, IA

Eating on the Run: Choices and Consequences; Minnesota Technical Institute; 1988 New Ulm, MN

Choices for Healthy Lifestyles Program: A Change of Plate; University of Minnesota Extension. 1988 Mankato, MN

Building Partnerships, 3-Day Workshop. "A Community Perspective." University of Minnesota, School of Public Health and American Dietetic Association Foundation. 1988 Minneapolis, MN

Figure 26-1. Sample Curriculum Vitae (cont.)
Reprinted with permission.

Linda Hachfeld, page 5

Recipes that Tell and Sell the Dietary Guidelines; Society of Nutrition
Educators 21st annual meeting -- "Meeting in the Marketplace."
1988 Toronto, Canada

A Change of Plate; American Heart Association--Southwest MN Division
annual meeting & dinner. 1988 Mankato, MN

Nutrition Puts the Bite on Cancer; American Cancer Society--MN Affiliate
and Mankato Technical Institute. 1988 Mankato, MN

The Power of Food; Mankato Chamber of Commerce, Leadership Forum.
1988.

HONORS

Minnesota Women in Business Advocate Award, Small Business Administration (SBA) 1993.

YWCA Community Leader Award, Mankato YWCA Leaderdinner XXI, 1993

Midwest Book Achievement (MBA) Award for COOKING ALA HEART, Midwest Independent
Publishers Association, 1993.

Benjamin Franklin Merit Award, Publishers Marketing Association (PMA),
1993 Appletree Press Catalog and 1991 GIFTS OF THE HEART

Woman of Achievement Award, YWCA Leaderdinner Award, 1993

Women in Business Advocate Award, U.S. Small Business Administration (SBA)
Small Business Advocate of the Year, 1993

Outstanding Services Award, American Heart Association--MN Affiliate, 1991

Certificate of Commendation for Community Health Promotion, Governor
of Minnesota, 1989

Secretary's Award for Excellence for Public Health, U.S. Department of
Health and Human Services, 1988

RYDY (Registered Young Dietitian of the Year) Award, Minnesota Dietetic
Association, 1981

Figure 26-1. Sample Curriculum Vitae (cont.)
Reprinted with permission.

Julie I. Taylor
5005 Maple Court
Chelsea, MI 48000
(313) 123-4567

EDUCATION:
Yale-New Haven Hospital Dietetic Internship - Generalist Program
Michigan State University - BS: Dietetics
Michigan State University - BS: Foods and Nutrition

Honors:
Community Service Scholarship

Certification:
Applied Food Service Sanitation Course. The Education Foundation of the National Restaurant Association. October, 1992

PROFESSIONAL EXPERIENCE:

Yale-New Haven Hospital
Community Nutrition
Efficiently managed and counseled outpatient services, including Radiation Therapy, Renal Stones & Bones, ENT, High-risk Pregnancy, Cranio-facial, and Pediatric Virology. Co-chaired, coordinated, and organized the National Nutrition Month (NNM) Health Fair — "Write Your Own Prescription. Prevention Through Nutrition." Collaborated with external hospital departments the following functions for the 800-participant NNM event; public relations advertising; community and patient food services; procurement and catering; and engineering. Participated in outpatient QA, developed educational materials, extensively participated in public-speaking engagements, and organized various community presentations.

Clinical Nutrition Management
Assisted with the cost-effective management and direction of inpatient, outpatient, and research nutrition services. Involved in departmental strategic planning, staffing, redesign, and policy and procedure review/development, and coordinated the resource information for the self-study report. Gained experience in the criteria-based performance appraisal system, clinical standards of care, and QA monitors.

Clinical Nutrition
Responsible for the effective nutritional management of patients in a tertiary-care hospital and trauma center. Skilled in prioritizing and classifying the patient population and assessing specific nutritional needs; providing appropriate recommendations for needed interventions, inclusive of enteral and parenteral nutrition support, and applying appropriate, cost-effective diet therapies. Obtained patient diet histories, preferences, and recalls, modified patient menus, and actively participated in the clinical QA program by assisting in the writing of the third-quarter report.

Food Service Systems Management
Participated in and supported the daily functions of food systems management, food production, patient food service, purchasing, and clinical operations management. Integrated menus into the food distribution and delivery system based on the standards of safety, sanitation, nutrition, competitive pricing, and efficiency. Managed inventory, purchasing, and forecasting congruent with operating goals. Conducted product tests and yield studies. Performed in the capacity of an assistant manager for Yale University Dining Halls, performing such tasks as menu forecasting, payroll, and menu and recipe analysis, and implemented numerous catering events.

Julie I. Taylor
Page 2

Clinical Nutrition Research
Developed menu and recipe formulations for research protocols using the ClinFo System. Integrated subjective and objective information into diets considering nutrition requirements, the parameters of the protocol, and study participant preferences.

Nutrition Counselor. Trim 4 Life
Counseled patients on various aspects of weight loss, including diet, exercise, and behavioral modification. Assumed managerial responsibilities, including operating expenses, inventory, and menu revisions.

Nutrition Aide. Cooperative Extension
Screened patients using anthropometric assessment, accurate food records, and socioeconomic status referring to appropriate community and government agencies.

PUBLICATIONS:
Gradwell EK. Thompson JI. Fairchild MM. Liskov TAP: The fine art of leadership among peers: a national nutrition month fair (Abstr). 76th Annual Meeting. The American Dietetic Association. Anaheim. CA. 1993.

Thompson. J: Food allergy vs food intolerance: what really is the difference? Food for Thought. Yale University Dining Halls. February 1993.

Thompson J: Learning to eat thin. Yale-New Haven Hospital. Good Consumer. 8(3): June 1993.

Thompson J: National nutrition month. Yale Health Care Student Council Bulletin. 1(4): 1993.

Thompson J: Liver transplant nutrition. Yale-New Haven Hospital. 1993.

PRESENTATIONS
Healthy Snacking. Volvo International Grassroots Program. New Haven. CT. August. 1993.

HIV Nephropathy. Clinical Case Study. Yale-New Haven Hospital. July. 1993.

The Food Guide Pyramid and the Importance of Choosing Low-Fat Foods for Disease Prevention. The Washington Magnet School. West Haven. CT. April. 1993.

Is the Food You Are Eating. Purchasing. and Preparing Healthy? Probus Community House. West Haven. CT. March. 1993.

Eating Your Way to a Healthy Heart. Yale University Dining Halls. February. 1993.

INSERVICES:
Kitchen First Aid and Safety. Yale University Dining Halls. February. 1993.

Reducing Your Blood Cholesterol Through Diet. Yale-New Haven Hospital. November. 1992.

PROFESSIONAL AFFILIATIONS
The American Dietetic Association
Connecticut Dietetic Association
Southern Connecticut Dietetic Association
Society for Nutrition Education

Figure 26-2. Sample Résumé

Kathy King Helm, RD

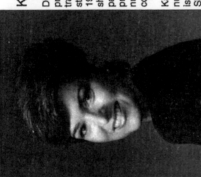

Discouraged with the lack of prevention being taught in traditional hospital settings, Kathy started her own private practice in 1972 in Denver. Since that date, she has counseled over 6,000 patients, and given over 500 presentations to the public, nurses, physicians, athletes and coaches.

Kathy specializes in preventive nutrition, weight loss, consumer issues, as well as sports nutrition. She was a nutritionist with the Denver Bronco Football Team, the Greenhouse spa in Dallas, associated with Neiman-Marcus, and the Lewisville, Texas, Sports Medicine Center.

The media has played a large role in Kathy's career. She started 18 years ago in Denver as a regular guest on "Blinky's Fun Club" and then became the "NoonDay" nutritionist on NBC-TV for four years. In 1989, she hosted her own weekly, nationally syndicated radio talk show from Dallas called "American Know How," which also featured Super Handyman Al Carrell and "Good Morning America's" Steve Crowley. She has guested on "Nightline," and NBC's magazine show "1986."

In September 1991, Kathy published the second edition of her popular book, *The Entrepreneurial Nutritionist.* She has authored numerous magazine articles and journal commentaries, as well as the consumer booklet "Let's Get To Know Vitamin Supplements." For several years Kathy reviewed diet books for the *Dallas Morning News.*

Kathy has served as the President of the Colorado Dietetic Association and two years on the Board of Directors of The American Dietetic Association. She now lives with her husband and two daughters, 10 and 5 years old, in Lake Dallas, Texas.

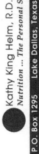

Kathy King Helm, R.D.
Nutrition ... The Personal Side

P.O. Box 1295   Lake Dallas, Texas 75065   (817)497-3558

SUSAN WILLIAMS, MS, RD, CNSD

CREDENTIALS

Susan Williams, MS, RD, CNSD, has been on the staff at Yale-New Haven Hospital since 1980, having served in the capacity of a Clinical Nutrition Specialist on several of the clinical services, including General Surgery, Cardiothoracic Surgery, Neurology and Neurosurgery, Plastic Surgery, and the Intensive Care Units.

She received her bachelor's degree in Dietetics at the University of Connecticut, Storrs, Connecticut, in the Coordinated Undergraduate Program in 1980, and her master's degree in Human Nutrition from the University of Bridgeport, Bridgeport, Connecticut, in 1988.

PROFESSIONAL MEMBERSHIPS

Ms. Williams is a member of The American Dietetic Association, the American Burn Association, the American Society of Parenteral and Enteral Nutrition, and CONN-SPEN, as well as the Dietitians in Nutrition Support ADA Dietetic Practice Group. She received certification in Nutrition Support from the American Society of Parenteral and Enteral Nutrition in 1980. Additionally, she has served as treasurer for the Southern Connecticut Dietetic Association from 1990 to 1992.

PROFESSIONAL RESPONSIBILITIES

In addition to her function of providing routine nutrition care to inpatients at Yale-New Haven Hospital, Ms. Williams has been a lecturer at Yale University Schools of Medicine, Nursing, and Public Health, as well as for the departments of surgery, nursing, and discharge planning. She serves as a member of the clinical faculty for the Yale-New Haven Hospital Department of Food and Nutrition Services accredited Dietetic Internship Program. She has presented several poster sessions at the annual meetings of both The American Dietetic Association and the American Society for Enteral and Parenteral Nutrition, and is completing a research paper for upcoming publication.

Figure 26-3. Sample Bio and Media Bio
Reprinted with permission.

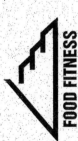

FOOD FITNESS

The Princeton Club already offers a variety of exercise options for everyone. Now the Princeton Club's **Food Fitness** program offers the other essential ingredient for a healthy lifestyle: healthy eating options for everyone. We all wish permanent weight control could be as simple as a crash diet. But just as there is no effortless way to exercise, there is no easy way to control your weight.

Most people know how to diet, but **Food Fitness** is about learning how to eat. Diets are temporary, but **Food Fitness** is a way of eating for a lifetime. Through this program you will find out how small changes in your eating habits can make a big difference to your weight and health. You will learn how to form new eating habits, ones that fit your lifestyle and that you can continue for life.

Food Fitness is based on real life situations, ones you encounter every day. The breakfast you didn't have time for becomes a donut in the middle of the morning. Your usual order just slips off your lips at the fast food drive up window. Familiar groceries appear in your cart as you weave up and down the aisles. The vending machine answers your stomach's rumbles in the middle of the afternoon. And the hand and mouth go into auto pilot with a bag of chips at the end of the day. **Food Fitness** will show how you can cope with these daily struggles.

Everyone has different reasons for being overweight. You may eat more when you are under stress. You may be too busy to think about what you should eat. You may not know how to change your eating habits. You may be unwilling to give up your favorite goodies. **Food Fitness** will show you that it is possible to eat tasty food, eat out, enjoy life, and still keep your weight under control, however stressful your life is.

Food Fitness includes:
- eight weekly classes taught by a registered dietitian
- a valuable food and fitness information kit
- an individual appointment with the dietitian, including computerized diet analysis
- fitness assessments at the beginning and end of the program
- unlimited use of the Princeton Club during the eight weeks
- $50 off for members

Whether you want to lose 5 pounds or 50 pounds, however many times you've tried to lose weight before, and however many times you've failed or gained it back, you can still be successful at eating well and living more healthfully. Diets bring to mind deprivation, misery, boredom, self-criticism, and failure. **Food Fitness** will show you that you can succeed at eating, feel good about yourself, and enjoy it too.

FOOD FITNESS SCHEDULE

Week 1 The Food Guide Pyramid
Shaping your eating habits.
What good food and fitness habits can do for you.

Week 2 Meals and Recipes
Substituting foods and ingredients to lose the fat and keep the flavor.

Week 3 For Those Who Don't Cook
Healthy eating habits using convenience foods, fast foods, vending machines, and cafeterias.

Week 4 Supermarket Tour
Making sense of food labels.

Week 5 Fitness and Food
Making sure you eat enough carbohydrates and fluid for your work outs.

Week 6 Eating Out
Deciding what to order from restaurant menus.

Week 7 Why We Eat What We Eat When We Eat It
Managing holidays, parties, friends, families, and other difficult situations.

Week 8 Foods We Need
Getting nutrients from food, rather than pills.
Focussing on eating rather than dieting.

Figure 29-1. Sample Brochure
Reprinted with permission of the Princeton Club.

Jane Jones, MS, RD
Ambulatory Nutrition Specialist
828 North Forrest Avenue • New Haven, CT 06504

September 12, 1995

John Smith, MD
Obstetrics and Gynecology
2 Church Street
New Haven, CT 06504

Dear Dr. Smith:

The Yale-New Haven Hospital Centers of Nutrition would like to extend its services to your OB-GYN patients. I have enclosed a package of information that describes our staff and services. Our program emphasizes a medically oriented approach providing in-depth initial nutrition assessment and long-term counseling. Patients are seen either individually or with family members. We welcome clients of all ages, and invite you to send your referrals for individualized nutrition care.

Some problems commonly encountered in our practice include prenatal nutrition, gestational diabetes, diabetes, hyperlipidemia, hypertension, obesity, diverticulosis, and food intolerance. Our centers are staffed by registered dietitians with advanced degrees in nutrition or public health. We work closely with the referring physician and endeavor to send timely correspondence reporting on patient progress.

I would be pleased to meet with you, your associates, and your staff at your convenience to discuss our program further and answer any questions you may have.

Sincerely,

Jane Jones

Jane Jones, MS, RD
Ambulatory Nutrition Specialist

Figure 30-1. Sample Introductory Letter

Jane Jones, MS, RD
Ambulatory Nutrition Specialist
828 North Forrest Avenue • New Haven, CT 06504

January 13, 1996

John Smith, MD
Obstetrics and Gynecology
2 Church Street
New Haven, CT 06504

Dear Dr. Smith:

Eating is an integral part of the holidays and weight loss is a challenge for the New Year. With counseling and literature from the Centers of Nutrition, your patients can enjoy traditions, holiday feasts, and celebrations without the extra calories, fat, and sugar.

At the Yale-New Haven Hospital Centers of Nutrition, we would like to concentrate our efforts during the New Year 1996 on reaching patients who, because of obesity, have an increased risk for high blood pressure, diabetes, and heart disease.

I have enclosed copies of our monthly consumer newsletter and would like to make these available to your patients. If you would like additional copies, please give me a call at 555-5555 or 555-3333.

I would also like to thank you for your continued support of the Yale-New Haven Hospital Centers of Nutrition. We remain committed to providing your patients with meaningful dietary counseling, whether it be for existing medical conditions or to promote wellness.

Sincerely,

Jane Jones

Jane Jones, MS, RD
Ambulatory Nutrition Specialist

Figure 30-2. Sample Follow-up Promotion Letter

L. Kathleen Mahan, R.D., C.D.E., Inc.

Consulting Nutritionist

120 Northgate Plaza, #101
Seattle, WA 98125
Tel (206) 363-5420
Fax (206) 363-0523

400 112th Avenue N.E., #110
Bellevue, WA 98004
Tel (206) 454-4644
Fax (206) 451-0214

October 4, 1993

Robert Kitchell, MD
1145 Broadway
Seattle, WA 98122

RE: SIMMONS, SUSAN
BD: 3/30/56

Dear Dr. Kitchell:

Thank you for referring your patient Susan Simmons to me for nutritional counseling for management of her overweight. I saw Susan for the first time on October 4th, 1993, and this letter summarizes my findings.

LAB DATA: Total serum cholesterol—185 mg/dl—8/19/93
HDL cholesterol—39 mg/dl
LDL cholesterol—122 mg/dl
Serum triglycerides—120 mg/dl

ANTHROPOMETRY: Height 63 7/8"
Weight 194 3/4 lb
Highest weight at adult height—present
Lowest weight at adult height—130-135 lb
Ideal body weight—130-135 lb
Assessment of body fatness—44.3%

NUTRITIONAL/SOCIAL HISTORY: Susan reports that she was normal weight as a child and as a teenager. Both parents are normal weight. One brother is slightly overweight. She easily maintained a weight of 130-135 lb in her early 20s until she married. She married at age 27 and gained about 10 lb in the next three years. At the conception of her first baby at age 30 she weighed 145 lb, and that baby was delivered at 26 weeks and died. When she got pregnant with her second baby shortly after, she weighed 160 lb and gained 30 lb during that pregnancy. She nursed that baby and dropped down to 168 lb, which she was at the beginning of her third pregnancy. She then gained about 22 lb up to a weight of 190 lb. She nursed that baby, dropped down to 172 lb one year later, and since that time, over the past three years, she has gained up to her present weight of 194 3/4 lb.

A several-day food record kept by Susan shows that she gets up at 6 o'clock and exercises at a gym. She then goes back home and gets her children ready for school for the next couple of hours. By the time she leaves the house at 9 or so, she has had a cup of cocoa. That is how she starts her day. She may have several pieces of chocolate candy throughout the day, and may have lunch at 11:30, when she gives her youngest lunch. That lunch is not really a lunch on her part, just eating off her youngster's plate. She has more high-sugar, high-fat snacks in the afternoon and makes a dinner for the family in the evening.

Susan reports that she is unaware of eating much, and the very habit of writing it down I think is going to help her.

VITAMIN/MINERAL SUPPLEMENTS: None.
ALLERGIES: None.
ALCOHOL: 1-2 glasses of wine per week.
CAFFEINE: Decaf coffee, caffeine free pop, hot chocolate three times a week: chocolate candy daily.
SALT/SODIUM: She does use a salt shaker; does not cook with salt.
SUGAR/SWEETENER: Adds artificial sweetener to her latte and coffee.
EXERCISE: Uses a stairmaster or stationary bicycle at the gym for 30 minutes three times a week.

ASSESSMENT: Susan admits she is overeating because of anxiety. She says she is not even aware that she is eating much of the time, and she certainly does not eat out of hunger. She is eating/nibbling a high-fat, high-sugar diet that is low in fruits, vegetables, and fiber. I am sure she will benefit from following a low-fat diet, in addition to her exercise, which she already has worked into her day. Susan seems very receptive to trying a low-fat diet combined with exercise.

RECOMMENDATIONS/PLAN:
1. Instruct Susan on a 20% calories from fat diet, with about 30 grams of fat a day.
2. Have Susan increase her exercise frequency to four times a week and increase the duration to 40 minutes for a greater fat-burning effect.
3. Have Susan increase the dietary fiber in her diet from about 12 grams a day to 20-25 grams.
4. Return visit in two weeks to assess progress from a food and activity record.

If you have any questions regarding Susan's nutritional care, please feel free to contact me.

Sincerely,

L. Kathleen Mahan

L. Kathleen Mahan, RD, CDE

Follow-up Letter to Referring Physician

LINDA McDONALD, MS, RD, LD
11102 Lakeside Forest Lane
Houston, TX 77042-1032
Telephone 713/978-6960
Facsimile 713/978-7044

PROPOSAL

Date: June 1, 1992

To: Dave Foreman
Director of Marketing
Guiltless Gourmet

From: Linda McDonald, MS, RD, LD

Proposal: Develop Recipes for Guiltless Gourmet Products

Objective: Encourage use of Guiltless Gourmet Products by providing recipes for point-of-purchase promotions, educational programs, packaging, and marketing literature.

Format: 3"x5" cards or pads. Graphic representation to be determined by marketing firm.

Contents: Eight recipes. nutrient analysis. and dietary exchanges.

Suggested
Recipes:

Party/Snack	Layered Dip
	Nachos
	Mexican Potato Skins
Soups	Tortilla Soup
	Bean Soup
	Potato Cheese Soup
Entrees	Taco Pie
	Chicken Casserole
	Pasta Sauce
	Omelette
Salads	Taco Salad
	Dressings

Procedure: 1. Submit recipe ideas for approval
2. Develop recipes
3. Test recipes
4. Computer-analyze recipes
5. Work with marketing firm on graphic presentation.

Time: One month

Cost: $1000 plus out-of-pocket expenses

LINDA McDONALD, MS, RD, LD
11102 Lakeside Forest Lane
Houston, TX 77042-1032
Telephone 713/978-6960
Facsimile 713/978-7044

May 26, 1992

David Foreman
Guiltless Gourmet
123 Chip Drive
Austin, Texas 77000

Dear Dave:

Thank you for the opportunity to visit, meet your staff, and observe the production of Guiltless Gourmet chips. Your products are right on target for the growth in health-conscious eating, and it is obvious that Guiltless Gourmet is successful and growing. Not only are your products tasty, but they are full of good complex carbohydrates and low in fat, cholesterol, and sodium.

As discussed, your emphasis on the health-conscious consumer and the use of the health professional as a tool for marketing your products fits some ideas I have had for promoting Guiltless Gourmet. Your products have proved useful when I have presented topics such as Low Fat Snacking, Holiday Survival Skills, and Heart Healthy Nibbles.

A registered and licensed dietitian can add authority and credibility to your products in our health-focused community. You can benefit from the following services:
1. Review promotional materials for accuracy of information and appropriate health-related language. This will be increasingly important as the new FDA labeling guidelines go into effect.
2. Act as a resource for your staff on health-related questions.
3. Represent Guiltless Gourmet at conventions and meetings and provide a network of qualified health professionals for local market areas.
4. Develop health-related promotional materials and programs, such as
   Guiltless Snacking Brochure – A marketing piece that includes snacking tips. comparison charts of Guiltless Gourmet products with regular products. recipes. and nutrient information for products.
   Recipes – Encourage the use of Guiltless Gourmet products with unique and tasty recipes for dishes such as taco pie. layered dips. casseroles. soups. Mexican favorites. and sauces.
   Guiltless Snacking Seminar – A Speaker's Kit for health professionals that can use Guiltless Gourmet products in seminars and classes. Kit will include lesson plan. handouts. tips for conducting tastings. and marketing tips.

Dave, you know that I have been excited about your products since the start of Guiltless Gourmet. I would welcome the opportunity to work with you as a consultant and suggest that we start with one project on a trial basis. Just let me know which project you are interested in and I will prepare a proposal.

Enclosed are sample materials developed for Tenneco Corporation's Fitness program. You are already familiar with my participation in the Houston Gourmet books. The enclosed resume will give you more information on my education and business experience.

Please call if you have any questions or need additional information. I look forward to working with Guiltless Gourmet and will call next week to discuss this with you further.

Sincerely,

Linda McDonald